Cancer in the Arab World

Humaid O. Al-Shamsi
Ibrahim H. Abu-Gheida
Faryal Iqbal
Aydah Al-Awadhi

Editors

Cancer in the Arab World

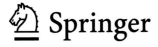 Springer

Editors
Humaid O. Al-Shamsi
Department of Oncology, Burjeel Cancer
Institute, Burjeel Medical City
Abu Dhabi, United Arab Emirates

College of Medicine, University of Sharjah
Sharjah, United Arab Emirates

Faryal Iqbal
Department of Oncology, Innovation and
Research Center, Burjeel Cancer Institute
Burjeel Medical City
Abu Dhabi, United Arab Emirates

Ibrahim H. Abu-Gheida
Department of Radiation Oncology, Burjeel
Cancer Institute, Burjeel Medical City
Abu Dhabi, United Arab Emirates

College of Medicine and Health Sciences
United Arab Emirates University
Abu Dhabi, United Arab Emirates

Aydah Al-Awadhi
Emirates Oncology Society
Dubai, United Arab Emirates

This book is an open access publication.

Publication of this book has been supported through an unrestricted educational grant provided by Merck to the Emirates Oncology Society/Emirates Medical association, Dubai, United Arab Emirates, The Emirates Society (http://www.eos.ae/) provided administrative and legal support to the editorial team.

ISBN 978-981-16-7944-5   ISBN 978-981-16-7945-2   (eBook)
https://doi.org/10.1007/978-981-16-7945-2

This Springer imprint is published by the registered company Springer Nature Singapore Pte Ltd.
The registered company address is: 152 Beach Road, #21-01/04 Gateway East, Singapore 189721, Singapore

Foreword

The Arab world was at the crossroads of the ancient trade routes and continues to be a central meeting point for civilizations due to its unique positioning and geography. This has contributed to its large cultural and population diversity and a distinctive admixture of local inhabitants and migrants. Arabs were collectively known for their passion to transmit their culture through their written records that have had an astounding impact on the arts and sciences as we know them today. Here, we have one more contribution from the region to be treasured for being the first and most comprehensive script highlighting the peculiarities of cancer and its treatment in the Arab world.

Despite considerable variations in resources and capabilities, the region has come a long way in offering state-of-the-art cancer prevention and management services for citizens and residents; with some countries even becoming destinations for medical care for the region and beyond. We were only able to achieve this through learning from experiences, setting achievable goals and objectives that address the needs of the highest priority, and most importantly, putting the patient at the center of everything we do. Advances in diagnosis and care are also largely attributed to a major transformation in strategic thinking towards multi-stakeholder collaboration and away from competition. Collaborative Multidisciplinary Tumor Boards (MTB) and Multidisciplinary Team (MDT) approaches where different specialized professionals are involved in patient care with the singular goal of improving treatment efficiency and treatment now forms the cornerstone at all major cancer centers in the region. Research and innovation are also becoming integral parts of regional healthcare systems, primarily directed towards building platforms for individualized care that will soon lead to the development of novel therapeutics that can address the individual patient needs in the region.

Cancer control planning without reliable data is prone to misdirected priorities and wasted investments. Knowing what to treat is fundamental, but how should it be done? This is where this publication fulfills an important function. The contents of this book represent an important step in supporting cancer teams as they seek the data needed to ensure that the best possible cancer prevention, control, and care measures are available for all populations in the region. This will make a major difference in the incidence, management, and the eventual elimination of cancer.

The editors of this book are experienced clinicians and researchers, who have provided a well-researched analysis. They are particularly commended for taking the initiative and pooling such an enormous amount of data from across the region, a task that does not come without its own barriers and challenges. More importantly, they have skillfully selected the partners for this task by collaborating with experienced physicians who have pioneered oncology practice in their respective Arab countries. This allows bridging published evidence with real-life insights across the covered topics and makes the findings in this book relevant to clinicians and all concerned with the care of patients with complex medical conditions. They have delivered a valuable resource for all stakeholders looking to understand the unique complexities and challenges of cancers in the Arab world. Given the increasing prevalence of cancers, this book provides the most recent data and clinical analysis that will enable the medical and cancer research communities to gain insights into clinical observations and practices and develop new locally-relevant therapeutic approaches. It will become a pillar for formulating future strategies for the control, prevention, and treatment of cancer.

Shamsheer Vayalil
VPS Healthcare
Abu Dhabi, UAE

Acknowledgment

Dedicated to My Creator and may God accept this work for his honorable sake

My father and my idol, the late Sheikh Zayed bin Sultan Al Nahyan, the founder and the late president of the UAE, may God have mercy on him, for his love for this good land and his belief in us (his people)

For the late Sheikh Hamdan bin Rashid Al Maktoum, the father of the Emirates Medical Association and for his support of sciences and research in the UAE and the region

My country and my leaders whom I do not have enough words to thank

The UAE armed forces that have taken care of and supported me during my 20 years of medical education and training, believing and trusting in me

To my late father, may God Almighty have mercy on him, who always blamed me for my long travel and absence away from him

To my dear mother, who planted the love of science and medicine since my childhood

To my dear wife and friend Khadija and my kids Sarah, Abdullah, Muhammad, Noor, Aseel, and Sama who were and still are my source of strength and inspiration

To my brother Hassan and my sisters for being away from them for many years and for their support and prayers for me ALL THE TIME

To Dr Parveen Wasi, my internal medicine program director during my residency for her support and pushing me to pursue research

To Dr Robert Wolff, Dr Bindi Dhesy, and Dr Peter Ellis for their support and mentorship during my fellowship and early career in oncology

To Dr Mouza AlSharhan, the president of the Emirates Medical Association, for her support for the EOS over the last many years

To Dr Shamsheer Vayalil for his continuous support to transform cancer care in the UAE and the region

To my dear friends: Sherif, Mitref, Abdullah, Khaled, and Tariq for being there for me at my downs and ups

To my friend and role model in science, medicine, and research, Dr Waleed Al-Hazzani

To my past, current, and future teachers and to everyone who supported me

To all my past and future patients: I promise you that I will take care of you as I take care of my own family

For humanity, believing in the Almighty saying: "We have sent you nothing but a mercy for the worlds."

Cancer that taught me a lot and which we will eliminate, God willing

Humaid Obaid Al-Shamsi
Nov 6, 2021

Contents

About the Editors

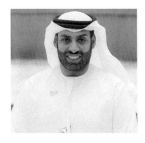

Humaid O. Al-Shamsi is the director of VPS oncology services in the United Arab Emirates, which is the largest cancer care provider network in the UAE. He is also the President of the Emirates Oncology Society and an adjunct professor at the College of Medicine—University of Sharjah. Prof. Al-Shamsi holds triple specialty board certifications in medical oncology from the UK, the USA, and Canada. He completed his Bachelor of Science and Bachelor of Medicine from Cork University, the National University of Ireland with honors in 2005. He then completed his internal medicine residency followed by a medical oncology fellowship, he then completed a subspecialty combined fellowship in gastrointestinal and palliative oncology at McMaster University in Canada in 2013. He then joined MD Anderson Cancer Center, The University of Texas, Houston, USA, as an assistant professor from 2014 to 2017. Prof. Al-Shamsi is the founder of Burjeel Cancer Institute at Burjeel Medical City in Abu Dhabi, UAE, which is the most comprehensive cancer center in the UAE. He has more than 70 peer reviewed articles and book chapters. His research focus is on precision medicine and health policies related to cancer care in the UAE and the Arab region. He was awarded the researcher of the year in 2020 and 2021 by the Emirates Oncology Society.

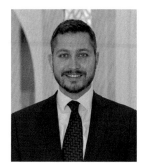

Ibrahim H. Abu-Gheida is the founding head of the Department of Radiation Oncology in Burjeel Medical City and an adjunct assistant professor in the United Arab Emirates University. Dr. Abu-Gheida completed his undergraduate training where he earned a Bachelor of Science with honors degree from the American University of Beirut. Following which Dr. Abu-Gheida completed his Medical School training at the American University of Beirut Medical Center. He continued and joined the Department of Internal Medicine at the American University of Beirut. Then did his training in the Department of Radiation Oncology at the American University of Beirut Medical Center, where he served also as the chief resident. During his training, Dr. Abu-Gheida completed a Harvard-affiliated NIH-funded research program as well. After his residency, Dr. Ibrahim went to Cleveland Clinic/Ohio, where he was appointed as an Advanced Clinical Radiation Oncology Fellow. Dr. Abu-Gheida went and joined the University of Texas MD Anderson Cancer Center. Dr. Abu-Gheida has many publications in prestigious medical journals including the American Society of Radiation Oncology official journal—International Journal of Radiation Oncology Biology and Physics, Nature, Journal of Clinical Oncology, and several others. He is also the primary author of several book chapters published in prestigious books. He also has been granted research awards during his residency.

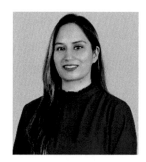

Faryal Iqbal holds an undergraduate degree in Molecular Biology and Biotechnology. Subsequently, she earned postgraduate qualification in Molecular Genetics from Pakistan, where she worked on finding the association between *XRCC1* gene polymorphism and radiation exposure in healthcare workers. She is currently working with an oncology specific research group and serving in the domains of scientific writing, data management, supervision of medical internees, and providing editorial assistance. Ms. Iqbal's research interests and publications encompass genetics and oncology. She intends to support research across the oncology key areas including prevention, diagnosis, and treatment. Her focus is on preparing for future adoption of genomic technology and increased use of genomic information as part of the cancer diagnostic and therapeutic pathways.

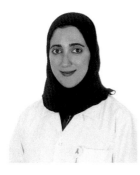

Aydah Al-Awadhi is a consultant medical oncologist, graduated in medical school from the United Arab Emirates University in 2012, then completed her internal medicine residency in the United States and completed her Medical Oncology and Hematology fellowship from the University of Texas, MD Anderson Cancer Center in 2019 and is American Board Certified in Hematology and Medical Oncology. She was awarded the Emirates Oncology Society (EOS) Member of the Year award, 2021. Dr. Al-Awadhi has published many articles and book chapters on breast cancer and oncology.

Chapter 1
Introduction

Humaid O. Al-Shamsi (iD), **Faryal Iqbal** (iD), **and Ibrahim H. Abu-Gheida**

1.1 Background

Stretching from Asia towards Africa and passing through the Middle East and the Arabian Gulf, Arab countries have been listed as a group of 22 Arabic speaking countries that have a population of approximately 620 million (Fig. 1.1) [1].

Arab countries share a considerable deal in terms of culture, yet there is great variability in their economic capabilities and growth. There is considerable heterogeneity between and within populations when it comes to disease epidemiology

H. O. Al-Shamsi (✉)
Department of Oncology, Burjeel Cancer Institute, Burjeel Medical City, Abu Dhabi, United Arab Emirates

Innovation and Research Center, Burjeel Cancer Institute, Burjeel Medical City, Abu Dhabi, United Arab Emirates

Emirates Oncology Society, Dubai, United Arab Emirates

University of Sharjah, Sharjah, United Arab Emirates
e-mail: humaid.al-shamsi@medportal.ca

F. Iqbal
Department of Oncology, Innovation and Research Center, Burjeel Cancer Institute, Burjeel Medical City, Abu Dhabi, United Arab Emirates
e-mail: faryal.iqbal@burjeelmedicalcity.com

I. H. Abu-Gheida
Department of Radiation Oncology, Burjeel Cancer Institute, Burjeel Medical City, Abu Dhabi, United Arab Emirates

Emirates Oncology Society, Dubai, United Arab Emirates

College of Medicine and Health Sciences, United Arab Emirates University, Abu Dhabi, United Arab Emirates

© The Author(s) 2022
H. O. Al-Shamsi et al. (eds.), *Cancer in the Arab World*,
https://doi.org/10.1007/978-981-16-7945-2_1

1

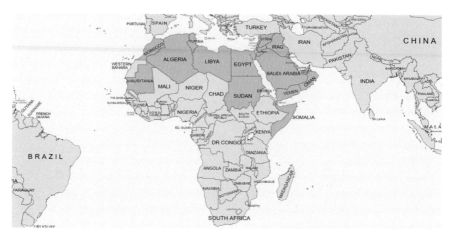

Fig. 1.1 Map representing the Arab countries. [Source: https://mapchart.net/]

and profile, although cancer burden remains significant across all countries. According to available data, cancer incidence rates are increasing due to developing age and population, with crucial consequences for the healthcare system and community [2].

1.2 Cancer Profile in the Arab World: An Overview

Cancer is a global public health issue. The most common cancers worldwide, in both genders, include breast, lung, colorectal, prostate, and stomach cancers. An analogous pattern exists in the Middle East and North Africa (MENA) region, whereas bladder and stomach cancers comprise the fifth and sixth most frequently occurring malignancies. In Gulf Cooperation Council (GCC) countries, colorectal, non-Hodgkin's lymphoma, lung, and liver cancers are most prevalent in males, whereas breast cancer, followed by thyroid, colorectal cancer and non-Hodgkin's lymphoma are most prevalent among females [3]. Cancer is the fourth leading cause of death in the Eastern Mediterranean Region (EMR), with approximately 419,000 deaths, in 2018; with breast, bladder, colorectal, liver, and lung cancers being the most prevalent. In EMR, the most frequent cancer cases among males include lung, liver, and prostate with 10.4%, 8.4%, and 8%, respectively; whereas the most predominant cancer cases among females include breast, colorectal, and cervical cancer with 34.7%, 5.7%, and 4.6%, respectively [1]. The EMR and GCC states demonstrate a startling growth in oncology patients' tally. Long-term estimation illustrates that by 2030, there would be a 1.8-fold spike in cancer incidence rate [4]. GLOBOCAN (2020) reported the rank of new cancer cases, among both genders and of all ages, in the Arab region (Table 1.1) [5].

Table 1.1 The rank of cancer cases in the Arab world [5]. Used with permission from the International Agency of Research on Cancer (IARC)/GLOBOCAN, 2020

	Country	1st	2nd	3rd	4th	5th
1	Algeria	Breast	Colorectum	Lung	Prostate	Bladder
2	Bahrain	Breast	Colorectum	Lung	NHL	Leukemia
3	Comoros	Cervix uteri	Prostate	Breast	Esophagus	Liver
4	Djibouti	Breast	Cervix uteri	Colorectum	NHL	Prostate
5	Egypt	Liver	Breast	Bladder	NHL	Lung
6	Iraq	Breast	Lung	Colorectum	Leukemia	NHL
7	Jordan	Breast	Colorectum	Lung	Bladder	Leukemia
8	Kuwait	Breast	Colorectum	Thyroid	Prostate	NHL
9	Lebanon	Breast	Lung	Prostate	Colorectum	Bladder
10	Libya	Breast	Colorectum	Lung	Bladder	Prostate
11	Mauritania	Breast	Cervix uteri	Prostate	Liver	Colorectum
12	Morocco	Breast	Lung	Colorectum	Prostate	NHL
13	Oman	Breast	Colorectum	NHL	Stomach	Leukemia
14	Palestine[a]	—	—	—	—	—
15	Qatar	Breast	Colorectum	Prostate	Leukemia	NHL
16	Saudi Arabia	Colorectum	Breast	Thyroid	NHL	Leukemia
17	Somalia	Breast	Cervix uteri	Colorectum	Prostate	Leukemia
18	Sudan	Breast	Colorectum	NHL	Prostate	Leukemia
19	Syria	Breast	Lung	Colorectum	Prostate	Leukemia
20	Tunisia	Breast	Lung	Colorectum	Bladder	Prostate
21	UAE	Breast	Colorectum	Thyroid	Leukemia	Prostate
22	Yemen	Breast	Colorectum	Leukemia	Stomach	NHL

Source: International Agency of Research on Cancer (IARC)/GLOBOCAN
[a]Palestine's report was unavailable

Population expansion, lifestyle modifications, industrialization, increase in lifespan, urbanization, and higher frequency of exposure to prospective causative factors are all expected to promote increased cancer incidence [1].

The observed variation in new cancer cases in the Arab world, which has been presented by different Arab countries in this book, reflects the fluctuating predominance and risk factors' distribution within and between Arab countries. This also suggests variation in delivery of efficient cancer control measures. The strategies should be introduced to lessen the disease burden in Arab countries to reflect the similarities and differences in cancer rates among the region.

1.3 Cancer Risk Factors

Although cancer etiology is multifactorial, an array of well-known risk factors has been contemplated as a major contributor to the advancement of cancer epidemiology (Table 1.2) [4, 6].

Table 1.2 Prevalent cancer risk factors

Element	Context
Tobacco	Incorporates the use of harmful substances such as benzene, chromium, cadmium, acrylonitrile, 4-aminobiphenyl, 2-naphthylamine, and benzo[a]pyrene [6]
Obesity	Excess weight escalates the production and circulation of estrogen and insulin. Subsequently, can trigger the cancer growth [6]
Air pollution	Some of the components that are responsible for air pollution include combustion products, industrial point sources in residential vicinity, radon, and organic fiber [6]
Genetics	Cancer predisposition in certain individuals can be caused by an error in genetic make-up of the corresponding individual. Sometimes, such changes can be inherited, and subsequently entire families are affected [6]
Infectious agent	Infectious agents can be the source of few cancers, e.g., *Helicobacter pylori* (HP) has been associated with the increased risk of stomach cancer nearly by 6-folds, *Human Papilloma Virus* (HPV) is the main cause of cervical cancer [6]
Occupational exposure	Some work-settings involve the risk of exposure to detrimental elements, e.g. diesel exhaust, solar radiation, wood dust, benzene, passive smoking, asbestos, polycyclic aromatic hydrocarbons, crystalline silica, cadmium, and nickel compounds, radon, chromium (VI), and formaldehyde [6]
Ionizing radiation	X-rays, γ-rays, and neutron radiations are carcinogenic to humans. Some of the ionizing radiation sources include natural terrestrial, cosmic background radiation, nuclear power production, atmospheric nuclear testing, nuclear accidents (e.g., Chernobyl), therapeutic usage of high-dose IR (radiotherapy for cancer treatment) [6]

1.4 Current Circumstantial Analysis

When compared with other MENA countries, Lebanon has a high Central Nervous System (CNS) cancer incidence rate in both genders. A study published in 2020 reported that males were more affected (34% increased risk) by CNS cancer compared with females in Lebanon. The association of various risk factors with the increased incidence of CNS cancers in the Lebanese community was observed. This includes pesticide exposure (agricultural workers are at high risk of such exposures due to their work-setting), ionizing radiations (CT scans), high level of uranium depletion (due to war and conflicts in the country), and genetic susceptibility [7].

In 2014, a study on high breast cancer incidence among Arab women showed obesity and strong family history were the prevailing risk factors in the community [8]. The significant economic progress in some parts of the Arab world has resulted in rapid urbanization in the region. Subsequently, lower physical activity, more accessibility to personal conveyance, and high caloric food intake have led to higher rates of obesity among the Arab population. Moreover, it was observed that women are more likely to become obese or overweight compared with men due to cultural norms [9].

From the hereditary cancer aspect, several Arab communities suffer from genetic disorders. This could be the result of increased inbreeding frequency (25–60% of all marriages are consanguineous, usually first cousin marriages). The absence of public health measures has aggravated the situation, along with legal, cultural, and religious limitations in the Arab world. Comprehensive research on familial cancers is needed in the Arab region, specifically broad-scale genetic screening programs coupled with genetic counseling. Few Arab countries (Saudi Arabia, Qatar, Egypt, and the United Arab Emirates) have launched their respective human genome project initiatives, which may pave the way to understanding of familial cancer genes [10].

Tobacco smoke is considered one of the most prevalent causes of lung cancer. Most Arab countries (Bahrain, Tunisia, Algeria, Morocco, and Libya) were able to illustrate a clear association between the risk of lung cancer and tobacco smoking prevalence in both genders. Few Arab countries, however, showed moderate (Egypt, Syria, and most GCC countries, except Bahrain) and low (Djibouti, Sudan, Yemen) cancer incidence rates despite high rates of smoking [11].

Asbestos exposure is associated with lung cancer, pulmonary fibrosis, and malignant pleural mesothelioma (MPM). In Egypt, mesothelioma cases represent 0.5% of all cancer cases. Studies from Lebanon, Jordan, and Tunisia have also reported the oncogenic effects due to asbestos exposure [11–13]. Considering the harmful effects of asbestos, the Government of Jordan issued a decree in 2005 to prohibit all kinds of asbestos [14].

A unified cancer control strategy is required at different community levels in the Arab region. Reducing exposure to avoidable risk factors can be the most effective strategy to control cancer. This can be achieved by adapting to an active lifestyle, following governmental policies, making healthy choices, and developing a commitment to maintain a better and healthier environment.

1.5   Oncology Care in the Arab World

1.5.1   Role of Cancer Registries

A cancer registry is an exclusive source of information. It is quite helpful for countries to develop strategies for cancer care and health programs. Several Arab countries have started to realize the importance of cancer registries which led to the establishment of the Gulf Center for Cancer Registration (GCCR), for the generation of population-based incidence data from GCC countries including Saudi Arabia, Bahrain, Kuwait, Qatar, the United Arab Emirates, and Oman. The registry started collecting data from 1st January 1998. The system works by assembling the data from the National Cancer Registry (NCR) of each individual country, followed by quality assurance measures. Data is received by GCCR in various formats (e.g., Epi-Info, Excel). Subsequently, GCCR converts all files to CanReg format (a validated software developed by the International Agency for Research on Cancer (IARC) to process cancer data) and then performs relevant analyses [15].

The most important element in cancer registration is to document mortality data, which can be affected by the extent to which the details have been provided and accuracy of the recorded cause of death along with completing the death registration process. These can vary significantly between countries and over time [6]. Most countries in the Arab world possess population-based cancer registries. However, all cancers are not well-documented and statistics for cancer mortality are also limited [4].

Comparative situational analysis can critically assess the cancer incidence, mortality, and survival patterns [6] in the Arab world, but this requires proper documentation for cancer mortality and morbidity rates to allow comparisons with Western countries.

1.5.2   Functionality of Oncology Societies in the Arab Region

The main responsibilities of cancer societies are to promote and foster the multi-dimensional care of cancer patients, by connecting practicing oncology professionals across all the disciplines (Fig. 1.2). Such associations support optimization of the expertise level among cancer professionals, augment the efficiency of cancer treatment, and strengthen collaborations with foreign oncology health bodies and encourage them to participate in Multidisciplinary Tumor Board Meetings (MDTs).

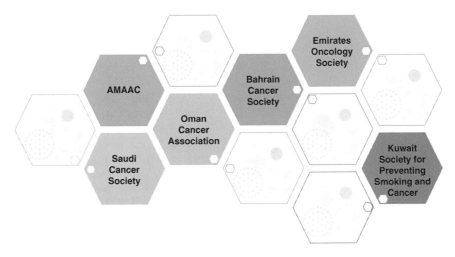

Fig. 1.2 Renowned cancer societies in the Arab world

1.6 Cancer Control Framework Recommendations

Various interventions can determine cancer outcomes, stretching from primary prevention to end-of-life care. A healthcare infrastructure that has been designed to deliver public health programs which can improve cancer outcomes along with turning down the cancer mortality rate (including clinical services for cancer diagnosed patients) is inevitably complex. This involves a broad range of highly competent professionals, together with input from their respective establishments at all stages of the healthcare journey [6].

Planned initiatives taken by healthcare authorities can lead to improved cancer outcomes among their country's population as well as at the individual's level. The following are excerpts from a study which suggested a complete range of interventions that can improve European cancer patients' outcomes [6]. The Arab world can also draw advantages by incorporating these suggestions into their healthcare infrastructure.

These recommendations include [6]:

- The population requires efficient cancer prevention, screening, and early diagnosis programs with the aim of achieving an overall reduction in cancer mortality rate.
- Individuals, who might have cancer, require a quick approach to appropriate professionals, for detailed examination, following proper clinical management.
- An effective cancer care system depends on a wide spectrum of cancer specialties, including multidisciplinary clinical professionals. This integrative approach executes the best plan for their respective patients' diagnosis, management, and support. Clinicians must also ensure safe and efficient treatment delivery to their patients.

- Diagnostic and treatment services should be accessible at all levels: primary, secondary, and tertiary. The majority of cancer patients reach out to different providers in the healthcare system during their treatment period. Hence, it is compulsory for the entire system to practice exceptional operational skills and develop the logical cancer care management plan.
- Effective communication and coordination skills among healthcare professionals must exist in the oncology care structure at every stage, to ensure the well-functioning delivery of cancer treatment.
- Complicated diagnostic interventions (like in lymphoma cases) or treatment (e.g., surgery, chemotherapy, or radiation for esophageal cancer cases) should be concentrated in a cancer-dedicated place, where all such essential expertise can be assembled in a cost-effective manner and the outcomes can be assessed persistently.
- The patients' views on therapeutic options along with the expected outcomes should be taken in consideration while making clinical decisions.
- A comprehensive cancer care plan should also implicate quality of life and psychosocial issues.

The need for high standard clinical cancer care services and a rise in patients' expectations for good outcomes has strained the entire healthcare system, even in countries with a strong economy. The growing expense of oncology treatments (including a speedy hike in anticancer drugs' cost) further increases the pressure on healthcare systems [6]. The Arab countries can cope with such a burden if they follow certain suggestions such as:

- Adopt systematic health technology assessment
- Assort the public health and clinical preferences
- Set the plan for the type of cancer treatment to be given and under what circumstances [6]

The aforementioned strategies, if applied in the Arab world, can support a framework for analytical decision-making, under inevitably limited resources.

The management of cancer patients can be reformed by advancing knowledge. Outstanding research determines the standard of care, and the significant relationship between research and the quality of patient care. Few studies have suggested that entities which take active part in clinical trials may generate improved outcomes. Advanced countries such as the United Kingdom and France have acknowledged this by extending links between clinical research, specifically Randomized Clinical Trials (RCTs) and oncology treatment systems. This kind of alliance is expected to improve cancer care delivery [6]. The field of cancer research has started developing in the Arab world. However, when compared with other regions, the total research output is nominal. Various gaps have been identified in a study that reviewed cancer research in the Arab World. The study found a deficiency in research that involves elderly individuals and analysis of certain risk factors, such as diet [3].

1.7 Cancer in the Arab World Book

There have been several articles, papers, and reviews that have attempted to quantify the cancer burden across the Arab region, yet these papers often target a specific site of cancer. So far, no comprehensive cancer analysis including epidemiological findings, oncology care services, education, and research for Arab countries has been presented. Hence, the editors came up with the notion of a book, entitled "Cancer in the Arab World." This book features general cancer care together with indications of challenges and suggested solutions for the Arab world.

The authors were invited to write about the general cancer care approach for their respective countries. Included countries were Algeria, Bahrain, Comoros, Djibouti, Egypt, Iraq, Jordan, Kuwait, Lebanon, Libya, Mauritania, Morocco, Oman, Palestine, Qatar, Saudi Arabia, Somalia, Sudan, Syria, Tunisia, the United Arab Emirates, and Yemen.

Moreover, eight special chapters were also included based on specific relevance and importance in the Arab region. These tackle common questions on breast and colorectal cancer, cancer care in conflict zones, palliative care, pediatric oncology, radiation therapy, challenges associated with medical tourism, and cancer research in the Arab World.

We do acknowledge that there were few countries for which we had difficulty in identifying authors or who had limited access to cancer related databases. Every author had gathered as much accessible and published data and relevant information from their respectful country as they could. However, there were several barriers related to the lack of data, or scattered information, or cancer statistics that have not been updated at the time of data collection.

The book analyzes the landscape of cancer care perspectives in Arab countries, to identify the gaps and opportunities in oncology care. This resource explores the issues associated with access and barriers to a high standard cancer care delivery throughout the region. The oncology field in the Arab world is complex. The cancer care burden in the region has been unevenly distributed based on gender, location, together with other various factors. Moreover, crises such as conflict zones and the growing number of immigrants have placed additional stress on oncology care organizations and providers in several countries.

1.7.1 Book Structure

This book attempted to incorporate the most crucial clinical service elements, recommended by the World Health Organization (WHO) for cancer control program [16]. An excellent approach to the complete spectrum of clinical services is important for prompt and suitable cancer diagnosis and treatment. Such services are crucial to timely curing cancer. The components have been elaborated under the aegis of more than 50 authors for their respective Arab countries (Fig. 1.3). Furthermore, in this volume, we tried to include the subjects that encompass the challenges in oncology core services, in accordance with the accessibility of the data for each country (Fig. 1.4). The cancer core services rely upon the center's capacity, and the allocation of healthcare facilities (stand-alone, union of health providers, or part of a larger hospital).

This project has been initiated to determine the void areas in cancer care prospects in the Arab world. It allows the readers to acquire a unique source of information to anyone tackling this subject in the region. Lastly, the book also aims to hopefully encourage all Arab countries to contribute and share cancer information among each other and internationally, to help analyze the areas that need to focus on cancer research and treatment in the future.

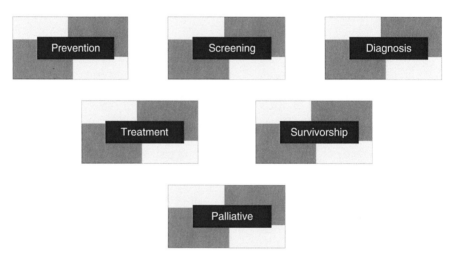

Fig. 1.3 Key cancer control components

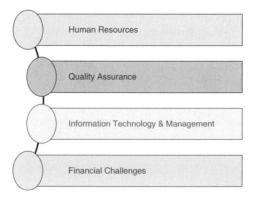

Fig. 1.4 Basic oncology core services

1.8   Closing the Gaps in the Cancer Care System

The comprehension of the shortfall in standards of current cancer services, along with other methods to improve the effectiveness and quality of the healthcare system, are the fundamental elements of any competent cancer control strategy. The oncology care system is complex as it requires multidisciplinary fields; hence, it poses critical challenges [16].

A broad range of differences, e.g., in education, availability of healthcare facilities, and quality of life has been observed among Arab countries, despite sharing a common language and culture. The Arab world stretches across an array of natural resources, from prosperous countries to the poverty, conflicts, and famine afflicted countries [17]. The chief target for the Arab region's healthcare authorities must be to transcribe the existing knowledge into an efficient plan of action at a population-level. Few approaches at the government level can steer cancer care services, subsequently producing good patients' outcomes in the Arab region (Fig. 1.5).

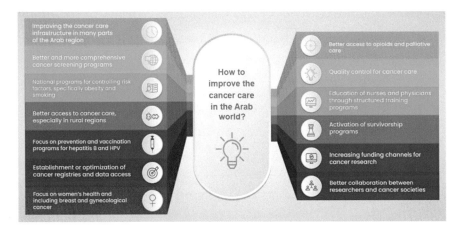

Fig. 1.5 Key suggestions to improve cancer care in the Arab world

1.9   Concluding Remarks

The cancer burden in the Arab region has been increasing. This chapter is a preface to the "Cancer in the Arab World" book. It presents the general cancer care approaches of included Arab countries. The illustration of complications and future perspectives in exceptional cancer care delivery along with the explanation of shortcomings in the respective countries has also been comprehended in this volume.

Conflict of Interest Authors have no conflict of interest to declare.

References

1. Siddiqui AA, Amin J, Alshammary F, Afroze E, Shaikh S, Rathore HA, Khan R. Burden of cancer in the Arab world. In: Handbook of healthcare in the Arab world. Springer; 2020. p. 495–519.
2. Salim EI, Moore MA, Al-Lawati JA, Al-Sayyad J, Bazawir A, Bener A, et al. Cancer epidemiology and control in the Arab world-past, present and future. Asian Pac J Cancer Prev. 2009;10(1):3–16.
3. Hamadeh RR, Borgan SM, Sibai AM. Cancer research in the Arab world: a review of publications from seven countries between 2000–2013. Sultan Qaboos Univ Med J. 2017;17(2):e147.
4. Arafa MA, Rabah DM, Farhat KH. Rising cancer rates in the Arab world: now is the time for action. East Mediterr Health J. 2020;26(6):638–40.
5. Ferlay J, Ervik M, Lam F, Colombet M, Mery L, Piñeros M, Znaor A, Soerjomataram I, Bray F. Global cancer observatory: cancer today. Lyon: International Agency for Research on Cancer; 2020. https://gco.iarc.fr/today. Accessed 21 Aug 2021
6. Coleman MP, Alexe DM, Albreht T, McKee M, World Health Organization. Responding to the challenge of cancer in Europe. Institute of Public Health of the Republic of Slovenia; 2008.
7. Salhab HA, Khachfe HH, Fares MY, Belkacemi Y, Hosseini H. Central nervous system cancers in the Middle East and North Africa (MENA) region: where does Lebanon stand. Chin Clin Oncol. 2020;9(2):36.
8. Elkum N, Al-Tweigeri T, Ajarim D, Al-Zahrani A, Amer SM, Aboussekhra A. Obesity is a significant risk factor for breast cancer in Arab women. BMC Cancer. 2014;14:788. https://doi.org/10.1186/1471-2407-14-788.
9. Alzaman N, Ali A. Obesity and diabetes mellitus in the Arab world. J Taibah Univ Med Sci. 2016;11(4):301–9.
10. AlHarthi FS, Qari A, Edress A, Abedalthagafi M. Familial/inherited cancer syndrome: a focus on the highly consanguineous Arab population. NPJ Genom Med. 2020;5(1):1–10.
11. Salim EI, Jazieh AR, Moore MA. Lung cancer incidence in the Arab league countries: risk factors and control. Asian Pac J Cancer Prev. 2011;12(1):17–34.
12. Kattan J, Faraj H, Ghosn M, Chahine G, Assaf E, Abadjian G, Khoury F. Mesothelioma-asbestos in Lebanon: a problem to be considered. Le Journal medical libanais - Leban Med J. 2001;49(6):333–7.
13. Bani-Hani KE, Gharaibeh KA. Malignant peritoneal mesothelioma. J Surg Oncol. 2005;91(1):17–25.
14. http://ibasecretariat.org/lka_asb_bans_jordan_rsa.php#1
15. Al Hamdan N, Ravichandran K, Al Sayyad J, Al Lawati J, Khazal Z, Al Khateeb F, et al. Incidence of cancer in gulf cooperation council countries, 1998-2001. East Mediterr Health J. 2009;15(3):600–11.
16. Gelband H, Jha P, Sankaranarayanan R, Horton S, editors. Cancer. disease control priorities. license: creative commons attribution CC BY 3.0 IGO, vol. vol 3. 3rd ed. Washington, DC: World Bank; 2015. https://doi.org/10.1596/978-1-4648-0349-9.

17. Waqas A, Mehmood S, Jawwad AM, Pittam B, Kundu S, Correia JC, AlMughamis N. Telemedicine in Arab countries: innovation, research trends, and way forward. Front Digit Health. 2021;2:58.

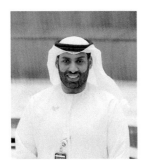

Prof. Humaid O. Al-Shamsi is the director of VPS oncology services in the United Arab Emirates, which is the largest cancer care provider network in the UAE. He is also the President of the Emirates Oncology Society and an adjunct professor at the College of Medicine—University of Sharjah. Prof. Al-Shamsi holds triple specialty board certifications in medical oncology from the UK, USA, and Canada. He completed his Bachelor of Science and Bachelor of Medicine from Cork University, the national university of Ireland with honors in 2005. He then completed his internal medicine residency followed by a medical oncology fellowship; he then completed a subspecialty combined fellowship in gastrointestinal and palliative oncology at McMaster University in Canada in 2013. He then joined MD Anderson Cancer Center, The University of Texas Houston, USA as an assistant professor from 2014 to 2017. Prof. Al-Shamsi is the founder of the Burjeel Cancer Institute at Burjeel Medical City in Abu Dhabi, UAE, which is the most comprehensive cancer center in the UAE. He has more than 70 peer reviewed articles and book chapters. His research focus is on precision medicine and health policies related to cancer care in the UAE and the Arab region. He was awarded the researcher of the year in 2020 and 2021 by the Emirates Oncology Society.

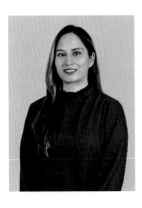

Ms. Faryal Iqbal holds an undergraduate degree in Molecular Biology and Biotechnology. Subsequently, she earned postgraduate qualification in Molecular Genetics from Pakistan, where she worked on finding the association between XRCC1 gene polymorphism and radiation exposure in healthcare workers. She is currently working with an oncology specific research group and serving in the domains of scientific writing, data management, supervision of medical internees, and providing editorial assistance. Ms. Iqbal's research interests and publications encompass genetics and oncology. She intends to support research across the oncology key areas including prevention, diagnosis, and treatment. Her focus is on preparing for future adoption of genomic technology and increased use of genomic information as part of the cancer diagnostic and therapeutic pathways.

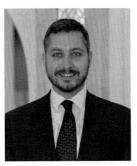

Dr. Ibrahim H. Abu-Gheida is the founding head of the Department of Radiation Oncology in Burjeel Medical City and an adjunct assistant professor at the United Arab Emirates University. Dr. Abu-Gheida completed his undergraduate training where he earned a Bachelor of Science with honors degree from the American University of Beirut. Following which Dr. Abu-Gheida completed his Medical School training at the American University of Beirut Medical Center. He continued and joined the Department of Internal Medicine at the American University of Beirut. Then did his training in the Department of Radiation Oncology at the American University of Beirut Medical Center, where he also served as the chief resident. During his training,

Dr. Abu-Gheida completed a Harvard-affiliated NIH-funded research program as well. After his residency, Dr. Ibrahim went to the Cleveland Clinic/Ohio, where he was appointed as an Advanced Clinical Radiation Oncology Fellow. Dr. Abu-Gheida went and joined the University of Texas MD Anderson Cancer Center. Dr. Abu-Gheida has many publications in prestigious medical journals including the American Society of Radiation Oncology official journal—International Journal of Radiation Oncology Biology and Physics, Nature, Journal of Clinical Oncology, and several others. He is also the primary author of several book chapters published in prestigious books. He also has been granted research awards during his residency.

Chapter 2
General Oncology Care in Algeria

Adda Bounedjar, Mohamed Aimene Melzi, Hassina Idir, and Nassiba Heba

2.1 Algeria Demographics

Cancer represents a particularly heavy burden because it causes more suffering and tragedy than any other disease at the personal and family level; it is also responsible for the greatest number of years of life lost. Finally, its particularly high and the constantly increasing financial burden risks unbalancing the entire financial structure of the health care system. In this chapter, we will review the state of cancer care in Algeria, after having first presented the determinants of health, i.e., the factors which influence the population's health status, few health indicators (mortality, morbidity, life expectancy) and finally risk factors (tobacco, obesity, diet, physical activity).

Since independence, the Algerian population has undergone a remarkable evolution in terms of demography; from 12 million inhabitants in 1966 to more than 43 million inhabitants in 2019 [1]. Figure 2.1 illustrates the evolution of the Algerian population between 1966 and 2019.

According to the report of the National Statistics Office published in 2020, the natural growth rate of the population is 1.93%, with a resident population in Algeria estimated at 43,900,000 inhabitants on January 1, 2021, including a male population of 50.7% and a median age of about 27.7 years (27.1 for men and 28.3 for women). The population aged over 60 years is estimated at 4,139,000 people, representing 9.5% of the total population [3]. Figure 2.2 shows the distribution of the Algerian population by age.

Life expectancy is estimated to be 77.2 years for men and 78.6 years for women (77.8 years in the overall population). A total of 198,000 deaths were recorded during 2019, with a crude mortality rate of 4.55%. Cancer deaths represent 12% of total deaths in 2016 [4].

A. Bounedjar (✉) · M. A. Melzi · H. Idir · N. Heba
Université Blida 1 Laboratoire de cancérologie, Faculté de Médecine, Blida, Algeria

Medical Oncology Department, Anti-Cancer Center, Blida, Algeria
e-mail: adda.bounedjar@univ-blida.dz

© The Author(s) 2022
H. O. Al-Shamsi et al. (eds.), *Cancer in the Arab World*,
https://doi.org/10.1007/978-981-16-7945-2_2

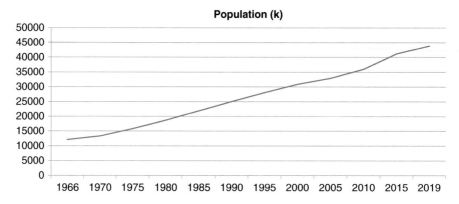

Fig. 2.1 Evolution of the Algerian population between 1966 and 2019 [1, 2]

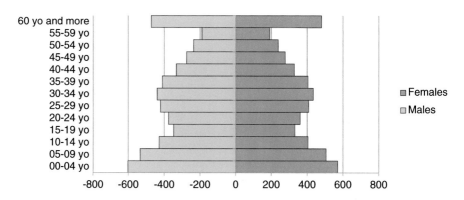

Fig. 2.2 Distribution of the Algerian population by age group and sex in 2019 [3]

2.2 Cancer Statistics in Algeria

2.2.1 Cancer Incidence in Algeria

A National Cancer Registry has been set up in the form of a network, comprising three regional registries covering the Center (13.5 million inhabitants), East (15.8 million inhabitants), and West (9.9 million inhabitants) regions, with coverage rates of 94.3%, 97%, and 86.6% respectively, and an overall coverage rate of 89.6% [1–3].

Algeria recorded 43,920 new cases of cancer in 2017, an incidence of 112.2 new cases per 100,000 inhabitants (93.7 new cases per 100,000 in men and 131.7 new cases per 100,000 in women [1–3]).

With an incidence of 14.2 new cases per 100,000 men, colorectal cancer is the most frequent cancer in men, followed by lung cancer (13.5 new cases per 100,000 men), prostate cancer (11.1 new cases/100,000 men), bladder cancer (10.16 new cases/100,000 men), and stomach cancer (8.4 new cases/100,000 men). The age of onset is 57, 62, 72, 65, and 60 years, respectively.

In women, the most common cancer is breast cancer with an incidence of 49.3 new cases/100,000 women, followed by colorectal cancer (12.9 new cases/100,000 women), thyroid cancer (9.3 new cases/100,000 women), cervical cancer (7.2 new cases/100,000 women), and stomach cancer (5.9 new cases/100,000 women). The median age of onset for women is 47, 65, 42, 62, and 65 years, respectively [5].

2.3   Oncology Care in Algeria

The fight against cancer in Algeria started during the French colonization. It was in 1928 that the first Anti-Cancer Center of Algiers was created, installed in the premises of the Mustapha Hospital. This center, if it had the merit to constitute the first link in the chain of anti-cancer fight in Algeria, could provide neither the screening nor the treatment of all the observed cancers.

In 1950, the Algerian center for the fight against cancer left the premises of the Mustapha Hospital to move into the buildings of the newly built Pierre and Marie Curie Center (CPMC). From January 1950 to December 1958 (9 years), 8706 cancers were registered in the central file of Algiers, divided according to ethnicity into:

- 5157 cases in the Muslim population, which amounted to 8,449,332 at the time
- 2164 cases in the population of European origin which amounted to 984,031
- 150 cases in the Jewish population

These few figures show that this anti-cancer fight was primarily aimed at the population of European origin and reached only very few Muslims.

After independence, with the development of medical knowledge and better health coverage in the country; the problem of caring for patients with cancer became a public health problem from 1975.

In terms of infrastructure for the treatment of cancer, apart from the CPMC, and until the early 2000s, there were only four Anti-Cancer Centers (ACCs) in Algeria (Algiers, Blida, Oran, Constantine), although the university departments of the various medical and surgical specialties took care of cancer patients within their specialties.

A reflection on what could be a national strategy to fight against cancer was emerging both in the medical community and the authorities in charge of health, to reduce mortality and cancer morbidity.

The epidemiological transition, which makes cancer one of the main causes of morbidity in the country, was however known: 42,720 new cases of cancer were recorded in 2015 in Algeria and 61,000 are expected in 2025 [5–7].

The construction of most of the Anti-Cancer Centers (ACCs) was relaunched in 2013, shortly before the National Anti-Cancer Plan, endowed with 185 billion dinars (about 1.6 billion euros at the time) until 2019 and placed under the supervision of the Presidency of the Republic, was adopted in 2015 [5].

2.3.1 National Cancer Control Plan 2015–2019

With cancer becoming a major public health problem, an anti-cancer plan was developed and implemented in 2014, with the objective of reducing mortality and morbidity of different types of cancers for the period 2015–2019. This plan was based on eight strategic axes [5] which are:

- Improving prevention against cancer risk factors
- Improving cancer screening
- Improving diagnosis
- Reinvigorating anti-cancer treatment
- The organization of the orientation, the accompaniment, and the follow-up of patients
- The development of the information and communication system
- Strengthening training and research
- The reinforcement of financing and care capacities

2.4 Cancer Risk Factors

The following are some known risk factors data [8].

- *Tobacco*: It is estimated that 11.22% of the population actively uses smoked tobacco (26.40% in men and 0.43% in women), with daily consumption in 94.81% of smokers (100% in women and 94.73% in men). The average age of smoking initiation is 19.13 years (18.83 years for women and 19.13 years for men). The average daily consumption is 14.77 cigarettes (9.91 cigarettes/day for women and 14.86 cigarettes/day for men).
- *Alcohol*: Alcohol consumption is found in 6.50% of the population (15.27% in men and 0.28% in women). The average consumption is 5.83 drinks/day.
- *Obesity*: Current data suggests that 55.90% of the population has a BMI ≥ 25 (66.52% of women and 41.29% of men). Global obesity (BMI ≥ 30) is found in 21.24% of subjects (30.08% of women and 9.07% of men). The frequency of obesity disease (BMI ≥ 40) is 1.14% with a clear female predominance (1.70% vs 0.38%). It is much more observed in urban areas (1.42% vs 0.65%).
- *Diet*: With a low consumption of fruits (0.6 per day vs. 2 recommended portions), vegetables (0.8 vs. 3 recommended portions), dairy products and animal proteins (1.3 vs. 2 recommended portions), and an excessive consumption of fatty and sugary foods (2.7 vs. 1 recommended portion) and cereals (3.8 vs. 3 recommended portions), the daily food consumption of the Algerian population is not in line with the international recommendations.
- *Physical Activity*: The most important part of the Algerian population's time is represented by low intensity physical activities, i.e., 14 h and 31 min per day (60.5% of the time), while moderate intensity activities represent only 8.35% of the time, i.e. 2 h per day. High intensity activities are very negligible and correspond to only 57 s per day.

2.5   Cancer Screening Programs

2.5.1   Cervical Cancer

A national cyto-diagnostic cervical cancer screening program has been implemented in collaboration with WHO since 1997 and HPV tests have been used since 2015 [8]. Currently, this cervical cancer screening consists of a request for a cervico-vaginal smear to women aged 25–65 years. The first smear is taken in the first year of marriage. It is followed by a second one a year later. If the two smears show no abnormalities, the woman is reassured and will only be asked for a follow-up smear once every 5 years [5]. Screening units located in the various gynecological facilities and departments at the university hospitals and local public health facilities are responsible for follow-up [9]. Smear tests are taken outside the menstrual period for all women, including those who are pregnant or in the menopause.

2.5.2   Breast Cancer

Algeria does not yet have an organized mass screening program for breast cancer, due to epidemiological particularities such as the young age of patients with a peak incidence before 50 years of age [10, 11] and technical difficulties related to the high breast density in Algerian women. Awareness campaigns on the interest in self-cleansing and the promotion of individual screening by mammography, especially among women at risk with a history of breast and/or ovarian cancer in the family, are organized through the media (press, billboards in public places, posters in waiting rooms of public and private health structures, etc.). These events multiply every year, especially during the month of October (pink October) with the participation of associations and private imaging centers.

2.5.3   Colorectal Cancer

The incidence of colorectal cancer in Algeria remains lower than those observed in Europe and the USA. Despite an annual increase of 7%, colorectal cancer screening in Algeria has remained controversial [12]. As the 2015–2019 national cancer program did not deem it necessary to include colorectal cancer as a priority, it was not until the publication of the results of the National Cancer Registry Network (as part of the First Atlas of Cancer in Algeria) in January 2017, that the Algerian National Cancer Screening Committee decided to introduce colorectal cancer screening in the objectives of the cancer plan, taking in consideration the incidence of colorectal (first and second place in men and women, respectively). This led to the launch of pilot studies in three wilayas of the country: Bejaia, Annaba, and Batna [13]. These studies use immunological tests to detect the presence of blood in the stool. A participation rate of 26% was obtained at a rate of 98% in the case of a positive test.

While some western countries (Europe and the USA) with a high incidence have implemented mass screening programs, in Algeria, recommendations and/or guidelines for oriented screening, i.e., individual screening for high-risk individuals, should be proposed at most. Other preventive measures include maintaining a correct body weight, practicing physical activity, minimizing red meat and alcohol consumption, and stopping smoking.

2.5.4 Prostate Cancer

To date, there is no organized screening for prostate cancer in Algeria. Only individual screening (voluntary) consisting of a rectal examination and Prostate Specific Antigen (PSA) test is recommended for men between the ages of 50 and 70, when life expectancy is estimated to be ≥10 years. Prostate cancer, which is continuously increasing in Algeria [14], is still diagnosed at a locally advanced and/or metastatic stage. In its objectives for 2015–2019, the cancer plan recommends the need to develop and ensure the dissemination by prescribers of clear information on the benefits and risks of individual screening for prostate cancer according to the modalities of management, as well as awareness and training of the attending physician [5]. At present, screening is carried out much more by associations or health structures at the initiative of isolated individuals.

Health professionals and the general population are exposed to a lot of alarming information about the frequency of cancers and their causes. This can lead to behavior without a rational basis. There is a need for a proper analysis of the data on the incidence of cancer and an assessment of the effect of the main causes identified, and of the means put in place by the country's health authorities for their management. Only based on this information, a validated strategy can be proposed for each of the major neoplastic sites.

2.6 Cancer Prevention Programs

A program of prevention (excluding vaccination) and control of risk factors is implemented within the framework of the multisectoral national strategic plan of integrated control of risk factors of non-transmittable diseases from 2015–2019 [8]. It is based on the following four main axes:

- Axis 1—Promotion of healthy nutrition, with the following objectives:

    - Promote nutrition for pregnant women, as well as exclusive breastfeeding up to 6 months and maintaining it up to 24 months
    - Promote healthy eating among children, youth, and adolescents in educational, school, and pre-school settings in order to reverse the trend of obesity

among children and adolescents, to reduce the prevalence of micronutrient deficiencies and to reduce the incidence of foodborne diseases
- Reduce the daily intake of salt, sugar, and fat in the general population
- Prevent obesity in the general population.

- Axis 2—The promotion of physical activity, the practice of sports and active mobility, with the following objectives:

  - Promote the practice of physical activity and sport
  - Promote active mobility

- Axis 3—Tobacco control, with the following objectives:

  - Strengthen tobacco control legislation and regulations in line with the provisions of the WHO Framework Convention on Tobacco Control
  - Create an environment conducive to reducing tobacco use
  - Provide smoking cessation assistance
  - Establish a comprehensive and permanent tobacco monitoring system

- Axis 4—The coordination framework, with the main objective of institutionalizing a multisectoral coordination framework, ensuring the implementation of actions to prevent risk factors for non-transmittable diseases.

  - Vaccination against hepatitis B was introduced in 2000, with a four-dose schedule: the first, at birth, followed by three doses at 2 months, 4 months, and then 12 months. But, to date, vaccination against HPV has not yet been implemented

2.7 Cancer Diagnosis

Algeria currently has 1400 radiologists, 2500 radiology rooms, 634 CT machines, 180 MRI machines, 2 PET scanners, 250 mammograms, with a total of 13 university hospital radiology services spread over the national territory.

Histopathology diagnosis is performed by the various public and private anatomical pathology departments, including 20 university hospital departments, providing standard and immunohistochemistry or in situ hybridization techniques. Reading committees for rare and atypical tumors have been set up since 2015 to improve the quality and response time of rare and/or complicated cases. Algeria also has five molecular biology platforms for the study of genetic mutations and genomic alterations of tumors, for therapeutic and scientific purposes [5, 6].

2.8 Treatment

Cancer treatment in Algeria is provided by 22 Anti-Cancer Centers, five of which belong to the public sector (liberal). Each center has a medical oncology department, radiotherapy with 52 linear accelerators, surgery, radiology, hematology, an analysis laboratory, and a pathological anatomy laboratory. There are also ten medical oncology departments, 22 surgical departments, and three hematology departments involved in cancer care and belonging to the various university hospitals and public hospitals in the country. A multidisciplinary discussion of rare and complicated cases is organized in multidisciplinary consultation meetings concerning digestive oncology; thoracic and urological oncology; neuro-oncology, sarcomas, head and neck cancers, and breast cancer.

2.8.1 Medical Oncology

Medical oncology is a specialty in full development in Algeria, with an increase of the future medical staff. The enumeration of medical oncologists was carried out by crossing files of practitioners provided by various organizations and learned societies, which allowed us to count approximately 1000 medical oncologists distributed on the whole territory. The duration of the training in this field is 4 years, with a total of 60 trainees counted in the fourth year.

2.8.2 Radiation Therapy

Currently, there are 600 active radiation oncologists. The initial training in radiotherapy takes place over 4 academic years. The number of trainees has been considerably growing in recent years, to keep up with the growing demand for new radiation therapy facilities and the acquisition of new equipment.

2.8.3 Surgery

Even if to date, there is no training in oncological surgery, surgical treatment is provided, depending on the neoplastic locations by organ specialists in university hospitals, Anti-Cancer Centers (CAC), and in the private sector also.

2.8.4 Pediatric Oncology

At present, there is no specialized training in pediatric oncology; the care of children and adolescents with cancer is done jointly by pediatricians and oncologists, either in pediatric or radiotherapy departments, in dedicated pediatric oncology units. The number of pediatricians trained in oncology is expected to increase with the creation of cross-disciplinary training in pediatric hematology and oncology.

2.8.5 Survivorship Track

The available data regarding cancer survivorship in Algeria suggests an estimated standardized net survival for adults (15–99 years) of 59.8% (95% CI: 48.6–71.1) for breast cancer, 58.5% (95% CI: 51.2–65.9) for prostate cancer, 57.2% (95% CI: 45.6–68.9) and 45.5% (95% CI: 36.3–54.8) for colon cancer and rectum cancer, respectively, 55.1% (95% CI: 49.8–60.4) for cervix cancer, 41.8% (95% CI: 22.2–61.4) for ovary cancer, and 14.8% (95% CI: 11.2–18.4) and 10.3% (95% CI: 6.7–14.0) for lung and stomach cancer, respectively [15].

2.8.6 Palliative Care Track

In Algeria, palliative care is still in the process of development, with only two units (the Anti-Cancer Center in Blida and the Pierre and Marie Curie Center in Algiers) currently treating patients with cancer at this stage of the disease. Palliative care in oncology is one of the objectives of the Cancer Plan, which has been gradually translated in recent years into various incentives for the organization and structuring of emerging units, thus increasing the possibilities for patients to benefit from it.

2.9 Research and Education

2.9.1 Clinical Trials and Research

At present, Algeria's participation in clinical trials represents 0.026% of the world's participation, with a total of 95 trials conducted until March 2021 [16]. Clinical trials in oncology represent 28.42% of all clinical trials conducted in Algeria, with a remarkable improvement from 10 trials in 2019 to 27 in 2021 [16, 17].

Interventional trials represent 62.96% of total trials, of which 70.59% are phase 3 (23.53% for phase 2 and 5.88% for phase 4). The total number of patients to be included in the 27 trials is 16,962, of which 52.8% are observational trials, 44.58% are phase 3, and 1.77% and 0.84% are phase 2 and 4, respectively [16]. Table 2.1 summarizes the clinical trials conducted in Algeria by cancer site.

More than 25% of the clinical trials in cancer in Algeria focused on breast cancer, with a total of 7317 patients to be included, i.e. 43.14% of the patients to be included in the clinical trials on cancer [16]. The number of patients to be included in clinical trials in Algeria is shown in Fig. 2.3.

Table 2.1 Clinical trials conducted in Algeria until March 2021 [16]

Trial Area	Number	Number of subjects
Breast cancer	7	7317
Prostate cancer	1	1533
Rectal cancer	2	434
Ovarian cancer	1	248
Nasopharyngeal cancer	2	141
Renal cancer	2	283
Lung cancer	1	919
Gastric cancer	1	1000
Multiple myeloma	2	2455
Thyroid cancer	1	667
Cervical cancer	1	40
Bone metastasis	1	650
Lymphoma	2	694
Others	3	581
Total	27	16,962

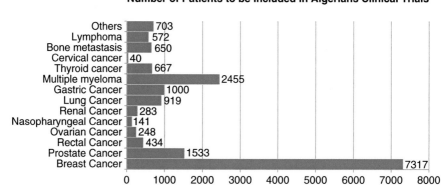

Fig. 2.3 Patients included in the clinical trials in Algeria in 2021 [16]

2.9.2 Scientific Publications

The scientific publications of Algeria have seen an interesting improvement in recent years, reaching 89 articles published in 2020 [18]. There are currently 1718 articles published by Algeria available on PubMed since 1963. The share of oncology in scientific publications represents 5.3%, corresponding to 91 articles since 1963 [18]. Figure 2.4 illustrates the evolution of Algerian oncology papers available on PubMed since 1963.

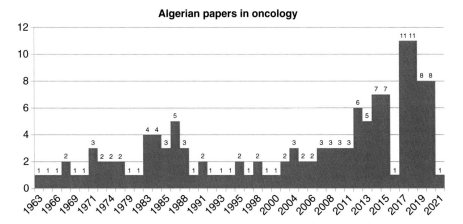

Fig. 2.4 Distribution of scientific publications from Algeria available on PubMed by year of publication since 1963 [18]

2.9.3 Training and Education

The training of medical personnel specialized in cancer (medical oncology, radiotherapy, and surgery) is ensured by 11 of the 14 faculties of medicine spread over the national territory. A total of 124 professors (medical oncology: 21.77%, radiotherapy: 9.68%, and surgery: 68.55%), 62 senior lecturers A (20.97% in medical oncology, 8.06% in radiotherapy, and 70.97% in surgery), 34 senior lecturers B (26.47% in medical oncology, 2.94% in radiotherapy, and 70.59% in surgery), and 197 assistant professors (20.90% in medical oncology, 10.66% in radiotherapy, and 62.44% in surgery) oversee providing the necessary medical education in cancer care. The Algerian faculties of medicine provide training for more than 1500 residents in the three specialties (24.4% for medical oncology, 8.49% for radiotherapy, and 67.11% for surgery), with more than 200 cancer specialists graduating each year (40.40% in medical oncology, 10.10% in radiotherapy, and 49.49% in surgery).

However, for medical oncology and radiotherapy, it is a training dedicated to cancerous disease, it is not a specific training in cancer surgery. Thus, any organ surgeon can manage a cancer patient in his or her specialty, which can be a loss of chance for the patient if the surgical procedure is incomplete or not indicated. In addition, in the Anti-Cancer Centers with a cancer surgery department, the surgeons are general surgeons who can manage cancers of the digestive tract, the gynecological sphere, and the thyroid. For cancers of other parts of the human body, it is always the surgical departments of specialties that are in charge.

2.9.4 Paramedical Training

Paramedical training is provided by 24 National Institutes of Higher Paramedical Training, seven paramedical training institutes, and one paramedical training school, spread throughout the country.

2.10 Cost Effective Cancer Care

The cost of cancer care in hospitals is about 500 million dollars. Cancer surgery represents more than one third of expenses. The remaining two thirds are represented by chemotherapy and radiation therapy since they are mostly given in multiple consecutive sessions. All treatment costs in the public sector are covered by the Algerian state with full medical coverage. Only 5% of the treatments are insured in the private sector and financed on an individual basis.

2.11 Challenges and Advantages

2.11.1 Access to Innovative Treatments

Algerian patients have free access to new technologies and innovative oncological treatments, such as monoclonal antibodies, tyrosine kinase inhibitors, and more recently immunotherapies, with a delay of around 2–3 years between obtaining the drug, Marketing Authorization in the USA and Europe, and registration of the drug in Algeria. This deadline is linked to the procedures for submitting and reviewing files at the level of the Ministry of Health.

2.11.2 Cancer Care

Cancer care in Algeria is financed by the Algerian state, free care has been a fundamental right since independence [5, 6].

2.12 The Future of Cancer Care in Algeria

The fight against cancer focuses on cancer care in general, with access to prevention, screening, palliative, and treatment services. The treatment of cancer continues to rest largely on three major modalities: surgery, radiotherapy, and systemic therapies, including chemotherapy and other approaches such as immunotherapy, targeted therapy, and gene therapy.

Future investment in the field of cancer should strengthen the impact of the national capacities; the performance should be more than ever on the agenda of the national health authorities to achieve two goals: reducing cancer related mortality and reducing cancer incidence.

The main objective is to stress the importance of being as close as possible to healthcare professionals and help them treat their patients better through training, not just new products, and technologies, to think about sustainable strategies that look towards the future lying in precision and individualized healthcare.

2.13 Conclusion

Colorectal, lung, prostate, and bladder cancers in men; breast, cervical, and thyroid cancers in women are the main cancers in adults in Algeria. Demographic changes in the population will have a major influence on the expected number of cancer cases in the future. In addition to the increase in cancer incidence due to demographic changes, changes in incidence and mortality rates for specific cancers will impact the future burden of these diseases. Since the implementation of the five-year plans to fight cancer, Algeria is catching up in terms of management of cancer patients, especially in terms of radiotherapy. Efforts remain to be made to develop multidisciplinary collaboration between the different specialists in charge of cancer disease, to introduce in the training cycle of surgery a subspecialty of cancer surgery after obtaining the surgeon's diploma, as it is done in most of the developed countries, to arrive at a care of cancer patients in dedicated centers provided with an adequate technical platform where the medical staff has an exclusive exercise in cancer care. Finally, to insist with the authorities to make the project of the Cancer Institute which was to be built in Oran and which would be the national reference center.

Conflict of Interest Authors have no conflict of interest to declare.

References

1. Statistiques rétrospectives 1962 - 2011. Algeria. Disponible sur: https://www.ons.dz/IMG/pdf/CH1-DEMOGRAPHIE.pdf
2. Berrah MK. Démographie Algérienne 2015. Algeria: National Office of Statistics; 2016 avr. Report no.: 740. Disponible sur: https://www.ons.dz/IMG/pdf/Demographie2015.pdf
3. Zidouni H. Démographie Algérienne 2019. Algeria: National Office of Statistics; 2020 avr. Report no.: 890/Bis. Disponible sur: https://www.ons.dz/IMG/pdf/demographie2019_bis.pdf
4. Belamri S. Causes médicales de décès (2015 - 2016). Algeria: National Institute of public Health; 2016. Disponible sur. http://www.insp.dz/images/PDF/Causes%20de%20deces/RAPPORT%202015-2016%20%203DC%20(2).pdf

5. Zitouni M. Plan national cancer 2015 - 2019. ANDS; 2014. Disponible sur: https://extranet.who.int/ncdccs/Data/DZA_B5_plan_national_cancer.pdf
6. Transition épidémiologique et système de santé 2007: Projet TAHINA. 2007.
7. Brehant J. Les centres anticancéreux en France et en Algérie. Bull Alger Carcinol. 1959;11(35):153–75.
8. Plan stratégique national multisectoriel de lutte intégrée contre les facteurs de risque des maladies non transmissibles 2015 - 2019.
9. Boublenza L, Moulessehoul S, Beldjillali H, Hadef K, Boulenouar F, Chabni N, et al. Analyse des activités de dépistage du cancer du col de l'utérus dans une région de l'ouest Algérien entre 2007 et 2011. J Afr Cancer Afr J Cancer. 2013;5(1):11–5.
10. Bounedjar A. Epidemiology and characteristic of breast cancer in CHU Blida, Algeria. 1.
11. Cherbal F, Gaceb H, Mehemmai C, Saiah I, Bakour R, Rouis AO, et al. Distribution of molecular breast cancer subtypes among Algerian women and correlation with clinical and tumor characteristics: a population-based study. Breast Dis. 1 juin 2015;35(2):95–102.
12. Abid L. Un dépistage du cancer colorectal est-il justifié en Algérie ? 2016. Disponible sur: http://www.santetropicale.com/santemag/algerie/poivue93.htm
13. Bouzid K, Mazouzi C. Organized screening for colorectal cancer in Algeria: first pilot study in North Africa. J Clin Oncol. 20 mai 2018;36(15_suppl):e15697.
14. Hamdi Cherif M, Zaidi Z, Abdellouche D, Hamdi S, Lakhdari N, Djema Bendjazia A, et al. Registre du cancer de Sétif (Algérie): incidence, tendance et survie, 1986–2005. J Afr Cancer Afr J Cancer. 2010;2(4):245–58.
15. Hamdi Cherif M, Bidoli E, Birri S, Mahnane A, Zaidi Z, Boukharouba H, et al. Cancer estimation of incidence and survival in Algeria 2014. J Cancer Res Ther. 2015;3(9):100–4.
16. Home - ClinicalTrials.gov. cité 3 mars 2021. Disponible sur: https://clinicaltrials.gov/ct2/home
17. Odedina FT, Shamley D, Okoye I, Ezeani A, Ndlovu N, Dei-Adomakoh Y, et al. Landscape of oncology clinical trials in Africa. JCO Glob Oncol. 2 juill 2020;6:932–41.
18. PubMed. cité 3 mars 2021. Disponible sur: https://pubmed.ncbi.nlm.nih.gov/

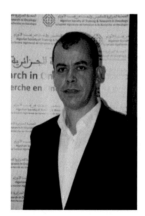

Adda Bounedjar is a Chairman of the Medical Oncology Department at Anti-Cancer Center, Blida, Algeria. He is a Professor of Medical Oncology at Blida 1 University. He is a President of the Algerian Society of Training and Research in Oncology (SAFRO) and a Vice president of the Arab Medical Association against Cancer (AMAAC). He is a chairman of Cancer Research Laboratory at Blida University. He is a member in the MENA-NCCN steering committee and of ASCO Clinical Practice Guideline Advisory, and he is also a member of several international research groups and scientific societies (ACHOG, ICRG, Saint Paul, AMCI, BGICC, ASCO, and ESMO). He has published some publications in international journals.

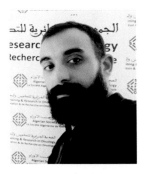

Dr. Mohamed Aimene Melzi, MD, is an assistant professor at the Faculty of Medicine of the Blida University 1 and a medical oncologist at the Medical Oncology Department of the Anti-Cancer Center of Blida. He is a cofounder and a member of the executive board of the Algerian Society of Training and Research in Oncology (SAFRO) and a member of the oncology team at the Cancer Laboratory of Blida.

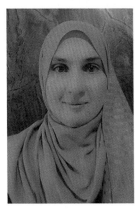

Dr. Hassina Idir is an assistant professor in medical oncology at the Medical Oncology Department of the Anti-Cancer Center of Blida, Algeria. She is affiliated to the Faculty of Medicine at Blida 1 university, Algeria. She served as a member of the executive board of the Algerian Society of Training and Research in Oncology (SAFRO).

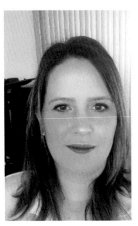

Dr. Nassiba Heba, MD, is a Medical Oncologist (since 2017). She has done advanced medical training and obtained several diplomas, including Cancer Supportive Care from Paris Descartes University, Geriatric Oncology from Toulouse University, Immuno-Oncology and Clinical Carcinology at the Gustave Roussy Institute, Paris Sud University, France. Dr. Heba has joined the Medical Oncology Department of the Anti-Cancer Center of Blida and helped for the foundation of the supportive care unit. She is a member of the Algerian Society of Training and Research in Oncology (SAFRO) and International Oncology Associations.

Chapter 3
General Oncology Care in Bahrain

Ravi Mohan Pedapenki and Ali Madan

3.1 Bahrain Demographics

The Kingdom of Bahrain is an island nation of about 800 sq km, the smallest among the Gulf Cooperative Council (GCC) region, rich in its culture and history. It has a population of about 1.56 million (according to the 2019 statistics). The native population is about 49% and Expatriates consist of 51% of the population. Bahrain has a universal health care system dating back to 1960 with all its citizens are provided with free health care by the government and to a certain extent subsidized to expatriates. With an average life expectancy of 77.7 years, (females 78.9 and males 76.9), The Kingdom of Bahrain has been ranked first in the Arab region as the healthiest country, and 36th in the world, among 169 countries around the world, based on various factors that reflect on health in general, and published by "Bloomberg" in a detailed report monitoring the health index globally in 2019 [1].

3.2 Cancer Statistics in Bahrain

The average annual crude cancer incidence rate is 86.3/100,000 for Bahraini males and 97.5/100,000 for Bahraini females (according to 2020 statistics). The average age-specific incidence rate of cancer is 136.4 and 135.8 per 100,000 Bahraini males and females, respectively, which is higher than GCC states and lower than Australia/New Zealand [2]. Lung cancer tops the list among males [3]. Breast, Lung, Colorectal, Bladder, and Prostate are the top five cancers among solid tumors;

R. M. Pedapenki (✉) · A. Madan
Department of Oncology-Hematology, Salmaniya Medical Complex, Ministry of Health, Manama, Kingdom of Bahrain

© The Author(s) 2022
H. O. Al-Shamsi et al. (eds.), *Cancer in the Arab World*,
https://doi.org/10.1007/978-981-16-7945-2_3

furthermore, Leukemias and lymphomas tops among the hematological malignancies. For females, breast cancer tops the list with an incidence of 53 per 100,000 population; it is second highest in the GCC only after Kuwait [4]. Lung cancer is the number one cause of death among males and breast cancer among females. The detailed list is given in Table 3.1 [5].

3.3   Oncology Care in Bahrain

Cancer treatment has been made available in the multi-specialty tertiary care hospital in the Ministry of Health facility at the Salmaniya Medical Complex (SMC), Manama, Bahrain since 1997, with a Radiotherapy unit. Subsequently, a chemotherapy unit and hemato-oncology services were added in 1999. General surgeons were offering the surgical management of solid tumors to a certain extent. Till then, the majority of the cases were referred for treatment abroad in Europe, the United States, India, and Singapore. After 2000, a greater number of Bahraini physicians got training abroad in oncological subspecialties including medical, radiation, and surgical oncology, and started treating cancer patients requiring multidisciplinary cancer care. Pediatric oncology and hemato-oncology services were available from 2000 onward. But most pediatric cancer patients were referred abroad for treatment till 2010. In early 2019, a new center was developed – Bahrain Oncology Center (BOC) on the premises of King Hammad university hospital (KHUH) with state-of-the-art equipment including the latest generation Linear accelerators, Brachytherapy, PET CT scans, PET MRI, and other Radio-nuclear pharmaceuticals. Apart from that, this facility also offers bone marrow/stem cell transplantation. From the diagnosis standpoint, most of the molecular testing is made available in this new facility [6]. No comprehensive cancer care facility is available in the private sector at present, but few multi-specialty hospitals provide surgical oncology, medical oncology services and palliative care. Bahraini citizens are treated free of charge, but expatriates are treated on payment to a certain extent for diagnostics and treatment in public hospitals.

3.4   Cancer Risk Factors

Cancer risk factors in Bahrain are similar to other GCC countries. Smoking is one of the most important risk factors, particularly among the young population. Obesity is another important risk factor; 33% of the Bahraini population is obese, particularly adolescents, which is one of the highest in the GCC. Due to consanguineous marriages, the prevalence of genetically transmitted cancers has been identified like BRCA 1 and 2. A government sponsored program of the genetic testing of all Bahraini citizens was started at the beginning of 2019 [7, 8].

Table 3.1 Incidence, mortality, and prevalence by cancer site in Bahrain 2018 (Source: Globocan 2020) [5]

Cancer	New cases				Deaths				5-year prevalence (all ages)	
	Number	Rank	(%)	Cum.risk	Number	Rank	(%)	Cum.risk	Number	Prop.
Breast	227	1	21.7	4.77	67	2	11.1	1.57	798	139.05
Lung	81	2	7.7	1.18	76	1	12.6	1.18	82	5.23
Colon	72	3	6.9	1.01	40	3	6.6	0.56	184	11.74
Non-Hodgkin lymphoma	61	4	5.8	0.88	23	11	3.8	0.44	181	11.55
Leukaemia	50	5	4.8	0.37	39	4	6.5	0.30	147	9.38
Bladder	47	6	4.5	0.68	25	9	4.1	0.34	142	9.06
Rectum	46	7	4.4	0.64	28	6	4.6	0.40	127	8.10
Prostate	39	8	3.7	1.16	14	13	2.3	0.30	124	12.49
Ovary	35	9	3.3	0.97	25	10	4.1	0.81	10	17.60
Thyroid	34	10	3.2	0.23	11	16	1.8	0.14	126	8.04
Brain, central nervous system	34	11	3.2	0.37	22	12	3.6	0.29	108	6.89
Liver	30	12	2.9	0.37	28	7	4.6	0.36	22	1.40
Pancreas	30	13	2.9	0.52	29	5	4.8	0.52	22	1.40
Stomach	30	14	2.9	0.39	27	8	4.5	0.39	48	3.06
Corpus uteri	29	15	2.8	0.58	8	22	1.3	0.16	97	16.90
Cervix uteri	19	16	1.8	0.46	12	15	2.0	0.37	59	10.28
Kidney	18	17	1.7	0.15	10	19	1.7	0.10	47	3.00
Lip, oral cavity	16	18	1.5	0.19	10	18	1.7	0.13	47	3.00
Multiple myeloma	13	19	1.2	0.14	12	14	2.0	0.13	35	2.23
Hodgkin lymphoma	13	20	1.2	0.08	4	25	0.66	0.04	52	3.32
Gallbladder	11	21	1.0	0.23	11	17	1.8	0.23	1	0.70
Larynx	10	22	0.95	0.16	8	21	1.3	0.14	30	1.91
Oesophagus	9	23	0.86	0.12	9	20	1.5	0.12	9	0.57
Testis	7	24	0.67	0.08	2	26	0.33	0.06	29	2.92
Nasopharynx	6	25	0.57	0.08	4	24	0.66	0.08	19	1.21
Mesothelioma	5	26	0.48	0.12	5	23	0.83	0.12	6	0.38
Anus	2	27	0.19	0.04	2	27	0.33	0.04	6	0.38
Vulva	1	28	0.10	0.02	1	28	0.17	0.02	4	0.70
Oropharynx	1	29	0.10	0.01	1	29	0.17	0.01	3	0.19
Melanoma of skin	1	30	0.10	0.01	1	30	0.17	0.01	3	0.19
Salivary glands	0	31	0	0	0	32	0	0	0	0
Kaposi sarcoma	0	32	0	0	0	33	0	0	0	0
Hypopharynx	0	33	0	0	0	34	0	0	0	0
Vagina	0	34	0	0	0	35	0	0	0	0
Penis	0	35	0	0	0	31	0	0	0	0
All cancer sites	1 048	–	–	11.49	603	–	–	7.82	2 828	180.47

3.5   Cancer Screening Programs

Cancer screening programs for breast and cervical cancers have been available for over a decade with mammography machines installed in some health centers in the country at primary care [9, 10]. PAP smear test is also available for women "at risk" in primary care. Prostate cancer screening is available in the tertiary care hospital at SMC for men at higher risk. Screening for colorectal cancer is also available at SMC.

3.6   Cancer Prevention Programs

Hepatitis B vaccination is undertaken at the primary care level. No vaccination program with HPV vaccine is available in public hospitals but it is optional and available in private hospitals [10].

3.7   Cancer Diagnosis

Imaging facilities of CT, MRI, Gamma cameras (scintillation cameras) are available in the tertiary care in SMC and at KHUH. PET/CT and PET/MRI are available only at KHUH. Organ-specific nuclear imaging is also available at KHUH. Laboratory Testing facility for Molecular testing, Cytogenetics and Genetic testing, e.g., KRAS, NRAS, BRAF, FISH, HER2, and hereditary cancer genetic tests are available at the tertiary hospitals of SMC and KHUH.

3.8   Treatment

3.8.1   Medical Oncology

Medical oncology and hemato-oncology departments in SMC and in BOC are active in providing treatment with cytotoxic chemotherapy and systemic treatment including immunotherapy, targeted therapy, and biological agents. Stem Cell Transplantation (autologous and allogeneic) facility is only available in BOC [11]. Medical oncology services are available in a few multi-specialty hospitals in the private sector. There are about 14 (3 Bahraini and all other expatriates) registered medical oncologists currently practicing in public and private hospitals [12].

3.8.2 Radiation Therapy

Currently, only one radiation oncology facility is functioning at BOC with four linear accelerators and one Gamma knife providing 3D, Intensity-Modulated Radiation Therapy (IMRT), Volumetric Modulated Arc Therapy (VMAT), Stereotactic Body Radiation Therapy (SBRT), and Stereotactic Radiosurgery (SRS) services. A dedicated brachytherapy unit is also functioning at the BOC. Currently, 12 registered radiation oncologists are practicing in public hospitals in BOC and SMC. None in the private sector.

3.8.3 Surgery

Many trained surgeons are providing services for specific cancers like breast cancers, gynecological cancers, thoracic, and head and neck cancers. Many of these qualified surgeons provide services in both public and private hospitals. Some of them are also offering laparoscopic and robotic surgeries (for radical prostatectomy). Hyperthermic Intraperitoneal Chemotherapy (HIPEC) is currently not available in Bahrain.

3.8.4 Pediatric Oncology

Pediatric oncology services have been available in Salmaniya medical complex since the early 2000 and at BOC since 2019. Both the centers are providing comprehensive treatment for pediatric cancers.

3.8.5 Survivorship Track

Survivorship from cancer tracks is maintained with annual functions of the survivors by the government as well as by the Bahrain cancer society. Post-treatment surveillance is carried out on these patients and for long-time survivors. Screening and surveillance for second cancers is regularly undertaken for these cancer survivors.

3.8.6 Palliative Care Track

Palliative and best supportive care is available at Salmaniya medical complex and at BOC with palliative care physicians, counselors, dietitians, psychiatrists, pain management, and social support teams. Regular palliative care clinics provide supportive care and pain management. Some of the patients are also provided with home care with the palliative team visiting the patient's residences. However, no hospice care center is available in Bahrain.

3.9 Research and Education

Currently, no oncology-related training programs are available in Bahrain. Bahraini doctors are sent abroad for specialized training in oncology. After obtaining the necessary qualification, these doctors typically work in public oncology facilities. Currently, both the oncology facilities are not involved in any international or national clinical trials. Regular national, regional international conferences and workshops are organized in Bahrain with public and private partnerships. There is a Bahrain Cancer Registry which is maintained by the Ministry of Health and cancer is a notifiable disease.

3.9.1 National Tumor Board (NTB)

The National Tumor Board (NTB) was established in early 2019 [13], where all cases of cancer, both from public and private hospitals are discussed for optimal multidisciplinary management. The meeting is organized twice a week at the BOC. Bahrain Cancer Society [14] was established in the late 1990s in the private sector, which organizes cancer awareness programs, educational events including organizing conferences, workshops, and other charitable programs in collaboration with the government oncology facilities.

There are few medical journals published from Bahrain. Bahrain Medical Bulletin is a popular medical journal in the country, but no specific oncological journal published. But every year few articles are published by Bahraini oncologists in national and international journals. Unfortunately, no basic research has been done so far on oncology in public hospitals.

3.10 Cost-Effective Cancer Care

Cancer treatment is expensive with the advent of new drugs and treatment modalities, it exhausts the health budget of the country [15]. Cancer care accounts for one-third of the health budget in Bahrain. To reduce the cost and to avoid human error, cases are discussed in the NTB for any change in the treatment modality following the current NCCN/NICE guidelines. Many generic molecules and biosimilars are incorporated into the pharmacy to cut short the cost of the treatment. Sometimes alternate therapies/molecules are used to reduce the financial burden.

3.11   Challenges and Advantages

Bahrain too comes across specific challenges in cancer care, particularly for the human resources of trained and qualified personnel [16]. The majority of the medical and radiation oncologists are expatriates, as few locals show interest in these challenging branches of oncology for training. Due to the social milieu, and taboo sometimes, patients' acceptance of a particular treatment modality is a daunting task. Many patients consult at an advanced stage of the disease when treatment is purely palliative. There is a considerable need for a greater number of facilities for palliative and supportive care, particularly a good hospice is the need of the hour as there are large numbers of terminally ill cancer patients.

The advantage is that the country is small in a compact area with a limited population, screening, surveillance, and follow-up are done effectively [1].

3.12   The Future of Cancer Care in Bahrain

With the new comprehensive cancer care center—Bahrain Oncology Center started functioning at the beginning of 2019, with its state-of-the-art equipment and qualified doctors in each subspecialty of oncology, there is great hope for cancer patients in Bahrain for *A HOLISTIC MANAGEMENT OF CANCER* in this center. Unfortunately, few of the Bahraini doctors are showing interest in the field of oncology, as a result, majority of the medical oncologists are expatriates. There is a need for more Bahraini doctors to be trained in oncology to fill the gap [16]. The available two public cancer care facilities need to increase the capacity to take the patient load [17]. More space and personnel are needed for palliative and supportive care. There is a strong need for a hospice center.

3.13   Conclusion

Bahrain, though a small country with a high incidence rate of cancer in the GCC, enjoys a high standard of health care. There is a comprehensive cancer center, Bahrain Oncology Center, which has been functioning since 2019. Salmaniya Medical Complex, a multi-specialty tertiary care center, takes care of cancer patients free of charge to all its citizens. Private hospitals treat a small number of cancer patients, both locals and expatriates. The majority of cancer caregivers are expatriates. There is a need for international collaboration for cancer research and clinical trials. The government must encourage local doctors to get trained in the field of oncology and its subspecialties, which are the needs of the hour. More beds are to be allocated for palliative care and hospice care.

Conflict of Interest Authors have no conflict of interest to declare.

References

1. www.bloomberg.com
2. Al Awadhi MA, et al. Bahrain Med Bull. 2016;38(1):30–4. https://doi.org/10.12816/0047384.
3. Shubbar AS, et al. Bahrain Med Bull. 2019;41(4):222–5.
4. Hamadeh RR, Abulfatih NM, Fekri MA, et al. Uni Med J. 2014;14(2):176–82.
5. Globocon Statistical Data October 2020, Arnold M, Rutherford M, Lam F, Bray F, Ervik M, Soerjomataram I. ICBP SURVMARK-2 online tool: international cancer survival benchmarking. Lyon: International Agency for Research on Cancer; 2019. http://gco.iarc.fr/survival/survmark
6. Salman bin Ateyatallah Al Khalifa et Editorial Bahrain Med Bull. 2018;40(4):205–6.
7. Taher A, et al. J Bahrain Med Soc Year. 2019;31(1):37–43.
8. https://www.moh.gov.bh/GenomeProject
9. info@bahraincancer.com
10. Mariam B, et al. Bahrain Med Bull. 2020;42(1):31–4.
11. https://www.moh.gov.bh/HealthInstitution/
12. NHRA. www.nhra.bh
13. AlNahdi E, et al. J Bahrain Med Soc. 2020;32(1):16–20.
14. https://www.newsofbahrain.com/bahrain/58991.html
15. http://www.iacr.com.fr/index
16. Sprakel J, et al. J Evid Based Med. 2019;12(3):209–17.
17. https://www.gulf-insider.com/bahrain-cabinet-stresses-to-recruit-more-bahraini-doctors/

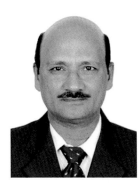

Dr. Ravi Mohan Pedapenki, 61, an Indian national, has been working as a consultant Medical Oncologist, Salmaniya Hospital, Ministry of Health, Government of Bahrain since December 2016. He obtained MBBS in 1983, MD in Internal Medicine in 1992 & Doctorate (DM- Medical Oncology), from the Cancer Institute, Chennai, India in 1997. He taught in various medical colleges in India for 25+ years and retired as a Professor of Medicine and Medical Oncologist from Guntur Medical College, Guntur, India. He taught for 2 years in the medical schools (AGU & RCSI) in Bahrain as a faculty. He has more than 20 publications and was a principal investigator in 40+ Cancer clinical trials.

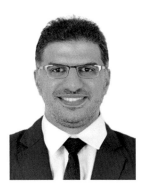

Dr. Ali Madan is a chief medical resident. He graduated from medical school with a high flayer certificate. He joined Salmaniya Medical Complex in the Kingdom of Bahrain in 2010. He has been working in the Oncology and palliative care department and has completed his training program.

Chapter 4
General Oncology Care in Egypt

Ahmed H. Ibrahim (iD) **and Emad Shash** (iD)

4.1 Egypt Demographics

4.1.1 Population

The Egyptian population is one of the largest in the Middle East and North Africa region. Egypt is home to a population of 99,842,504, according to the latest official census in January 2020 [1]. The population in Egypt represents 1.29% of the global population. It is ranked 14th in the list of countries sorted by population [2]. The rural areas encompass 57.2% of the total population, while the urban regions have 42.8%, where the percentage of males is 51.5%, and the percentage of females is 48.5%. Egypt is characterized by an expansive population pyramid with a youth bulge (Fig. 4.1a, b). It is estimated that 50.6% of the population is under the age of 24 years and only 5.3% are above the age of 65 years [4]. Cairo is the most populous city with about 9.9 million inhabitants. Ninety-five percent of the population density lives along the Nile valley [1].

A. H. Ibrahim
Ain Shams University, Cairo, Egypt

Medical Oncology Department, Shefaa- El Orman Hospital, Luxor, Egypt

E. Shash (✉)
Medical Oncology Department, Shefaa- El Orman Hospital, Luxor, Egypt

Medical Oncology Department, National Cancer Institute at Cairo University, Cairo, Egypt
e-mail: emad.shash@nci.cu.edu.eg

© The Author(s) 2022   41
H. O. Al-Shamsi et al. (eds.), *Cancer in the Arab World*,
https://doi.org/10.1007/978-981-16-7945-2_4

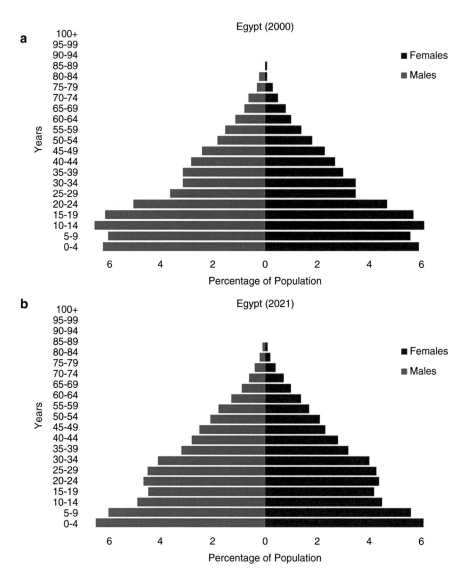

Fig. 4.1 (**a**) Population distribution in Egypt by age and sex in 2000 [1, 3]. (**b**) Population distribution in Egypt by age and sex in 2021 [1, 3]

4.1.2 Regions

Egypt has an area of approximately one million square kilometers. It is ranked 31st in the list of countries sorted by population [5]. Most of the Egyptian land is in the Northeastern part of Africa. Only the Sinai Peninsula is in the southwestern part of the Asian continent. Egypt has 27 governorates and is divided into four main geographical regions: the Nile River and Delta, the Sinai Peninsula, the Eastern Desert, and the Western Desert.

4.1.3 Economy

Egypt had an estimated Gross Domestic Product (GDP) of 363,092 million US dollars and an estimated GDP per capita of 3613 US dollars in 2020 [6]. Egypt is a developing country, with a Human Development Index (HDI) of 0.707 in 2019, which classifies it as a 'High Development Country' and ranks 116th out of 189 countries [7].

4.1.4 Government

Egypt is a presidential republic. The current president of Egypt is Abdel Fattah el-Sisi, in-house, since May 2014. Egypt is ruled by a new constitution, approved by referendum in January 2014. The constitution states that Egypt is a democratic state with a division of power between the bicameral parliament (composed of the House of Representatives and the Shura Council), the Government and the Judicial system [8].

4.1.5 Life Expectancy

The average life expectancy of Egyptians has increased over the past decades. In 2020, the life expectancy at birth was 73 years (74.3 for males; 75.5 for females) [1], and the life expectancy at age 65 was 14.1 years [4]. In 1990, the average life expectancy at birth was only 63.5 years.

4.2 Cancer Statistics in Egypt

In 2019, 324,949 patients with malignant neoplasms were being treated in Egypt at the states' expense [1]. As estimated by Global Cancer Observatory (GLOBOCAN) in December 2020, the most prevalent cancers in Egypt are (5-year prevalence of all ages) [9]: breast (61,160), liver (28,977), bladder (26,986), Non-Hodgkin Lymphoma (19,096), leukemia (14,274), brain, and Central Nervous System (11,470), and prostate (10,523); with a total of 278,165 for all cancers. The highest incidence numbers for specific cancer cases in Egypt in 2020 were: liver (27,895), breast (22,038), bladder (10,655), Non-Hodgkin Lymphoma (7305), lung (6538), leukemia (5231), and prostate (4767); with a total of 134,632 for all cancers (Fig. 4.2a). The specific cancer distribution in males and females is shown in Fig. 4.2b and in Fig. 4.2c, respectively [9].

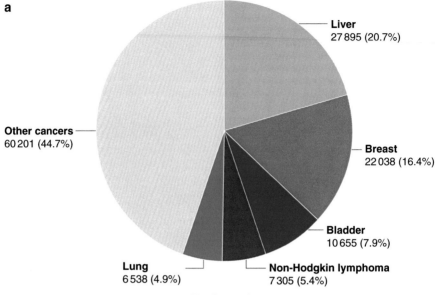

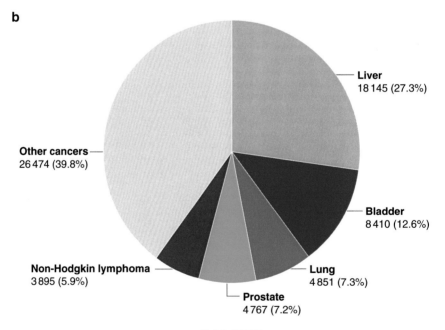

Fig. 4.2 (**a**) Number of new cases in 2020, both sexes, all ages (GLOBOCAN) [9]. (**b**) Number of new cases in 2020, males, all ages (GLOBOCAN) [9]. (**c**) Number of new cases in 2020, females, all ages (GLOBOCAN) [9]

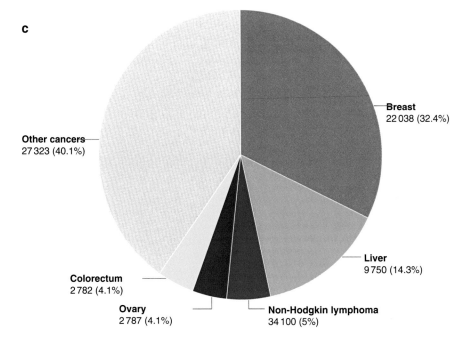

c

Breast
22 038 (32.4%)

Other cancers
27 323 (40.1%)

Liver
9 750 (14.3%)

Colorectum
2 782 (4.1%)

Ovary
2 787 (4.1%)

Non-Hodgkin lymphoma
34 100 (5%)

Total: 68 090

Fig. 4.2 (continued)

The highest mortality numbers for 2020 in Egypt were: liver (26,523), breast (9148), bladder (6170), lung (5817), Non-Hodgkin Lymphoma (4078), leukemia (3858), and brain and Central Nervous System (3686); with a total of 89,042 for all cancers [9].

A gradual increase in mortality numbers over the years can be seen in the WHO Cancer Mortality database report for 2015 (Tables 4.1 and 4.2) [10].

4.3   Oncology Care in Egypt

Cancer care in Egypt is provided by the Ministry of Health (MoH), university hospitals, Non-Governmental Organizations (NGOs), military and police oncology units, and the private sector.

There are 11 oncology centers supervised by the Ministry of Health, which contain 943 beds. The number of all physicians registered in the ministry is 120,606. Yet, there is not an official count of the number of oncologists [1].

University hospitals are major elements of the healthcare sector. There are 24 public medical schools, ten private medical schools, and 109 university hospitals covering most of Egypt. Each medical school has an oncology department with a radiotherapy unit, nuclear medicine, surgical oncology, and chemotherapy unit.

Table 4.1 Number of deaths, all cancers, females, all ages, WHO cancer mortality database [10]

Year	Deaths	Crude rate	ASR(W)	Cumulative risk
1955	1043	9.14	14.78	–
1956	1125	9.59	14.73	–
1957	1068	8.86	13.19	–
1958	1245	10.05	15.02	–
1959	1346	10.57	15.75	–
1960	1354	10.35	14.67	–
1961	1348	10.03	13.93	–
1962	1454	10.53	14.49	–
2000	6773	19.82	25.21	–
2001	7764	22.29	28.14	–
2002	8446	23.81	29.82	–
2003	9130	25.27	31.61	–
2004	9530	25.92	32.29	–
2005	9904	26.46	32.82	–
2006	10219	26.84	33.08	–
2007	10149	26.20	32.08	–
2008	10915	27.68	33.72	–
2009	11357	28.28	34.22	–
2010	12042	29.40	35.57	–
2011	12370	29.58	35.50	–
2014	14321	32.02	38.26	–
2015	14533	31.78	37.78	–

Table 4.2 Number of deaths, all cancers, males, all ages—WHO cancer mortality database [10]

Year	Deaths	Crude rate	ASR (W)	Cumulative risk
1955	1596	13.51	25.93	–
1956	1791	14.76	26.59	–
1957	1583	12.69	21.76	–
1958	1845	14.39	25.35	–
1959	1951	14.80	25.45	–
1960	1999	14.75	24.93	–
1961	2092	15.02	25.31	–
1962	2360	16.50	26.02	–
2000	9544	27.54	40.08	–
2001	10851	30.72	44.21	–
2002	11538	32.04	46.14	–
2003	12716	34.65	49.70	–
2004	12957	34.64	49.71	–
2005	13136	34.48	49.33	–
2006	13474	34.73	49.16	–
2007	13514	34.22	48.23	–

Table 4.2   (continued)

Year	Deaths	Crude rate	ASR (W)	Cumulative risk
2008	14262	35.47	49.52	–
2009	15139	36.95	51.63	–
2010	15651	37.44	52.40	–
2011	16283	38.13	53.14	–
2014	18547	40.59	55.85	–
2015	17855	38.22	52.77	–

Examples include [11]: Cairo University hospitals (Kasr El Ainy), Ain Shams University hospitals (El-Demerdash), Alexandria University hospitals, El-Mansoura University hospitals, and Asyut University hospitals.

"National Cancer Institute (NCI)" is an organization affiliated with Cairo University. The primary institute is in the heart of Cairo and has been operating since 1969. In 2012, The "National Cancer Hospital and Institute: Breast Cancer Hospital" started operating in the First Settlement, New Cairo, to cover the increased demand caused by the increased breast cancer incidence in Egypt [9]. A third hospital "New National Cancer Institute 500500" is currently under construction, expected to open in 2023. It is located at Sheikh Zayed City, Giza. The hospital will have 1020 beds in the inpatient department, 500 beds in the day-care department, 60 operating theaters, 15 radiotherapy machines, and a research center [12].

Charity hospitals play a major role as cancer treatment can be very expensive for many. Shefaa El-Orman Hospital is a big comprehensive center in upper Egypt. The number of beds in the inpatient unit at the adult cancer hospital is 150, and 26 beds in the Intensive Care Unit (ICU). A children's cancer hospital has recently opened on February 23, 2021. It includes 100 beds in the inpatient department and 20 beds in the ICU unit [13].

In Cairo, Children's Cancer Hospital Egypt 57,357 is a child cancer hospital founded in 1999 and operated in 2007. It is located at El-Sayeda Zinab distract, Cairo. It has reported an average overall survival rate of 72% and it received 3355 new patients in 2020 [14].

Baheya Hospital is a specialized hospital for breast cancer. It is located at El-Haram, Giza. The hospital reported the monthly rate as screening 3000 women, 3000 chemotherapy sessions, and 1000 radiotherapy sessions [15].

The Non-Governmental Organizations (NGOs) are also active players in the health field in Egypt, as they help by increasing the awareness of the disease, offer financial, professional aid and psychological support to breast cancer survivors. Examples of NGOs: Breast Cancer Foundation of Egypt, operating since 2004, Egyptian Society of Women's Health and CanSurvive.

Other providers are military and police oncology units that treat both military and civilian patients, private cancer centers, and oncology clinics inside private hospitals.

4.3.1   Liver Cancer

Liver cancer, especially Hepato-Cellular Carcinoma (HCC), is a significant health burden in Egypt, which ranks above the 90th percentile worldwide in liver cancer incidence. There is a strong male predominance of 45.9% in comparison with 22.7% for females [16, 17]. Male predominance is presumably due to higher exposure of males to HCV. Some authors attributed this difference to the fact that males were more affected by schistosomiasis. Hence, males were the main target of parenteral anti-schistosomal therapy campaigns, causing iatrogenic transmission of infection [18].

4.3.2   Breast Cancer

Breast cancer is the leading malignancy among females in Egypt [9]. The most common tumor histology is infiltrating duct carcinoma (83.2%), followed by infiltrating lobular carcinoma (9.1%) and medullary carcinoma (3.2%). The most prevalent type is luminal A subtype (41.2%), followed by triple-negative subtype (28.5%), then Her2-expressing subtype (19.4%), and luminal B subtype (13.9%) [19]. The reasons for this trend are not clear yet. It is possible that different environmental factors affecting the younger generation lead to this consequence. Examples of these factors are the delayed age of marriage (i.e., late age of first birth), the smaller number of offspring and delayed age of breastfeeding (as more young women are educated and working than before) can be responsible for this trend.

4.3.3   Bladder Cancer

Egypt has a very high prevalence rate of bladder cancer compared to global rates. In 1987, Egypt was ranked the top worldwide in bladder cancer mortality rate (Age-specific mortality rate of 10.8 per 100,000 in males) [20]. Over the past 26 years, a significant change in the histopathological types of bladder cancer in Egypt has been noticed. The relative frequency of Transitional Cell Carcinoma (TCC) increased from 22% in 1980 to 73% of bladder diagnosed in 2005, while Squamous Cell Carcinoma (SCC) decreased from 78% of diagnosed bladder tumors in 1980 to 27% of diagnosed bladder tumors [21]. A significant decrease in the relative frequency of bladder cancer at the National Cancer Institute in Cairo was also noted [20]. Even though, bladder cancer remains the second most common cancer among Egyptian males [9, 22]. There is a strong male predominance of the disease with 4:1 male to female ratio [21, 23]. This may be due to higher rates of schistosomiasis hematobium among male farmers who are more exposed to the Nile water [24].

4.4   Cancer Risk Factors

4.4.1   Liver Cancer

The global burden of diseases study in 2015, reported the etiological factors for HCC in Egypt as HCV (63%), HBV (13%), alcohol (12%), and other factors (12%) [25]. This significantly high prevalence of viral Hepatitis C among the Egyptian population is linked to HCC. 92.5% of anti-HCV-positive Egyptians are found to be infected with Genotype 4 (Genotype 4a alone constitutes about 63% of Hepatitis C genotypes) and are thus less responsive to interferon therapy [26–29]. A two-fold increase in HCC incidence rate in the last two decades was reported among chronic liver disease patients in Egypt, accompanied by a significant decline of HBV and a slight increase of HCV as risk factors [26]. HCV is the main risk factor for HCC, as a study reported, anti-HCV antibodies in 71% of HCC cases [27].

The high prevalence of viral Hepatitis B and C has been largely attributed to iatrogenic transmission of infection in mass treatment campaigns of schistosomiasis in the 1960s through 1980s [30]. Environmental factors, especially aflatoxins, have also been linked with the high prevalence of liver cancer in Egypt [31], and have been shown to contaminate more than 20% of silage, due to improper grain storage [32].

4.4.2   Bladder Cancer

Schistosoma-Associated Bladder Cancer (SABC) is different from non-Schistosoma-Associated bladder carcinoma, and it is often regarded as a separate type of bladder cancer. Schistosoma hematobium's eggs trigger a chronic local inflammatory response in the urinary bladder leading to the formation of "sandy patches." This chronic wear and tear process triggers the release of various carcinogenic compounds. It should be noted, however, that a latent period of 20–30 years exists between the peak of the schistosomal catch of infection and the manifestation of SABC. This explains why the incidence rate is highest among 40–59 year-old patients (42% of cases), while the schistosomal peak is during their 30s. Egypt has been largely successful in controlling schistosomiasis. Starting from the early 1920s, tartar emetic was the only available treatment. This has lowered the disease prevalence to around 50% [33]. The Snail Control program was initiated in the late 1930s, aimed at interrupting the life cycle of the parasites by destroying their snail host [34]; however, the prevalence hardly changed [35]. The major shift happened after the approval of praziquantel in 1980, especially when the National Schistosomiasis Control Project (NSCP) supplied ten million children in school-age in rural Egypt and all residents of more than 500 villages were at high risk of infection with praziquantel. This success changed the prevalence of schistosomiasis from 20% to 10% in 1999 and then lowered again to 3.5% in 2002 [36]. Also, there is an emerging trend whereby the proportion of SABC is decreasing in comparison to TCC. Hence, Egypt is becoming more "Westernized" in terms of its bladder carcinoma subtypes [20, 37]. Another risk factor for bladder cancer is cigarette smoking, which increased the risk of bladder urothelial carcinoma as male smokers had a 1.8-fold higher risk of urothelial carcinoma than males who never smoked [37]. The prevalence of smoking among the Egyptian population in 2010 was 22% [38] and is thought to be increasing [39]. Its prevalence could explain why bladder cancer remains among the top killers in Egypt.

4.5 Cancer Screening Programs

In September 2018, the government announced, "100 Million Healthy Lives," the initiative of President Abdel Fatah el-Sisi to eradicate Hepatitis C and detection of Non-Communicable Diseases. It is an initiative that is targeted for screening and documentation of the exact number of current HBV, HCV, hypertension, and diabetes mellitus patients in the Egyptian population. It was expanded by launching a sub-campaign "Egyptian Women's Health Initiative," a three-phase project, aiming at early detection of breast cancer by screening 28 million women [40]. One of the initiatives' goals is to link all oncology centers that provide breast cancer management service in a single network to ensure the integration between institutions and the high quality of the service provided [40].

Currently, there is no national screening program for cervical cancer as Papanicolaou (PAP) smear screening for cervical cancer is arguably cost-ineffective, given the relatively low rates of cervical cancer screening among Egyptian females in comparison to western countries [41]. By 2015, only 0.3% of the Egyptian females had a Pap smear [42]. Moreover, the new HPV vaccine, which was released in 2007, is very expensive and it is doubtful that it can be integrated into Egypt's compulsory vaccination schedule any time soon. And the same could be stated about colon or prostate cancer screening programs.

However, many local initiatives provide this screening tool. The first locally organized service to offer regular screening to women was established at the Ain Shams University, in the Early Cancer Detection Unit (ASU-ECDU), in 1981 [43]. After this initiative, other universities and teaching hospitals in different governorates have started similar units.

4.6 Cancer Prevention Programs

4.6.1 Anti-Schistosomiasis Campaigns

Aiming to eradicate the high prevalence of schistosomiasis hematobium; the government founded 172 bilharzia centers, 449 bilharzia groups, and 1624 bilharzia units in Egypt [1]. There are regular local campaigns in areas with a reported recent increase in the number of new cases.

4.6.2 Anti-HCV and HBV Campaigns

As is mentioned earlier, hepatocellular carcinomas' prevalence in Egypt is significantly high as compared with global rates. Hence, prevention of its top etiological factors in Egypt, i.e., HBV and HCV, is a priority.

The Egyptian National Committee for the Control of Viral Hepatitis (NCCVH) started the national treatment program for HCV in 2007, based on sofosbuvir, pegylated-interferon, and ribavirin regimen [44].

MoH set up a web-based registry to arrange patient appointments and visits, and to record their patient data using a central database. A total of 49,630,319 individuals from a target population of 62.5 million (79.4%), spontaneously participated in the screening between October 1, 2018, and April 30, 2019. The overall HCV seroprevalence in the 48,345,948 individuals tested was 4.61%. 1,148,346 (76.5%) had viremia, and 91.8% of those with viremia had started their treatment. 465,992 of patients who started their treatment, reached the 12-week follow-up after the end of therapy. 386,103 of these 465,992 patients (82.9%) had a known treatment outcome, and 381,491 (98.8%) of those with a known outcome had a sustained virologic response. NCCVH worked on making oral Direct-Acting Antivirals (DAAs), available for the national treatment program at affordable prices. The cost of the HCV testing and treatment component of the program amounted to $207.1 million. The cost of screening a patient with HCV viremia is $85.41, and the cost of screening and curing a patient is $130.62 [45, 46].

Hepatitis B vaccination has become mandatory for all newborns in Egypt, as the hepatitis B vaccine (HB-Vaccine) was included in the compulsory vaccination program for Egyptian children in 1992 [47]. It is part of the "Expanded Programme on Immunization", planned to be given in 3 doses for all newborns at 2, 4, and 6 months after birth. Some studies showed that the hepatitis B coverage rate was markedly increased from 91% in 1996 to 97.3% by 2005 [48, 49].

4.7   Cancer Diagnosis

Carcinogenesis is a multi-step process that may be silent through most of its natural history. This fact is often more complicated in Egypt. A retrospective, multicenter study, held in two pediatric oncology units found that delay in diagnosis is correlated to socio-economic status, parental education, and family, being worse in lower-income families and among illiterate individuals [50]. Application of Guideline-Directed Management and Therapy (GDMT) faces technical and financial limitations. The absence of rich, nationwide medical literature limits standardization and validation of diagnostic protocols designed specifically for Egyptian patients.

Cancer diagnosis involves multiple modalities such as biochemical markers, imaging modality, and histopathological examination. The combination of these methods usually leads to accurate preoperative staging and risk-stratification. However, few cancers are still staged surgically. Post-treatment diagnosis of recurrence remains underestimated in Egypt, with some cases passing undiagnosed due to patients' preferences in a quiet end of life.

4.7.1   Imaging

A variety of imaging modalities are used to screen or diagnose cancer in Egypt, starting from x-ray, which may show an accidental discovery of a mass that necessitates further assessment to detect its nature. Continuing with Computed Tomography (CT) scan and Magnetic Resonance Imaging (MRI), both can be enhanced by an external contrast. For breast cancer, mammograms and bilateral ultrasound are the most used modalities for screening. Positron Emission Tomography (PET) scan is used for the detection of remote metastases, especially for bony lesions. CT and MRI are accessible almost everywhere in Egypt. However, PET scans are only available in large centers. The financial cost of them is to be paid either by the patient's own money, health insurance, or by the government for specific cases.

4.7.2   Molecular Testing

There are several technologies for the detection of sequence variations that have been developed and used in the oncology field in Egypt. There are three main groups of these technologies: Polymerase Chain Reaction (PCR), Hybridization, and Next-Generation Sequencing (NGS).

A tumor biopsy, followed by molecular testing is a common procedure in the daily practice of oncology medicine in Egypt. It is broadly used to detect hereditary cancers and select the most effective treatment based on the molecular characteristics of the tumor biopsy.

4.7.3 Cytogenetics and Genetic Testing

Cytogenetics testing for chromosomal aberrations and their corresponding fusion genes in specific cancers as Acute Myeloid Leukemia (AML), is a novel field in Egypt. It is still only available in major institutions such as NCI and university hospitals.

Since the introduction of advanced Fluorescence in Situ Hybridization FISH-based methods in the late 1980s, they greatly improved the cytogenetic analysis of hematopoietic and solid tumors. Several chromosome alterations are specific to a particular disease, such as the Philadelphia chromosome which is the translocation between chromosomes 9 and 22 in Chronic Myeloid Leukemia (CML), resulting in the BCR-ABL fusion protein.

Genetic testing for hereditary cancers and acquired mutations is available in university hospitals and central private hospitals. Examples include BRCA1 and BRCA2 mutations in breast cancer hospitals, Philadelphia chromosome mutations in leukemia cases and KRAS mutations in colorectal cancer.

4.8 Treatment

In Egypt, matching with the global trend, cancer care is progressively becoming a matter of multidisciplinary management. This reduces discrepancies in classification, management and improves the quality and prognosis. However, this approach still faces technical and financial problems, limiting its nationwide implementation. Cancer treatment involves oncological surgeries, radiation therapy, medical oncology, palliative care, and pain management. Cancer patients may deal with one or more medical specialties during their treatment journey, which demands data-driven practices to support faster decision-making [51].

4.8.1 Medical Oncology

Medical oncologists carry most of the burden of cancer management. They are responsible for stabilizing patients' other conditions—with the help of internists—before, through, and after the therapeutic plan, in addition to, choosing the medical plan and administering the selected chemotherapy. To specialize in medical oncology in Egypt, medical graduates must apply for the Egyptian fellowship in medical oncology. Fellowship's duration is 5 years, 2 years of general internal medicine training, and 3 years of specialty training. The capacity of the fellowship's training program in 2020 was 50 doctors, and 150 in 2021.

Cancer care is always a multidisciplinary process that necessitates the cooperation of medical oncologists, surgical oncologists, and radiation therapists. For example, breast cancer patients need a throughout risk stratification to choose the best treatment modality. Some patients may need neo-adjuvant chemotherapy and/ or hormone therapy. Others may undergo surgery directly, either Breast Conservative Surgery (BCS) or mastectomy, some patients may need radiotherapy either ordinary regimens or Accelerated Partial Breast Irradiation (APBI).

4.8.2 Radiation Therapy

Radiation-based surgical knife modalities include Stereotactic Radiosurgery (SRS), Gamma knife systems, Linear Accelerator (LINAC) systems and Proton beam therapy or cyclotron. Radiation therapy modalities include Fractionation, 3D Conformal Radiotherapy (3DCRT), Intensity-Modulated Radiation Therapy (IMRT), and Image-Guided Radiotherapy (IGRT).

To specialize in radiotherapy in Egypt, medical graduates must apply for the Egyptian fellowship in radiotherapy. Fellowship's duration is 4 years of specialty training. The capacity of the fellowship's training program in 2020 was 28, and 46 in 2021.

4.8.3 Surgery

Surgery always walks hand in hand with medical intervention. This can be noticed in liver cancer patients, who can be treated surgically with either liver transplantation, or surgical hepatectomy. However, due to the limited supply of organs and advanced cirrhosis, many patients are not eligible for surgery and many of them opt for Radiofrequency Ablation (RFA) or Trans-arterial chemoembolization (TACE). Also, bladder cancer patients in Egypt are treated with either radical cystectomy or Transurethral resection of the bladder (TURBT) if resectable, or with cisplatinum-based multi-agent chemotherapy, if unresectable.

4.8.4 Pediatric Oncology

All university hospitals in Egypt have specialized pediatric oncology units. There are specialized hospitals in pediatric oncology such as Shefaa El-Orman Hospital and Children's Cancer Hospital Egypt 57,357. In 57,357 hospitals, 59% percent of patients had solid tumors and 41% had hematopoietic cancers. The most common cancers were leukemia, lymphoma, CNS tumors, and neuroblastoma [52].

4.8.5 Survivorship Track

As a part of the management plan, those with reported good outcomes are set on a follow-up plan, ranging between 2 and 5 years on average. Regular checkup dates include full physical examination, laboratory, imaging investigations, and counseling for lifestyle modifications and psychological support. Patients are advised to seek help immediately if any new symptom is developed.

Psycho-oncological service remains a cornerstone in management. In a recent meta-analysis study, it became evident that 38.2% of cancer patients suffered from any type of mood disorder, and 31.6% suffered from depression or anxiety, which is underestimated in Egyptian oncological care [53]. Palliative care and End-of-life care (EOLC) is a growing medical specialty in Egypt. However, it also faces a few financial and technical limitations [54].

4.8.6 Palliative Care Track

Palliative care is care given to improve the quality of life of patients in terminal stages. It targets several physical symptoms such as pain, fatigue, loss of appetite, nausea, vomiting, shortness of breath, and insomnia. This can be done using non-therapeutic doses of chemotherapy and/or radiotherapy. Surgery is also an option for oncological emergencies such as spinal cord compression. Emotional and spiritual support is also given to patients and their families to cope with the difficulties of the situation.

4.9 Research and Education

The main academic research and education sector in Egypt is covered by public and private universities. There are 24 public and ten private medical schools in Egypt. Each is run by a varsity of academic staff who publish hundreds of publications annually. In addition to teaching thousands of undergraduate and postgraduate medical personnel. The number of medical graduates in December 2019 was 7–8 thousand [55].

Theodor Bilharz Research Institute in Warrak district, Giza, Egypt is an institute primarily focused on schistosomiasis prevention and control. The institute was founded in 1964, after an agreement between the Federal Republic of Germany and the Egyptian Government [56]. There are high prevalence and incidence rates of schistosomiasis in Egypt as mentioned earlier, which is responsible for the high incidence rate of Transitional Cell Carcinoma (TCC). Successful management of schistosomiasis and breaking its life cycle, especially the freshwater snail—the intermediate host—will subsequently cause a noticeable decrease in Transitional Cell Carcinoma (TCC) incidence rate.

Although Theodor Bilharz Research Institute was mainly founded to control schistosomiasis, the institute's mission is to control endemic tropical diseases in Egypt such as viral hepatitis and to be a leading center in research and training. The institute has 300 hospital beds and is managed by manpower of 482 researchers [57].

Few charity hospitals have their research centers, such as Shefaa El-Orman Hospital, Children's Cancer Hospital Egypt 57,357, and Baheya Hospital. They run both clinical and academic trials, benefiting from the high number of patients registered in each hospital, opening the door for more future private-funded trials.

The Egyptian Cancer Research Network launched on November 5, 2016, is a collective of research professionals, groups, organizations, and institutions involved in Cancer research in Egypt. The goal of the network is to connect oncology researchers in Egypt and to facilitate the conduction of large-scale multicenter [58].

4.10   Cost-Effective Cancer Care

Being a developing country, assuring cost-effectiveness is an important side of the healthcare sector in Egypt. Especially for oncology patients, as managing their condition is almost always very expensive.

A study that used Egypt as a case study for hepatitis C screening and treatment in the developing countries found implementing hepatitis C screening and treatment of non-symptomatic, average-risk Egyptian adults would be cost-saving with triple-therapy and very cost-effective with dual-therapy [59].

4.11   Challenges and Advantages

Some of the challenges faced by the Egyptian healthcare system are mentioned as follows:

- Affected by the sustained increase in incidence rates of neoplasms in the Egyptian population through the years; the health sector is facing many challenges especially with the number of facilities and manpower needed to operate them and provide the standard quality of care.
- Mostly guided by local institutional guidelines for cancer management, providing the same medical service in all regions can be quite challenging. Hence, the need to adhere to a unified national guideline is becoming a priority for the healthcare sector in Egypt.

- As shown in the WHO Cancer Mortality database's report for 2015 [10], there has been a sustained increase in the mortality rate in Egypt since the 1950s; further work should be conducted to investigate this trend. On one hand, it may be due to the increase in population number and consequently, the increase in population at risk which caused the increase in incidence rates. On the other hand, it may be caused by strict and more accurate documentation and advanced screening and investigative tools. Other occult factors may also be responsible.
- One of the challenges facing cancer care in Egypt is the late stage at first presentation, leading to reduced effectiveness of therapy and higher morbidity and mortality rates. For example, one of the most important reasons is the lack of health awareness in Egyptian women about the early warning signs of breast cancer and the importance of early consultation. Eighty-five percent of Egyptian women were found to have insufficient knowledge about the disease in some studies [60].
- As a developing country, the expensive cost of cancer treatment is a magnificent problem. It can be an obstacle in the road of providing newly released treatment modalities.
- Many facilities do not integrate a multidisciplinary team approach into their cancer management plans. Its implementation should be taken into consideration to improve the quality of healthcare.

4.12 The Future of Cancer Care in Egypt

Cancer care in Egypt is a progressive sector due to the ongoing increase in the number of oncology-specialized hospitals, in addition to receiving more attention from both the government and the community, subsequently increasing the fund given to healthcare-providing hospitals and institutes and research cuts. Yet, more focus should be given to the prevention and screening of specific types of cancers that do not have an existing system.

4.13 Conclusion

Egypt has the potential to become an eminent country in the field of oncology. Having the required manpower, growing infrastructure, and endemic diseases and factors that are rarely found in advanced countries, which is an excellent opportunity for research. More oncology-specialized hospitals, trained oncologists, and medical personnel will be needed to keep up with the actively growing Egyptian population and subsequently, the prevalence of cancers.

Conflict of Interest Authors have no conflict of interest to declare.

References

1. Central Agency for Public Mobilization and Statistics (CAPMAS) A. 2020 electronic statistical yearbook. 2020. http://www.capmas.gov.eg/book.aspx. Accessed 25 Jan 2021.
2. United States Census Bureau, 2020. https://www.census.gov/popclock/world/eg#world-footer. Accessed 25 Jan 2021.
3. U.S. Census Bureau. International data base (IDB), Egypt section in 2021 and 2000. 2021. https://www.census.gov/data-tools/demo/idb/#/country?YR_ANIM=2021&FIPS_SINGLE=EG&dashPages=BYAGE&ageGroup=5Y. Accessed 6 Jul 2021.
4. United Nations, Department of Economic and Social Affairs, Population Division. World population prospects 2019. Volume II: demographic profiles.
5. World Factbook area rank order. 2021. Cia.gov. Accessed 25 Jan 2021.
6. Ministry of Finance, Arab republic of Egypt. The Financial Monthly. 2020;15(13).
7. United Nations Development Programme. Human development report 2020. The next frontier: human development and the anthropocene.
8. Egypt's Government Cabinet. https://www.cabinet.gov.eg. Accessed 26 Jan 2021.
9. Global Cancer Observatory (Globocan), Egypt fact sheet. 2020. https://gco.iarc.fr/today/data/factsheets/populations/818-egypt-fact-sheets.pdf
10. International Agency for Research on Cancer (IARC). WHO cancer mortality database. http://www-dep.iarc.fr/WHOdb/WHOdb.htm
11. Egyptian Supreme Council of Universities. University Hospitals. 2021. https://scu.eg/pages/university_hospitals. Accessed 1 Feb 2021.
12. Al-Bawaba news, official statement from the Minister of High Education. 2020. https://www.albawabhnews.com/4164757. Accessed 3 Feb 2021.
13. Dar El Orman. Shefaa El Orman Hospital project. 2021. https://dar-alorman.com/Projects/Details/1. Acecessed 2 Feb 2021.
14. 57357 Children's Cancer Hospital Foundation – Egypt portal. 2021. https://www.57357.org/en/about-57357/future-growth-plan/. Accessed 2 Feb 2021.
15. Baheya Hospital website. 2021. https://baheya.org/en/about. Accessed 2 Feb 2021.
16. Parkin DM, Whelan SL, Ferlay J, Teppo L, Thomas DB. Cancer incidence in five continents, volume VIII. IARC scientific publication no 155. IARC; 2002.
17. Ray SC, Arthur RR, Carella A, Bukh J, Thomas DL. Genetic epidemiology of hepatitis C virus throughout Egypt. J Infect Dis. 2000;182(3):698–707.
18. Mohamoud YA, Mumtaz GR, Riome S, Miller D, Abu-Raddad LJ. The epidemiology of hepatitis C virus in Egypt: a systematic review and data synthesis. BMC Infect Dis. 2013;13(1):1–21.
19. El-Hawary AK, Abbas AS, Elsayed AA, Zalata KR. Molecular subtypes of breast carcinoma in Egyptian women: clinicopathological features. Pathol Res Pract. 2012;208(7):382–6.
20. Møller H, Heseltine E, Vainio H. Working group report on schistosomes, liver flukes and Helicobacter pylori. Meeting held at IARC, Lyon, 7–14 June 1994. Int J Cancer. 1995;60(5):587–9.
21. Felix AS, Soliman AS, Khaled H, Zaghloul MS, Banerjee M, El-Baradie M, El-Kalawy M, Abd-Elsayed AA, Ismail K, Hablas A, Seifeldin IA. The changing patterns of bladder cancer in Egypt over the past 26 years. Cancer Causes Control. 2008;19(4):421–9.
22. Ibrahim AS, Khaled HM, Mikhail NN, Baraka H, Kamel H. Cancer incidence in Egypt: results of the national population-based cancer registry program. J Cancer Epidemiol. 2014;2014:437971.
23. Kahan E, Ibrahim AS, Najjar KE, Ron E, Al-Agha H, Polliack A, El-Bolkainy MN. Cancer patterns in the Middle East special report from the Middle East Cancer Society. Acta Oncol. 1997;36(6):631–6.
24. Kyritsi F, Loffredo CA, Zheng YL, Philips G, Amr S. Urinary bladder cancer in Egypt: are there gender differences in its histopathological presentation? Adv Urol. 2018;2018:3453808.
25. Akinyemiju T, Abera S, Ahmed M, Alam N, Alemayohu MA, Allen C, Al-Raddadi R, Alvis-Guzman N, Amoako Y, Artaman A, Ayele TA. The burden of primary liver cancer and underlying etiologies from 1990 to 2015 at the global, regional, and national level: results from the global burden of disease study 2015. JAMA Oncol. 2017;3(12):1683–91.

26. El-Zayadi AR, Badran HM, Barakat EM, Attia ME, Shawky S, Mohamed MK, Selim O, Saeid A. Hepatocellular carcinoma in Egypt: a single center study over a decade. World J Gastroenterol: WJG. 2005;11(33):5193.
27. El-Zayadi AR, Abaza H, Shawky S, Mohamed MK, Selim OE, Badran HM. Prevalence and epidemiological features of hepatocellular carcinoma in Egypt—a single center experience. Hepatol Res. 2001;19(2):170–9.
28. Kouyoumjian SP, Chemaitelly H, Abu-Raddad LJ. Characterizing hepatitis C virus epidemiology in Egypt: systematic reviews, meta-analyses, and meta-regressions. Sci Rep. 2018;8(1):1–7.
29. Abdel-Hamid M, El-Daly M, Molnegren V, El-Kafrawy S, Abdel-Latif S, Esmat G, Strickland GT, Loffredo C, Albert J, Widell A. Genetic diversity in hepatitis C virus in Egypt and possible association with hepatocellular carcinoma. J Gen Virol. 2007;88(5):1526–31.
30. Rao MR, Naficy AB, Darwish MA, Darwish NM, Schisterman E, Clemens JD, Edelman R. Further evidence for association of hepatitis C infection with parenteral schistosomiasis treatment in Egypt. BMC Infect Dis. 2002;2(1):1–7.
31. Abdel-Wahab M, Mostafa M, Sabry M, El-Farrash M, Yousef T. Aflatoxins as a risk factor for hepatocellular carcinoma in Egypt, Mansoura Gastroenterology Center Study. Hepato-gastroenterology. 2008;55(86–87):1754–9.
32. El-Shanawany AA, Mostafa ME, Barakat A. Fungal populations and mycotoxins in silage in Assiut and Sohag governorates in Egypt, with a special reference to characteristic Aspergilli toxins. Mycopathologia. 2005;159(2):281–9.
33. Khalil M. The history and progress of anti-ankylostomiasis and anti-bilharziasis work in Egypt. 1924, 6.
34. Farley J. Bilharzia: a history of imperial tropical medicine. Cambridge University Press; 2003.
35. Cline BL, Richards FO, El Alamy MA, El Hak S, Ruiz-Tiben E, Hughes JM, McNeeley DF. 1983 Nile Delta schistosomiasis survey: 48 years after Scott. Am J Trop Med Hyg. 1989;41(1):56–62.
36. Salem S, Mitchell RE, El-Alim El-Dorey A, Smith JA, Barocas DA. Successful control of schistosomiasis and the changing epidemiology of bladder cancer in Egypt. BJU Int. 2011;107(2):206–11.
37. Zheng YL, Amr S, Doa'a AS, Dash C, Ezzat S, Mikhail NN, Gouda I, Loay I, Hifnawy T, Abdel-Hamid M, Khaled H. Urinary bladder cancer risk factors in Egypt: a multicenter case–control study. Cancer Epidemiol Prevent Biomark. 2012;21(3):537–46.
38. Fouad H, Commar A, Hamadeh RR, El-Awa F, Shen Z, Fraser CP. Smoking prevalence in the Eastern Mediterranean Region. East Mediterr Health J. 2020;26(1):94–101.
39. Fouda S, Kelany M, Moustafa N, Abushouk AI, Hassane A, Sleem A, Mokhtar O, Negida A, Bassiony M. Tobacco smoking in Egypt: a scoping literature review of its epidemiology and control measures. East Mediterr Health J. 2018;24(02):198–215.
40. Egyptian Presidency Portal. Egyptian women's health initiative. 2021. https://www.presidency.eg/en/%D8%A7%D9%84%D8%B1%D8%A6%D8%A7%D8%B3%D8%A9/%D9%85%D8%A8%D8%A7%D8%AF%D8%B1%D8%A9-%D8%B1%D8%A6%D9%8A%D8%B3-%D8%A7%D9%84%D8%AC%D9%85%D9%87%D9%88%D8%B1%D9%8A%D8%A9-%D9%84%D8%B9%D9%85-%D8%B5%D8%AD%D8%A9-%D8%A7%D9%84%D9%85%D8%B5%D8%B1%D9%85%D8%B1%D8%A3%D8%A9-%D8%A7%D9%84%D9%85%D8%B5%D8%B1%D9%8A%D8%A9/. Accessed 1 Feb 2021.
41. Abd El All HS, Refaat A, Dandash K. Prevalence of cervical neoplastic lesions and human papilloma virus infection in Egypt: national cervical cancer screening project. Infect Agent Cancer. 2007;2(1):1–4.
42. El-Zanaty Associates, Ministry of Health and Population. Egypt health issues survey. Cairo and Rockville, MD: Ministry of Health and Population and ICF International; 2015.
43. Fahim HI, Faris R, Arab SE, Sammour MB. An epidemiologic study of Papanicolaou smear data at Ain-Shams University Hospitals. J Egypt Public Health Assoc. 1991;66(1-2):97–111.
44. Elsharkawy A, El-Raziky M, El-Akel W, El-Saeed K, Eletreby R, Hassany M, El-Sayed MH, Kabil K, Ismail SA, El-Serafy M, Abdelaziz AO. Planning and prioritizing direct-acting antivirals treatment for HCV patients in countries with limited resources: lessons from the Egyptian experience. J Hepatol. 2018;68(4):691–8.

45. Waked I, Esmat G, Elsharkawy A, El-Serafy M, Abdel-Razek W, Ghalab R, Elshishiney G, Salah A, Abdel Megid S, Kabil K, El-Sayed MH. Screening and treatment program to eliminate hepatitis C in Egypt. N Engl J Med. 2020;382(12):1166–74.
46. Rashed WM, Kandeil MA, Mahmoud MO, Ezzat S. Hepatocellular carcinoma (HCC) in Egypt: a comprehensive overview. J Egypt Natl Canc Inst. 2020;32(1):1–1.
47. Ministry of Health and Population (MOHP). Ministry of Health and Population/Child Survival Project: the expanding programme of immunization in Egypt; 1984–1994. MOHP/EPI: Egypt. 1995.
48. Saad A, Safi-El-Dine A, AI El-Sham K. The trend of mandatory vaccination among children in Egypt. Open Vaccine J. 2009;2(1):77–84.
49. Salama II, Sami SM, Said ZN, El-Sayed MH, El Etreby LA, Rabah TM, Elmosalami DM, Hamid AT, Salama SI, Mohsen AM, Emam HM. Effectiveness of hepatitis B virus vaccination program in Egypt: multicenter national project. World J Hepatol. 2015;7(22):2418.
50. Abdelkhalek ER, Sherief LM, Kamal NM, Soliman RM. Factors associated with delayed cancer diagnosis in Egyptian children. Clin Med Insights Pediatr. 2014;8:CMPed-S16413.
51. Elzomor H, Taha H, Nour R, Aleieldin A, Zaghloul MS, Qaddoumi I, Alfaar AS. A multidisciplinary approach to improving the care and outcomes of patients with retinoblastoma at a pediatric cancer hospital in Egypt. Ophthalmic Genet. 2017;38(4):345–51.
52. Soliman R, Elhaddad A, Oke J, Eweida W, Sidhom I, Mahmoud S, Abdelrahman H, Moussa E, Sedki M, Zamzam M, Zekri W. 19 Childhood cancer health outcomes in Egypt: ten-year real-world evidence from children's cancer hospital 57357–Egypt (CCHE) and comparison with results from England. BMJ Evid Based Med. 2019;24:A14–5.
53. Mitchell AJ, Chan M, Bhatti H, Halton M, Grassi L, Johansen C, Meader N. Prevalence of depression, anxiety, and adjustment disorder in oncological, haematological, and palliative-care settings: a meta-analysis of 94 interview-based studies. Lancet Oncol. 2011;12(2):160–74.
54. Silbermann M, Pitsillides B, Al-Alfi N, Omran S, Al-Jabri K, Elshamy K, Ghrayeb I, Livneh J, Daher M, Charalambous H, Jafferri A. Multidisciplinary care team for cancer patients and its implementation in several Middle Eastern countries. Ann Oncol. 2013;24:vii41–7.
55. El-Youm El-Sabaa News. Official statement from the head of the training sector at the Ministry of Health. 2019. https://www.youm7.com/story/2019/12/17/8/4549444. Accessed 7 Feb 2021.
56. Council of Research Centers and Institutes website, Theodor Bilharz Research Institute Section. http://www.crci.sci.eg/?page_id=596. Accessed 7 Feb 2021.
57. Theodor Bilharz Research Institute website. https://www.tbri.gov.eg/index.aspx. Accessed February 7, 2021].
58. The Egyptian Cancer Research Network website. http://www.egycrn.net/. Accessed 7 Feb 2021.
59. Kim DD, Hutton DW, Raouf AA, Salama M, Hablas A, Seifeldin IA, Soliman AS. Cost-effectiveness model for hepatitis C screening and treatment: implications for Egypt and other countries with high prevalence. Glob Public Health. 2015;10(3):296–317.
60. Allam MF, Abd Elaziz KM. Evaluation of the level of knowledge of Egyptian women of breast cancer and its risk factors. A cross sectional study. J Prev Med Hyg. 2012;53(4):195–8.

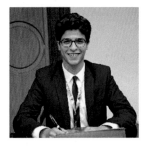

Dr. Ahmed H. Ibrahim , M.B.B. Ch, is a medical intern at Ain Shams University, in Egypt, and a medical oncology intern at Shefaa Al Orman hospitals, in Egypt.

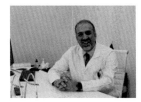

Dr. Emad Shash , M.B.B. Ch, MSc., M.D. is currently the Medical Director and General Manager of the Breast Comprehensive Cancer Hospital at the National Cancer Institute, Cairo University. He is a visiting Medical Oncology consultant and Breast Cancer Program Director at Shiffaa Al Orman Cancer Hospital, Luxor since 2016. Dr. Shash is a consultant and lecturer faculty member of Medical Oncology, at the National Cancer Institute, Cairo University. Dr. Shash has published well-recognized reviews and original articles, in national and international journals in the field of medical oncology and cancer education. He is the Associate Editor of the prestigious Journal of the Egyptian National Cancer Institute.

Chapter 5
General Oncology Care in Iraq

Nada A. S. Al Alwan

5.1 Iraq Demographics

The Republic of Iraq lies in western Asia encircling the Mesopotamian plain. It has an area of 437,072 km^2; fed by the Euphrates and Tigris rivers. The population, estimated to be 40,384,685, continues to grow at a rate of 2.4% per year and the fertility rate is 3.9%. Almost 70% lives in urban areas and only 5% are over 60 years old with a life expectancy at birth reaching 72 years. There are 18 governorates in Iraq, including three in the Kurdistan Region (KRG). The capital, Baghdad, is the second largest city in the Arab World, following Cairo with a population of eight million [1–4].

The fifth largest proven conventional oil reserve globally, with 141 billion barrels, is present in Iraq, which is considered the third largest oil exporters [4]. Owing to the continuous conflicts over the past four decades, merely 30–40% of the countries have been properly explored. In 2019, the Gross Domestic Product (GDP) grew by an estimated 4.4% due to improved security conditions, higher oil prices, and increased agricultural production. The GDP in Iraq was worth 234.09 billion US dollars in 2019, according to official data from the World Bank and projections from Trading Economics (https://tradingeconomics.com/iraq/gdp); representing 0.20% of the world economy [1, 4, 5].

N. A. S. Al Alwan (✉)
National Cancer Research Center, College of Medicine, University of Baghdad, Ministry of Higher Education and Scientific Research, Baghdad, Iraq
e-mail: nadalwan@bccru.uobaghdad.edu.iq

H. O. Al-Shamsi et al. (eds.), *Cancer in the Arab World*,
https://doi.org/10.1007/978-981-16-7945-2_5

5.2   Cancer Statistics in Iraq

It has been estimated that the highest incidence of cancer within the coming 15 years will be registered in the Eastern Mediterranean Region (EMR) for reasons attributed to population growth, aging, lifestyle modification, urbanization, and exposure to carcinogens [19]. The types and burden of cancers are variable in different countries in the region [20]. In Iraq, the Ministry of Health (MOH) established the Iraqi Cancer Registry (ICR) in 1974 in collaboration with the International Agency for Research on Cancer (IARC), France. Since then, several reports have been published recording the ICR for the years (1976–1985), (1986–1988), (1989–1991), (1992–1994), (1995–1997), (1998–1999), followed by successive reports yearly. The pooled data from all governorates are registered by well-trained staff, instructed on Cancer Registry Program 4 (Can Reg 4) and ICD-O code, who work at the cancer registry units in the major hospitals [21, 22]. The filled forms are referred at three-month intervals to the cancer registry section of the Iraqi Cancer Board (ICB); where they are checked for accuracy and completeness, then introduced in the Alphabetical Index into the system to prevent duplication [23].

The age-standardized incidence and mortality rates of cancer among the Iraqi population in 2018 as displayed in the Global Cancer Observatory [24] are 105.5 and 64.7, respectively (Table 5.1). The latest ICR [25] has illustrated that the total number of new cancer cases during 2018 was 31,502, with an incidence rate of 82.6/100,000 population; 43% occurred in males and 57% in females (Table 5.2). The top registered cancers were breast cancer (19.7%), bronchus and lung (8.2%), colorectal (6.1%), leukemia (6.0%), and urinary bladder (4.9%) (Table 5.3, Fig. 5.1). Among males, the top three cancers were bronchus and lung (13.4% with an incidence of 9.5/100,000 male population), followed by urinary bladder (8.6%) and leukemia (7.8%). On the other hand, the top three cancers among females were breast (34.1% with an incidence of 32.3/100,000 female population), thyroid gland (6.1%), and colorectal (5.1%). Among children, the total number of cancers was 1715, representing 5.44% of total cases of cancer at all age groups. The most prevalent childhood malignancy was leukemia (3.6%) followed by Brain/CNS (1.9%) and Non-Hodgkin Lymphoma (0.9%) [25].

Overall, the most common causes of malignant related deaths in Iraq were due to cancers of the bronchus and lungs (18.9%), breast (12.3%), and leukemia (12.1%) (Fig. 5.2) [25].

Table 5.1 Incidence, mortality, and prevalence of cancer in Iraq by cancer site [24]

Cancer	New cases				Deaths				5 year prevalence, all ages	
	Number	Rank	%	Cum. Risk	Number	Rank	%	Cum. Risk	Number	Prop.
Breast	5141	1	20.3	4.03	1727	2	11.9	1.4?	13006	66.9
Lung	2123	2	8.4	1.36	2066	I	14.2	1.32	2039	5.18
Leukemia	1614	3	6.6	0.48	132?	3	9.1	0.41	4437	11.28
Bladder	1454	4	5.7	0.89	596	6	4.1	0.33	3465	8.81
Brain/nervous system	1342	5	5.3	0.50	1085	4	7.5	0.45	3189	8.11
Non-Hodgkin lymphoma	1250	6	4.9	0.49	476	10	3.3	0.21	3013	7.66
Colon	926	7	3.7	0.49	528	8	3.6	0.27	1888	4.80
Stomach	791	8	3.1	0.40	750	5	5.2	0.38	1006	2.56
Hodgkin lymphoma	650	9	2.6	0.16	168	16	1.2	O.0	1934	4.92
Thyroid	631	10	2.5	0.22	69	23	0.48	0.03	1823	4.63
Prostate	556	11	2.2	0.80	159	19	I	0.14	1051	5.28
Liver	539	12	2.1	0.32	538	7	3.7	0.32	443	1.13
Ovary	534	13	2.1	0.42	362			0.34	1279	6.59
Kidney	530	14	2.1	0.23	195	15	1.3	0.10	1214	3.09
Pancreas	503	15	2.0	0.31	500	9	3.4	0.31	380	0.97
Larynx	491	16	2.0	0.32	360	12	2.5	0.24	1189	3.02
Rectum	409	,,	1.6	0.19	235	14	1.6	0.11	847	2.15
Gall bladder	293	18	1.2	0.18	253	13	1.7	0.16	329	0.84
Cervix uteri	244	19	0.96	0.20	159	18	I.I	0.15	612	3.15
Oral cavity	237	20	0.94	0.13	146	20	1.0	0.08	568	1.44
Corpus uteri	215	21	0.85	0.22	60	24	0.41	0,01	552	2.84
Multiple myeloma	187	22	**0.74**	0.11	143	21	0.98	0.09	374	o.95
Nasopharynx	1'4	23	0.69	0.07	125	22	0.86	O.O<i	487	1.24
Testis	173	24	0.68	0.08	32	30	0.22	0.03	551	2.77
Esophagus	172	25	0.68	0.10	165	17	I.I	0.10	165	0.42
Melanoma of skin	96	26	0.38	0.04	34	29	0.23	0.02	239	0.61
Salivary glands	96	27	0.38	0.05	57	25	0.39	0.03	223	0.57
Anus	56	28	0.22	0.03	so	26	0.34	0.03	119	0.30
Hypopharynx	51	29	**0.20**	0.03	28	31	0.19	0.01	81	0.21
Oropharynx	40	30	0.16	0.02	38	27	0.26	0.02	99	0.25
Kaposi sarcoma	40	31	0.16	0.02	23	32	0.16	0.01	92	0.23
Mesothelioma	36	32	0.14	0.02	35	28	0.24	0.02	39	0.10
Vulva	23	33	0.09	0.02	16	33	0.11	0.01	66	0.34
Vagina	18	34	0.07	0.02	12	34	0.08	0.02	44	0.23
Penis	5	35	0.02	0.01	3	35	0.02	0.00	13	0.07
All cancer sites	**25320**			**11.1**	14524			**7.07**		**139.32**

Table 5.2 Distribution and incidence rates/100,000 population of new cases of cancer by gender, ICR, Iraq, years 1994–2018 [25]

Year	Male no.	%	Female no.	%	Total no.	%	IR[a]
1994	4230	54.4	3555	45.6	7785	100	38.91
1995	4344	54.7	3604	45.3	7948	100	44.69
1996	4466	53.5	3894	46.5	8360	100	45.69
1997	4521	52.7	4071	47.3	8592	100	45.67
1998	4774	52.9	4259	47.1	9033	100	45.74
1999	4556	50.9	4380	49.1	8936	100	43.95
2000	5376	49.4	5512	50.6	10,888	100	52.00
2001	6758	50.6	6574	49.4	13,332	100	61.83
2002	6964	49.8	7021	50.2	13,985	100	62.97
2003	5698	50.6	5550	49.4	11,248	100	49.17
2004	7525	51.8	6995	48.2	14,520	100	61.63
2005	7505	49.5	7667	50.5	15,172	100	54.26
2006	7377	48.5	7849	51.5	15,226	100	52.84
2007	6656	46.8	7557	53.2	14,213	100	47.88
2008	6589	46.5	7591	53.5	14,180	100	44.46
2009	7201	47.3	8050	52.7	15,251	100	48.16
2010	8544	46.3	9938	53.7	18,482	100	56.89
2011	9352	46.2	10,926	53.8	20,278	100	60.82
2012	9268	43.9	11,833	56.1	21,101	100	61.69
2013	10,568	45.4	12,740	54.6	23,308	100	66.41
2014	11,411	44.5	14,187	55.5	25,598	100	71.10
2015	11,205	44.4	14,064	55.6	25,269	100	68.41
2016	11,194	43.8	14,362	56.2	25,556	100	67.45
2017	12,502	43.1	16,521	56.9	29,023	100	78.14
2018	13,612	43.0	17,890	57.0	31,502	100	82.62

[a]Incidence rate

Table 5.3 Distribution of the top ten cancers in Iraq, ICR, 2019 [25]

	Top ten cancers/all	No.	%
1	Breast	6206	19.70
2	Bronchus and lungs	2579	8.19
3	Colorectal	1936	6.15
4	Leukemia	1899	6.03
5	Urinary bladder	1542	4.89
6	Brain and CNS tumors	1541	4.89
7	Thyroid	1413	4.49
8	Non-Hodgkin lymphoma	1268	4.03
9	Skin	1142	3.63
10	Prostate	1023	3.25
Total top ten	20,549	20,549	65.23
Total other sites	10,953	10,953	34.77
Grand total	31,502	31,502	100

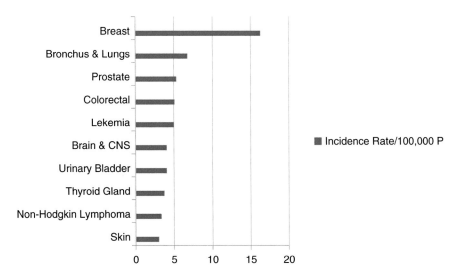

Fig. 5.1   Incidence rate/100,000 population of the top ten cancers in Iraq, IRC, 2019 [25]

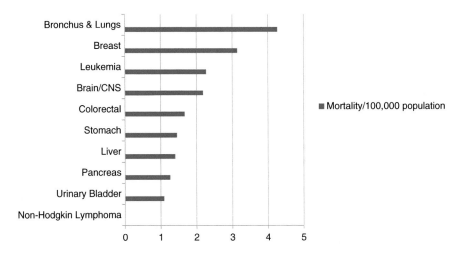

Fig. 5.2   Mortality rates: top ten cancers in Iraq/100,000 populations, ICR, 2018 [25]

5.3   Healthcare System in Iraq

Before 1980, the United Nations (UN) reported that Iraq had the most robust health-care system in the Middle East with respect to its infrastructure, competent special-ists, and free universal health service coverage [6]. The consequences of the successive wars, sanctions, civil conflicts and political instability yielded a shortage in the medical resources, expertise, and funds [4–8]. Currently, the government spends 6–7% of its GDP on the health sector, providing free of charge services to all citizens through a network of Primary Health Care Centers (PHCC) and public hospitals. Specialized care is also presented by private hospitals, the costs of which are met out-of-pocket as the health insurance program has not initiated yet in Iraq [1, 3].

The latest Annual Statistical Report of the Ministry of Health/Environment (MOH) in Iraq (http://www.moh.gov.iq/arabic) has displayed that there are 286 governmental hospitals, 143 private hospitals, and 2808 PHCC; the PHCC and units serve 0.7/10,000 populations. The number of hospital beds per capita is 1.3/1000 population, of which 70–75% are in general hospitals and 25–30% in specialized clinics and centers. Currently, there are 37 functioning medical colleges distributed at the government and private levels. The rates of physician, paramedical, and nursing staff are equivalent to 0.93, 2.3, and 2.2/1000 population, respectively. The adult mortality rate/1000 population is 2%. The main registered causes of death among the population are ischemic heart disease (12%), followed by cancer (9%) and cerebrovascular accidents (8%) [1, 9].

5.4 Oncology Care in Iraq

At the beginning of the twentieth century, Baghdad was a pioneer among the Arab World in cancer management. X-ray machines were introduced in the Radiology Institute of Baghdad since 1920, followed by installing cobalt-60 units in the 1950s, Cs-137 for brachytherapy in the 1960s, and linear accelerators in the 1970s [10]. Between 1950 and 1980, Iraq hosted many patients and students from neighboring countries, providing quality healthcare and medical education [11, 12]. During the gulf wars (1990, 2003), Iraq was exposed to various ammunitions of massive destruction, which raised the debate upon their probable carcinogenicity. The UN sanction (1990–2003) imposed an embargo on a range of diagnostic and therapeutic cancer equipment, including linear accelerators, certain chemotherapy drugs and radioisotopes, suspecting that they might be converted into chemical weapons [8, 13].

With the objective of addressing the cancer burden in Iraq, the MOH established the "Iraqi Cancer Board" (ICB) in 1985, which is represented by various specialties from different governorates. The ICB consists of specific functional units to coordinate their relevant programs, i.e. registration, prevention, early detection, treatment, palliative care, and research. In 2010, members of the ICB designed a "National Cancer Control Plan" (NCCP) for Iraq [14], in accordance with the cancer control strategy, recommended by the World Health Organization (WHO) [15–17]. Ongoing efforts have been exerted to ensure translation of the NCCP into implemented financed, evidence-based actions. Documentation of the cancer data is carried out through the national population based "Iraqi Cancer Registry" (ICR), which pools information on newly diagnosed cancer cases from medical record departments of all hospitals and laboratories (public and private) of the governorates.

Excluding the Kurdistan Region (KRG), currently there are about 35 public cancer care facilities, i.e., hospitals, centers, and units, distributed over the Iraqi governorates (10 of which are in the capital), comprising approximately 2000 beds. The largest public tertiary hospital in Baghdad, the "Medical City Teaching Complex"

(MCTC), includes four specialized cancer centers. KRG established "Zhianawa Cancer Center" in Sulaymaniyah equipped with brachytherapy, and "Hiwa Cancer Hospital." The latter is considered the second largest provider of public oncology care following "Al-Amal National Cancer Center" in Baghdad [5, 18]. Nowadays, Iraq is investing in the private health sector to upgrade cancer services and save the money it spends yearly on the medical evacuation program.

5.5 Cancer Risk Factors

The prevalence of tobacco smoking exceeds 30% among men in the EMR [26]. World Health Organization (WHO) estimated that tobacco-related cancer deaths have reached 18.4% [27]. The latest population based "STEPS Survey of Non-Communicable Disease" (NCD) risk factors carried out on 4071 Iraqi adults revealed that 38.0% of men and 1.9% of women were current smokers of tobacco. The daily tobacco users constituted 19.6% of the Iraqi adult population (36.1% men, 1.8% women). About 0.4% of men were users of smokeless tobacco. Six in ten smokers had tried to stop smoking 1 year before the survey. Approximately, 56% and 52% of adults were exposed to second-hand smoke at the workplace and at home, respectively. The average monthly expenditure on cigarette smoking was (34485) Iraqi dinars in 2015, whereas the cost of 100 packs of manufactured cigarettes, as a percentage of per capita GDP, was 2.4% [28, 29].

The same STEPS survey [28] displayed that 33.5% of the adult population in Iraq were obese (25.6% men, 42.6% women), while 65.4% were overweight (58.7% men, 73.1% women). Overall, 47% have experienced insufficient physical activity (34.9% men, 60% women). The median time spent on average activity per day was 25 min, whereas 82.3% did not engage in any physical activity. It has been recently estimated that about 50% of men and 35% of women in the EMR are currently overweight or obese [30]. Studies on alcohol consumption have demonstrated that 97.8% of Iraqi adults were lifetime abstainers (95.8% men, 100% women), only 0.6% were current drinkers [2, 28].

5.6 Cancer Screening Programs

In 2001, a "National Program for Early Detection of Breast Cancer" in Iraq was initiated by the MOH through establishing four main specialized referral training centers for early detection in Baghdad, Basra, and Mosul, in addition to specialized clinics in the major hospitals of each governorate. The main objectives of the program are early detection of breast cancer, reduction in cancer-related morbidity and mortality, and public promotion of cancer prevention and control [8, 17, 33–36]. The Ministry of Higher Education and Scientific Research (MOHESR) supported MOH by developing a "National Cancer Research Program" in 2010, focusing on breast cancer and a "National Cancer Research Center" (NCRC) in 2012. In addition to the research and training activities, the NCRC of Baghdad University has launched several awareness campaigns among the society on early detection of the disease [38]. Chaired by community leaders, a series of educational seminars were carried out covering almost all Universities, Ministries, Council of Ministers, Iraqi Parliament; and extended to reach the rural areas. Under the supervision of WHO/IARC, the NCRC developed an online information system database for patients with breast cancer. Numerous implemented activities of the aforementioned programs were sponsored by WHO, through provision of some urgently needed equipment and facilitating training of the staff running the breast cancer centers and clinics [8, 17, 36, 39, 40]. Although cervical cancer is not common in Iraq, yet there are sporadic activities for screening through Pap smears. It has been reported that 9.9% of Iraqi women (aged 30–49 years) had a Pap smear test at least once in a lifetime [28, 37]. Currently, there are active plans to initiate screening for colorectal and cervical cancers in Iraq.

5.7 Cancer Prevention Programs

The International Union against Cancer (UICC), World Cancer Declaration Target Report [31], shows that Iraq has made significant progress in key preventive areas including:

- Implementation of tobacco control legislation in accordance with the WHO MPOWER tool [32].
- Existence of national regulations on the prohibition of public availability of alcohol [2, 28].
- Launching national public mobilization campaigns on tobacco control, promotion of physical activity and healthy diet. Anthropometric measurements and obesity screening have been introduced in schools [2, 28].
- Implementation of the WHO STEP wise surveillance survey on the NCD risk factors [28, 31].
- Reduction of stigma and myths around breast cancer through public awareness campaigns reaching rural areas. Initiation of breast cancer early detection programs supported by research projects [8, 17, 33–36].

5.8 Cancer Diagnosis

5.8.1 Imaging

It has been registered in 2019 that there are 152 Computed Tomography (CT) scans and 90 Magnetic Resonance Imagining (MRI) machines, constituting 3.9 and 2.3/100,000 population, respectively [1]. Positron Emission Tomography/Computed Tomography (PET/CT) is available in the Medical City Teaching Hospital and in private oncology centers in Baghdad, Najaf, and Erbil. There are five Gamma Cameras in Baghdad and Gamma knife procedures are readily practiced in Erbil [1]. Excluding Baghdad and Erbil, there is very limited access to nuclear medicine diagnostic and treatment facilities.

5.8.2 Laboratory

Iraq is in the process of establishing accreditation for cancer diagnosis according to the international standards, in collaboration with IAEA, WHO, and the Royal College of Pathologists through adopting Good Laboratory Practice (GLP).

5.8.3 Cytogenetic and Molecular Genetics

The "Iraqi Center for Research on Cancer and Medical Genetics," affiliated to Mustansiriya University since 1995, focused on the study of the genetic material in cancer cells and carried out the transplantation of human and animal cells, in vivo and vitro. In 2016, the MCTC organized a plan of action to upgrade the genetic test procedures in different fields, focusing on hematology. The prevalence of BRCA1 and BRCA2 as common founder mutations among Iraqi families at risk of breast cancer was explored [54]. Great efforts were placed to ensure the availability of the requested resources, including sufficient infrastructure, competent trained manpower, logistics and financial support. During 2019, several advanced genetic tests were introduced in the diagnostic service for the first time in Iraq to serve leukemia patients. The provided examinations included, but not limited to, the molecular genetic tests for AML patients, i.e., FL3, NPM1, PML-RARA mutations for APL, JAK2 mutations for MPN, BCR-ABL quantitative assessment for CML patients, in addition to assays for MPL and CALR mutations. At a subsequent stage, cytogenetic tests were provided to the clinical laboratory service in the "Center of Hematology," MCTC, complementing the molecular genetics through adding cytogenetic analysis of chromosomal translocations in AML and MDS and baseline analysis of Philadelphia chromosome for patients with CML.

5.9 Treatment

5.9.1 Medical and Radiation Oncology

Oncology care is provided through specialized oncology and radiotherapy hospitals. Clinical oncologists are licensed by the Ministry of Health to perform chemotherapy and radiotherapy. It has been recorded that out of 11,585 specialized physicians in Iraq, there were 128 medical or radiation oncologists [41]. Excluding KRG, 72 medical oncologists and 58 radiation oncologists have been officially registered at the present time in the Iraqi MOH, whereas 75 postgraduate medical students are completing their board-certified studies in oncology and radiotherapy. In addition, there are 42 oncology physicians currently running the cancer care facilities in KRG. Nevertheless, the total number in most governorates is still lower than that requested to reach a coverage rate of 80% and is obviously far less than the international recommendations on oncology consultant staffing [42]. This shortage emphasized the urgent need for the MOH and MOHESR in Iraq to invest in qualifying human resources in all aspects of cancer care [12, 42, 43].

5.9.2 Medical Oncology

The MOH imports cancer drugs and medical equipment through the "State Company for Marketing Drugs and Medical Appliance" (KIMADIA) and distributes throughout all governorates, where chemotherapy is administered at specialized public tertiary hospitals and cancer centers free of charge [44]. As the provision of affordable access to cytotoxic medicine is a major challenge in the cancer care of patients in middle- and low- resource settings, WHO developed its "Model Lists of Essential Medicines," to support countries in prioritizing their reimbursable medicine [45]. Within the past decades, many of the essential cancer drugs were in short supply in Iraq. The situation improved recently when the government increased the allocated budget to the MOH [1, 4, 5]. The UICC declared that Iraq has made progress towards achieving the world cancer control targets through improving the free access to accurate diagnosis and multimodal treatment of cancer, adding that almost 80% of the treatment protocols are covered and the waiting lists for radiotherapy in the cancer centers have been significantly shortened [31].

5.9.2.1 Hematopoietic Stem Cell Transplantation

The first published article on Hematopoietic Stem Cell Transplantation (HSCT), submitted by the "Iraqi Bone Marrow Transplantation Center" in 2016, had reported 88% survival rate in lymphoma patients [50]. The same year witnessed the start-up of the first HSCT center in KRG, as a capacity-building collaborative project, initiated by the "Hiwa Cancer Hospital" and the Italian Agency for Development Cooperation [51]. To perform 1200 cases of HSCT in Iraq, around 100 BMT-specialized single bedrooms are needed. At the present time, the "Specialized Bone Marrow Transplant Center," affiliated to the MCTC in Baghdad, comprises four fully equipped rooms; yet the number is scheduled to reach 25, within the coming 2 years. Autologous SCT has been initiated in Iraq since 2013, more than 180 transplantation procedures have been performed mainly on lymphoma and myeloma patients. Allogeneic SCT is not yet available in Iraq, the MOH is still sending the patients outside Iraq for such procedures. The main challenge remains in ensuring high-quality post transplantation follow-up to avoid mortality complications, specifically, in the absence of some advanced diagnostic and therapeutic equipment requested for immune-compromised patients.

5.9.3 Radiation Therapy

Progress in radiation oncology has been proceeding in Iraq through continuous establishment of specialized centers and rehabilitation of the staff. Within the past 5 years, national societies for radiation/clinical oncology and medical physics have been established. Currently, there are 21 Mega Voltage Machines in Iraq, six in Baghdad [1]. A high dose rate Brachytherapy has been functioning in Zhianawa Cancer Center. The directory of Radiotherapy Centers has revealed the registered public oncology facilities within the corresponding governorates [46]:

- Baghdad: Al-Amal National Oncology Hospital, Kadhimiya Teaching Hospital, and Medical City Radiotherapy and Nuclear Medicine Center
- Babylon: Babylon Oncology Center, Marjan Hospital, and Al Imam Jaafar al-Sadeq Hospital
- Basra: Children Specialist Hospital, Educational Oncology Centre, and Basra Hospital
- Erbil: Rizgary Teaching Hospital—Oncology Center
- Karbala: Holy Karbala Hospital
- Maysan: Al Maysan Hospital and Maysan Oncology Center
- Mosul: Hazim Al-Hatiz Radiotherapy and Nuclear Medicine Hospital
- Holy Najaf: Al Najaf Hospital, Oncology Specialists Centre, and Middle Euphrates Cancer Centre
- Dhi Qar: Al Naseriya Hospital
- Al-Anbar: AlRamadi Hospital and Ramady General Hospital
- Sulaimaniya: Zhianawa Cancer Center and Hiwa Cancer Hospital.

5.9.4 Surgery

Cancer patients receive surgical treatment by specialized surgeons, following international guidelines, in tertiary public hospitals and private centers. Robotic surgery has not been commonly practiced in Iraq yet. Postgraduate studies in the fields of surgical oncology have been initiated within the past few years by the Arab and Iraqi Boards for Health and Medical Specializations.

5.9.5 Pediatric Oncology

In 2010, the first "Children Cancer Hospital" in Iraq was opened in Basra as the largest state of the art referral specialty care facility. It includes 101 beds, imaging department with MRI, automated laboratories and oncology departments provided with linear accelerators. Within the MCTC in Baghdad, the 240 bed "Children's Welfare Hospital" offers public services by a competent specialized multi-disciplinary team for diagnosis and treatment of childhood neoplasms. The oncology unit receives an average of 300 new malignant cases per year. Improvement in childhood cancer services was achieved over the past two decades through better availability of WHO essential chemotherapy drugs, introduction of advanced diagnostic/screening tools and bone marrow transplant services, provision of satellite telemedicine e-learning training program, in collaboration with Sapienza University in Rome, fostering consultation and quality control, using Tele-Pathology, introduction of ATRA, adapted APL protocols, strengthening research in coordination with Japanese institutes and promote training in accredited international centers [47–49].

5.9.6 Survivorship Track

The diagnosed cases of cancer have been officially registered in the ICR. Survivorship is estimated through follow-up of cancer patients and routine review of the related death records. In 2020, the Global Cancer Observatory reported that the age-standardized mortality rate in Iraq was 90.5 and 81.2 for males and females, respectively, while the risk of dying from cancer before the age of 75 was 9.7%.and 8.7% for males and females, respectively [24].

5.9.7 Palliative Care Track

In general, access to palliative care in the EMR has been hampered due to deficient national policies, low financial resources, lack of trained staff, and limited access to pain relieving drugs [52, 53]. Pain management units have been established in most tertiary hospitals of the Iraqi governorates during the past 15 years. In cases of cancer, prescription of morphine and other opioids is the responsibility of the examining oncologists, who refer patients to these clinics, where they are comprehensively assessed through history, clinical, laboratory, and imaging examinations. In 2016, a 2-year fellowship in pain management was initiated by the MOHESR for certified

Iraqi Board specialists. The curriculum includes intensive training in pain management clinics, followed by theoretical and practical examinations.

5.10 Research and Education

5.10.1 Research

In general, numerous research studies on the burden of cancer in Iraq have been published by Iraqi specialists in international peer reviewed journals, and are readily available online. Among the specialized journals are the Iraqi Journal of Cancer and Medical Genetics, started in 2010.

5.10.1.1 The Iraqi Regional Comparative Breast Cancer Research Project

Emphasizing the role of research as one of the basic pillars in the adoption of a national cancer control strategy, a National Breast Cancer Research Program was established by the Iraqi MOHESR in 2009, from which stemmed the NCCR in 2012. Following a visit to Lyon, the Founding Director of NCRC, author of this chapter, organized an online information system for breast cancer patients in coordination with the screening unit of IARC. In the same year, the WHO office of EMR, planned to utilize that database model to compare the demographic characteristics, clinicopathological presentations, and management outcomes of breast cancer patients in the region through developing a "Regional Comparative Breast Cancer Research Project" [8, 17, 36, 39]. The first consultative meeting was organized by WHO/EMRO in Egypt (2012), in collaboration with the Iraqi NCRC, IARC, IAEA and Susan G. Komen, to discuss the plan of action for that project. A detailed proposal was submitted to IARC for ethical approval and sponsorship following the second regional meeting which was carried out in 2015, through coordination between WHO/EMRO, IARC, NCRC (Iraq), and King Hussain Cancer Center (Jordan), with the participation of eight countries including Iraq, Jordan, Egypt, Lebanon, Sudan, Saudi Arabia, Oman, and Kuwait.

A *Memorandum of Understanding* has been developed recently between IARC and the Iraqi Cancer Board in Iraq. The objectives are to conduct high-quality, evidence-based research in cancer prevention and control, focusing on registration, descriptive epidemiologic studies, training, and biological material transfer. The scheduled activities include building capacity in the cancer registry through developing a detailed plan for 2020–2023, providing software for Can Reg5 users, utilizing the WHO standard population guidelines to strengthen quality control, designing a standard operating manual for complete resources, and finally disseminating the results on international databases and evaluating the activities of the NCCP.

5.10.2   Education and Training

5.10.2.1   Local Education and Training

The Iraqi Board for Medical Specialization [55] grants a certified Board in Oncology for postgraduate students. In general, the officially registered educational training programs belonging to the Iraqi MOHESR and MOHE, i.e., Dip., MSc, PhD, Iraqi Board, Arab Board for Health Specialization [56] and Kurdistan Board of Medical Specialties [57], graduate hundreds of oncology specialists annually, yield numerous studies on cancer care. Hopefully, this will help in addressing the shortage of oncology physicians. Many of the teaching hospitals in Iraq are recognized training centers by the Arab League Council in various medical specialties. The syllabus of these training programs requires subsequent evaluations, enrollment in recognized international centers, and submission of a thesis or peer-review publications for final graduation [58].

5.10.2.2   International Collaborations and Country Program Frameworks

In addition to the educational and training opportunities on cancer control offered through WHO and IARC, IAEA signed a Country Program Framework (CPF) with the Republic of Iraq in 2017 for the years (2018–2023). The CPF focused on building the capacity of the health sector, particularly on nuclear medicine and radiotherapy. Previously, the Iraqi Atomic Energy Commission was responsible for all nuclear activities in medicine, general healthcare, production of radioactive isotopes and pharmaceuticals for both diagnostic and therapeutic purposes. At present, due to the harmful consequences of wars and instability, IAEA has been supporting Iraq to ensure rehabilitation with respect to the maintenance of medical equipment, used in radiotherapy. The core program includes provision of requested equipment and sponsoring training programs on quality assurance. The project involves collaboration with IAEA/PACT (Program of Action for Cancer therapy) and WHO to implement the Iraqi NCCP. The Capacity Building Program executed its first activities in 2017, through training Iraqi pathology leaders in the UK, under the supervision of the Royal Colleges [59].

5.11 Cost-Effective Cancer Care

Excluding the private sector, the whole spectrum of cancer care services (including diagnostic imaging and laboratory tests, chemotherapy, radiotherapy, other relevant drugs, and medical appliances) is being provided by MOH freely without any charges in specialized oncology hospitals and cancer centers. Article 31 (1) of the Iraqi Constitution guarantees citizens the right to health care and commits the state to maintain public health freely through provision of prevention and treatment in hospitals and health institutions. Article 31 (2) guarantees individuals and entities the right to build hospitals, clinics, or private health care centers under state supervision [1, 4, 5, 44]. Currently, MOH is collaborating with the private sector to cover the requested cancer care specifically in the field of treatment. Purchasing internationally approved generic chemotherapy drugs supported in lowering the overall costs.

5.12 Challenges and Advantages

The economy of Iraq is mainly run by the government with limited role of the private sector. Over 90% of Iraq revenues and 65% of its GDP come from the oil sector. Decades of conflict, sanctions, and economic planning yielded a culture of government reliance for livelihoods [1, 4]. As an upper middle-income country, the health sector is still facing considerable challenges because of political instability and security issues. Financial allocations are urgently needed to strengthen the existing cancer care infrastructure, the surveillance and quality assurance systems, and to build the capacity of the human resources. Currently, the Iraqi health system is stepping forward, in collaboration with the private sector, international organizations (i.e., WHO, IAEA, and IARC) and foreign strategic financial investors, transitioning from emergency response to developmental reconstruction and rehabilitation in order to address the health needs of millions of vulnerable Iraqis and refugees (http://www.emro.who.int/media/news/statement-on-iraq-by-dr-ahmed-al-mandhari.html).

5.13 The Future of Cancer Care in Iraq

Nowadays, there are significant investment opportunities in the healthcare sector of Iraq. The MOH, aware of the challenges facing the system, has developed plans to overcome the existing obstacles. The current 4-year governmental program has approved the purchasing of 20 advanced linear accelerators, to be distributed among the radiotherapy centers all over the governorates. New specialized oncology centers are scheduled for construction during the coming year. The private sector is actively cooperating with MOH, to strengthen cancer care in Iraq. Andalus Specialized Cancer Treatment Center in Baghdad is well equipped with PET and cyclotron 8300-tonne particle accelerator, providing sophisticated private oncology services. Several charities have started to invest in the field of oncology to support the public cancer control activities, such as the Society for Cancer and Friends, Mosul Oncology Society, the Iraqi Medical Physics Society, and the Breast Cancer Society of Iraq.

Currently, WHO is assisting MOH in the institutionalization of a National Health Account to support in the development of healthcare policy financing systems and social insurance through compiling relevant data on the country's health expenditures [60]. In 2020, WHO has planned a mission on cancer control, in collaboration with IEA/PACT and IARC, to aid the ICB in implementing the following:

- Update the NCCP for the years (2020–2024).
- Assess and endorse the national strategy for prevention and control of NCDs.
- Evaluate the budget specified for the ICB and coordinate with the relevant stakeholders.
- Review the essential medical list focusing on cancer drugs and assess the access to chemotherapy.
- Evaluate the status of the universal health coverage for cancer and support the role of private sectors.
- Strengthen the ICR through assessing the registration of mortality coverage and surveillance systems.
- Specify international advisers to upgrade skills of the Iraqi staff in implementing the NCCP.

5.14 Conclusion

Iraq is emerging from the deep economic strains and decades of conflicts through accelerating progress to address the accumulated development and healthcare deficit. The government has actively planned to upgrade the capacity of its health sector, to ensure that specialized oncology services are delivered freely to all Iraqis on a sustainable basis. Recently, the UICC declared that Iraq has made progress towards the world cancer control targets through improving free access to accurate diagnosis and multimodal treatment of cancer. Hundreds of cancer specialists have been graduated annually by the MOHESR and MOHE to compensate for the shortage in oncology physicians. Together with the private sector, several charities have started to invest in the field of oncology to support public efforts. Currently, international organizations including WHO, IARC, and IAEA are actively collaborating to scale up cancer care and to support the implementation of the NCCP, focusing on cancer registration, prevention, early detection, treatment, palliative care, and research.

Conflict of Interest Authors have no conflict of interest to declare.

Acknowledgement The author would like to thank the following cancer care managers for their assistance in providing relevant information, namely Ass. Prof. Khudair Al Rawaq (Secretary General, ICB); Prof. Muhammed Saleem, Prof. Mazin Al Jadiry, Prof. Salma Al Haddad, Dr. Muhammed Ghanim, and Dr. Ayad Abbas (MCTC, MOH); Dr. Basak Tahir, Dr. Haja Abdulla, and Dr. Tamara Al Mufty (KRG, MOH).

References

1. Annual Statistical Report 2019. Planning Directorate, Ministry of Health/Environment, Republic of Iraq, 2019. https://moh.gov.iq/upload/upfile/ar/1070.pdf. Accessed 25 Oct 2020.
2. Eastern Mediterranean Region: framework for health information systems and core indicators for monitoring health situation and health system performance 2018/WHO Regional Office for the Eastern Mediterranean.
3. World Health Organization, Eastern Mediterranean Region: Key Statistics from WHO Global Health Observatory, Country Office Website, Iraq 2020. WHO, Office for the Eastern Mediterranean. https://www.who.int/countries/irq. Accessed 25 Oct 2020.
4. DFAT Country Information Report IRAQ, Department of Foreign Affairs and Trade, Australian Government, 2020.
5. Country Policy and Information Note. Iraq: Medical and Healthcare Issues, Version 1.0, Home Office, UK; 2019.
6. United Nations, World Bank, Joint Iraq Needs Assessment 2003. Available at: http://siteresources.worldbank.org/IRFFI/Resources/Joint+Needs+Assessment.pdf. Accessed 26 Oct 2020.
7. Schweitzer M. Iraq's public healthcare system in crisis. EPIC. 2017. https://www.epic-usa.org/healthcare-in-crisis/. Accessed 25 Oct 2020.
8. Alwan NAS, Kerr D. Cancer control in war-torn Iraq. Lancet Oncol. 2018;19(3):291–2.
9. Ministry of Health and Environment, Baghdad, Republic of Iraq. http://www.moh.gov.iq/arabic. Accessed 25 Oct 2020.
10. Al-Ghazi M. Cancer care in a war zone: radiation oncology in Iraq. Int J Radiat Oncol Biol Phys. 2016;96(2 Suppl):E413. https://doi.org/10.1016/j.ijrobp.2016.06.1668. Accessed 24 Oct 2020
11. Al Hilfi TK, Lafta R, Burnham G. Health services in Iraq. Lancet. 2013;381(9870):939–48. https://doi.org/10.1016/S0140-6736(13)60320-7. Accessed 23 Oct 2020
12. Mula-Hussain L, Alabedi H, Al-Alloosh F, Alharganee A. Cancer in war-torn countries: Iraq as an example. In: Laher, editor. Handbook of healthcare in the Arab world. Cham: Springer; 2019. p. 1–14. https://doi.org/10.1007/978-3-319-74365-3_152-1. Accessed 25 Oct 2020.
13. Skelton M. Health and health care decline in Iraq: the example of cancer and oncology. Costs of War. 2013. Available at: https://www.academia.edu/4725776/Skelton_M._Health_and_Health_Care_Decline_iin_Iraq-The_Example_of_Cancer_and_Oncology_costsofwar.org. Accessed 24 Oct 2020.
14. Iraqi National Cancer Control Program Five Year Plan (2010–2014), 2nd ed. Iraqi cancer board, Baghdad: Ministry of Health; 2010.
15. World Health Organization. Strategy for cancer prevention and control in the eastern Mediterranean region 2009—2013; WHO, Office for the Eastern Mediterranean, 2010.
16. Romero Y, Trapani D, Johnson S, et al. National cancer control plans: a global analysis. Lancet Oncol. 2018;19(10):E546–55. https://doi.org/10.1016/S1470-2045(18)30681-8. Accessed 22 Oct 2020

17. Alwan N. Establishing guidelines for early detection of breast cancer in Iraq. Int J Adv Res. 2015;3(12):539–55.
18. Skelton M, Mula-Hussain LY, Namiq KF. Oncology in Iraq's Kurdish region: navigating cancer, war, and displacement. Journal of Global Oncology. 2017;4:1–4.
19. Pourghazian N, Sankaranarayanan R, Alhomoud S, Slama S. Strengthening the early detection of common cancers in the eastern Mediterranean region. East Mediterr Health J. 2019;25(11):767–8.
20. Lyons G, Sankaranarayanan R, Millar AB, Slama S. Scaling up cancer care in the WHO eastern Mediterranean region. East Mediterr Health J. 2018;24(1):104–10. https://doi.org/10.26719/2018.24.1.104.
21. Hussain RA, Habib OS. Cancer registration in Basrah-southern Iraq: validation by household survey. Asian Pac J Cancer Prev. 2016;17:197–200.
22. Abood SF, Al-Timimi A, Al-Dahmoshi HO, et al. Malignancy registered in Babylon oncology center (1990-2015). Ann Oncol. 2016;27(Suppl. 6):v462–8.
23. Annual Report, Iraqi Cancer Registry 2016. Iraqi Cancer Board, Ministry of Health and Environment, Republic of Iraq; 2018.
24. Global Cancer Observatory: Cancer Today. International Agency for Research in Cancer, France. https://gco.iarc.fr/today/data/factsheets/populations/368-iraq-fact-sheets.pdf. Accessed 26 Oct 2020.
25. Annual Report, Iraqi Cancer Registry 2018. Iraqi Cancer Board, Ministry of Health and Environment, Republic of Iraq; 2019.
26. Fouad H, Commar A, Hamadeh RR, et al. Smoking prevalence in the eastern Mediterranean region. East Mediterr Health J. 2020;26(1):94–101.
27. Iraq Country Profile. Baghdad: WHO Office; 2017. https://www.who.int/gho/countries/irq/country_profiles. Accessed 24 Oct 2020.
28. WHO STEPS Survey, Chronic Disease Risk Factor Surveillance, IRAQ 2015/WHO Regional Office for the Eastern Mediterranean; 2015.
29. GYTS Global youth tobacco survey, fact sheet, IRAQ 2015/WHO regional Office for the Eastern Mediterranean and Center for Disease Control and Prevention, 2015.
30. Amin J, Siddiqui AA, Al-Oraibi S, et al. The potential and practice of telemedicine to empower patient-centered healthcare in Saudi Arabia. Intern Med J. 2020;27(2):151–4.
31. World Cancer Declaration Progress Report 2016, International Union against Cancer (UICC) 2017. https://issuu.com/uicc.org/docs/uicc_worldcancerdeclaration_progres/46. Accessed 23 Oct 2020.
32. Tobacco Control Laws, legislations by country, IRAQ, Campaign for Tobacco-Free Kids, 2020. https://www.tobaccocontrollaws.org/legislation/country/iraq/summary. Accessed 25 Oct 2020.
33. Alwan NAS, Al-Attar WM, Al Mallah N. Baseline needs assessment for breast cancer awareness among patients in Iraq. Int J Sci Res. 2017;6(1):2088–93.
34. Alwan N, Al-Attar W, Eliessa R, et al. Knowledge, attitude and practice regarding breast cancer and breast self-examination among a sample of the educated population in Iraq. East Mediterr Health J. 2012;18(4):337–45. WHO, Eastern Mediterranean Regional Office
35. Von Karsa L, Qiao Y, Ramadas K, et al. Prevention/screening implementation. In: Stewart BW, Wild CP, editors. World cancer report 2014. Lyon: WHO, International Agency for Research on Cancer; 2014.
36. Alwan N. Iraqi initiative of a regional comparative breast cancer research project in the Middle East. J Cancer Biol Res. 2014;2(1):1016–20.
37. Alwan NAS, Al-Attar WM, Al Mallah N, Abdulla K. Assessing the knowledge, attitude and practices towards cervical cancer screening among a sample of Iraqi female population. Iraqi J Biotechnol. 2017;16(2):38–47.
38. The National Cancer Research Center, University of Baghdad, MoHESR, Iraq. http://www.bccru.baghdaduniv.edi.iq. Accessed 27 Oct 2020.

39. Alwan NAS. Breast cancer among Iraqi women: preliminary findings from a regional comparative breast cancer research project. J Global Oncol. 2016;2(5):255–8.
40. Alwan NAS, Kerr D, Al-Okati D, et al. Comparative study on the clinicopathological profiles of breast cancer among Iraqi and British patients. Open Publ Health J. 2018;11:3–17.
41. Annual Statistical Report 2017. Planning directorate, Ministry of Health/Environment, Republic of Iraq, 2018.
42. The Royal College of Radiologists. Scotland clinical oncology workforce census 2018 summery Report. London: The Royal College of Radiologists 2019. https://www.rcr.ac.uk/system/files/publication/field_publication_files/clinical-radiology-uk-workforce-census-report-2018. pdf. Accessed 25 Oct 2020.
43. Mula-Hussain L, Al-Ghazi M. Cancer care in Times of War: radiation oncology in Iraq. Int J Radiat Oncol Biol Phys. 2020;108(3):523–9.
44. The State Co. for Marketing Drugs and Medical Appliances, KIMADIA, Ministry of Health/Environment, Republic of Iraq 2020. http://demo.kimadia.iq/en/article/view/8. Accessed 24 Oct 2020.
45. Robertson H, Barr R, Shulman LN, Forte GB, Magrini N. Essential medicines for cancer: WHO recommendations and national priorities. Bull World Health Organ. 2016;94:735–42. https://doi.org/10.2471/BLT.15.163998.
46. DIRAC (DIrectory of RAdiotherapy Centres), Country: IRAQ. International Atomic Energy Agency (IAEA), Vienna, Austria 2020. Available at: https://dirac.iaea.org/Data/Operator?country=IRQ. Accessed 27 Oct 2020.
47. Phelps HM, Al-Jadiry MF, Corbitt NM, et al. Molecular and epidemiologic characterization of Wilms tumor from Baghdad, Iraq. World J Pediatr. 2018;14(6):585–93.
48. Moleti ML, Al-Jadiry MF, Shateh WA, et al. Long-term results with the adapted LMB 96 protocol in children with B-cell non Hodgkin lymphoma treated in Iraq: comparison in two subsequent cohorts of patients. Leuk Lymphoma. 2019;60(5):1224–33.
49. Testi AM, Al-Hadad SA, Al-Jadiry MF, et al. Impact of international collaboration on the prognosis of childhood acute promyelocytic leukemia in Iraq. Haematologica. 2006;91(4):509–12.
50. Hammadi AM, Azeez WA, Jasim FH, et al. First report on stem cell transplant from Iraq. Exp Clin Transplant. 2017;15(1):133–5.
51. Majolino I, Othman D, Rovelli A, et al. The start-up of the first hematopoietic stem cell transplantation Center in the Iraqi Kurdistan: a capacity-building cooperative project by the Hiwa cancer hospital, Sulaymaniyah, and the Italian Agency for Development Cooperation: an innovative approach. Mediterr J Hematol Infect Dis. 2017;9(1):e2017031. https://doi.org/10.4084/MJHID.2017.031.
52. Lyons G, Sankaranarayanan R, Millar AB, Slama S. Scaling up cancer care in the WHO eastern Mediterranean region. East Mediterr Health J. 2020;4(1):104–10. https://doi.org/10.26719/2018.24.1.104. Accessed 26 Oct 2020
53. Fadhil I, Lyons G, Payne S. Barriers to, and opportunities for, palliative care development in the eastern Mediterranean region. Lancet Oncol. 2017;18(3):e176–84.
54. Ghanim M, Alwan NAS, McDonald F. Low prevalence of BRCA1 and BRCA2 common founder mutations among Iraqi breast cancer cases and at risk families. J Cancer Sci Res. 2016;2(7):047.
55. The Iraqi Board for Medical Specialization. Baghdad: Ministry of Higher Education and Scientific Research. https://www.iraqiboard.edu.iq. Accessed 27 Oct 2020.
56. The Arab Board for Health Specialization in Iraq. Baghdad: Ministry of Health/Environment. Available at: https://www.arab-board.org/en. Accessed 27 Oct 2020.

57. Kurdistan Board of Medical Specialties. Erbil, Kurdistan: Ministry of Higher Education and Scientific Research. https://www.facebook.com/KurdistanBoard. Accessed 27 Oct 2020.
58. Mula-Hussain L, Shamsaldin AN, Al-Ghazi M, et al. Board-certified specialty training program in radiation oncology in a war-torn country: challenges, solutions and outcomes. Clin Transl Radiat Oncol. 2019;19:46–51.
59. The Royal College of Pathologists (RCPath): International Pathology Day: A Look Back at the Year with the International Team, 2018, UK. https://www.rcpath.org/discover-pathology/news/international-pathology-day-a-look-back-the-year-with-the-international-team.html. Accessed 25 Oct 2020.
60. World Health Organization, Regional Office for the Eastern Mediterranean, Iraq|Programme areas|Primary Health Care. http://www.emro.who.int/irq/programmes/primary-health-care.htm. Accessed 27 Oct 2020.

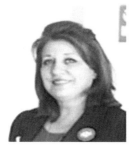

Nada A. S. Al Alwan, M.D, Ph.D., is the Health Advisor to the Presidency of the Iraqi Republic, Professor of Pathology at Baghdad University (since 2001), and the Founding Director of the National Cancer Research Center (2012–2019). She organized the National Cancer Research Program and led the Medical Committee of the Iraqi Scientific Research Council (2010–2019). Prof. Alwan served earlier as the Executive Director of the National Breast Cancer Early Detection Program and the Manager of its Referral Training Center (2001–2017). She has published 106 peer-reviewed articles focusing on cancer control and acted as a regional advisor to WHO, IAEA, and IARC.

Chapter 6
General Oncology Care in Jordan

Sami Khatib and Omar Nimri

6.1 Jordan Demographics

The Hashemite Kingdom of Jordan is an Arab country in the levant region of western asia. Jordan is bordered by Syria on the North, Palestine (west bank) to the west and Iraq, Saudi Arabia on the east south frontiers. The Dead Sea is located along its western borders and it is the deepest inhabitation on earth below sea level. Jordan is advantageously located at the crossroads of Asia, Africa, and Europe. The country was allocated into 12 governorates. Amman, the capital of the country, is the most populous city as well as the country's economic, political, and cultural center.

After experiencing a period of fast population growth from 2000 to 2020, which increased the population by over five million people, the Jordan population is expected to continue growing. The population is expected to peak at 14.15 million people by 2050. In 2015, a true census showed Jordan inhabited with around nine and half million dwellers, where three million are non-Jordanians and refugees [1]. Jordan is home to Palestine refugees given Jordanian citizenship; Jordan also hosts around 1.4 million Syrian refugees who fled to the country due to the Syrian Civil War since 2011. Yemenis, Libyan, and thousands of Lebanese refugees live in Jordan. Up to one million Iraqis came to Jordan following the Iraq War in 2003; their counts are much less now [2].

Figures 6.1 and 6.2 show Jordan's demographic figures and health indicators [2]. Jordan is classified as a country of "high human development" with an "upper middle income" economy. In the most recent update, Jordan has been reclassified from upper-middle-income to lower-middle-income [3].

S. Khatib
Clinical Oncologist, Arab Medical Association Against Cancer (AMAAC), Amman, Jordan

O. Nimri (✉)
Cancer Prevention Department, Jordan Cancer Registry, Ministry of Health, Amman, Jordan
e-mail: onimri@moh.gov.jo

Population	2015 census: 9,531,712
	2019 estimate: 10,392,309
Density	116/km^2 (300/sq mi)
Growth rate	2.05% (2017 est.)
Birth rate	23.9 births/1,000 population (2017 est.)
Death rate	3.4 deaths/1,000 population
Life expectancy	74.8 years (2017 est.)
- male	73.4 years
- female	76.3 years
Fertility rate	2.7 children born/woman (2018 est.)
Age structure	
0-14 years	34.68%
15-64 years	61.87%
65 and over	3.45%

Sex ratio	
Total	1.02 male(s)/female (2016 est.)
At birth	1.06 male(s)/female
Under 15	1.05 male(s)/female
15-64 years	1.00 male(s)/female
65 and over	0.89 male(s)/female
Nationality	
Nationality	Jordanians
Major ethnic	Arab
Minor ethnic	Armenians, Chechens, Circassians
Language	
Official	Arabic
Spoken	Arabic, English

Fig. 6.1 Demographics of Jordan [2]. Copyright to Demographics of Jordan, wikipedia.org/wiki/Demographics_of_Jordan#Population_growth_rate

Health — الصحة

مؤشرات صحية مختارة، 2017-2019*
Selected Health Indicators, 2017-2019

Indicator	2019	2018	2017	المؤشر
No. of Hospitals	118	116	116	عدد المستشفيات
No. of Beds	14,536	14,701	14,779	عدد الأسرّة
Population Per Bed	726	701	680	عدد السكان لكل سرير
No. of Pharmacies	3,176	3,019	2,838	عدد الصيدليات
Population Per Pharmacy	3,323	3,415	3,542	عدد السكان لكل صيدلية
**Physicians Per (0000)	24.8	19.8	22.5	الأطباء لكل (10000) مواطن*

** Source: Jordanian Medical Syndicate.   ** المصدر: نقابة الأطباء الأردنيين.

الإدخالات في مستشفيات وزارة الصحة، 2017-2019*
Admissions at the Ministry of Health Hospitals, 2017-2019

Particulars	2019	2018	2017	التفاصيل
Admissions (000)	412.1	401.6	388.2	الإدخالات (بالألف)
Discharged Alive (000)	404.7	394.8	381.7	الإخراجات أحياء (بالألف)
Surgical Operations (000)	99.1	97.9	90.6	العمليات الجراحية (بالألف)
Deliveries (000)	74.6	78.8	80.5	حالات الولادة (بالألف)
Beds Annual Occupancy Rate	69.0	69.2	66.2	معدل إشغال الأسرّة السنوي

Fig. 6.2 Selected health indicators [1]. Copyright to dos.gov.jo/DataBank/JordanInFigures-Jorinfo_2019.pdf (dos.gov.jo)

المشتغلون في المهن الطبية والمساعدة في وزارة الصحة، 2016-2019*

Medical and Related Professional Employees at the Ministry of Health, 2016-2019

Particulars	2019	2018	2017	2016	التفاصيل
No. of Physicians	5,694	5,838	4,924	4,798	عدد الأطباء
No. of Dentists	725	743	752	782	عدد أطباء الأسنان
No. of Pharmacists	827	805	734	723	عدد الصيادلة
No. of Nurses (Male & Female)	8,336	8,578	7,571	7,987	عدد الممرضين والممرضات
No. of Midwives	1606	1612	1,467	1,531	عدد القابلات القانونيات

*Source: Ministry of Health.

Department of Statistics, Jordan

* المصدر: وزارة الصحة.

دائرة الإحصاءات العامة، الأردن

Fig. 6.2 (continued)

6.2 Cancer Statistics in Jordan

Jordan cancer statistics were obtained from the hospital-based registry; the only data source on cancer patients was from the main Ministry of Health referral hospital, "Basheer Hospital" where cancer patients were treated.

Later, Jordan Cancer Registry (JCR), a population-based cancer registry, was established in 1996 under the jurisdiction of the Ministry of Health (MOH), by the order of His Excellency the Minister of Health. JCR is a unit of the Cancer Prevention Department in the Non-Communicable Disease Directorate. Cancer notification has been compulsory since 1996 through a ministerial decree. JCR monitors cancer incidence rates and cancer trends in Jordan. The aim of JCR is to provide national cancer incidence data to the public in a timely and accurate manner. JCR also provides data for clinical and epidemiological research. The JCR cancer data collected from all health sectors in the country have more than 95% coverage.

Annual cancer incidence report for both Jordanian and non-Jordanians is released showing the epidemiology of the cancer burden in the kingdom for a specific period (1 year), and the last issued report is of the 2016 data, which shows the following cancer figures in Fig. 6.3.

The total number of cancer cases registered for the year 2016 was 8152 cases; out of them, 5999 cases were Jordanian (73.6%) and the other 2153 were among the non-Jordanian population (26.4%). The crude incidence rate among males was 80.2 and in females, it was 94.5; and it was 87.2 for both genders/100,000 population [4]. Standard rates were 135.6 for both genders. 131 for males and 138.2 for females/100,000. The median age at diagnosis was 59 for males and 53 years for females. Pediatric cancers accounted for 236 of both genders, which is 3.9% of the total cancers registered among the Jordanian population [4]. The crude incidence

No of cases	Male	Female	Total
Total cases	3889	4263	8152
Jordanian.	2815	3184	5999
Non-Jordanian.	1069	1084	2153
Pediatric age group o < 15 years-Jor.	138	98	236
Crude incidence Rate-Jor.	80.2	94.5	87.2
Age standardized Rate-Jor.	131	138.2	135.6
Median age at diagnosis-Jor.	59	53	56

Fig. 6.3 Summary of Number of cancer cases in Jordan −2016 data. (Jordan Cancer Registry) [4]. The 21st annual report of 2016 data. Copyright of this figure to Jordan cancer Registry, Report

Table 6.1 Number of cancer and crude incidence rates by governorates and gender, 2016 [4]

Governorate	Male		Female		Total		
	N	CR	N	CR	N	CR	%
Amman	1600	72.3	1863	97.7	3463	84.1	57.7
Balqa	159	58.6	177	75.6	336	66.5	5.6
Zarka	317	42.7	330	49.9	647	46.1	10.8
Madaba	66	64.2	67	73.1	133	68.4	2.2
Central region	2142	64.4	2437	84.2	4579	73.6	76.3
Irbid	351	37.3	381	43.3	732	40.2	12.2
Mafraq	80	27.4	61	22.3	141	24.9	2.4
Jarash	40	31.6	70	59.8	110	45.1	1.8
Ajloun	36	38.6	51	58.1	87	48.1	1.5
North Region	507	34.9	563	41.5	1070	38.1	17.8
Karak	64	37.6	78	50.2	142	43.6	2.4
Tafiela	25	48.3	25	53.0	50	50.5	0.8
Maan	24	31.0	25	35.4	49	33.1	0.8
Aqaba	37	33.8	38	45.2	75	38.8	1.3
South Region	150	36.7	166	46.5	316	41.3	5.3
Out side	16		18	97.7	34		0.6

Crude incidence Rate (CR, crude rate)/100,000 pop
The 21st annual report of 2016 data. Copyright of this table to Jordan cancer Registry Report

rates in the different governorates by gender are shown in Table 6.1 which shows the high rates in the central region compared with both northern and south regions of the Jordanian population. The top 10 cancers and their ranks among the male and female population are shown in Figs. 6.4 and 6.5. The top 10 pediatric cancers are shown in Fig. 6.6.

The number of deaths due to cancer was 3084 (16.2%) out of the 19,676 registered mortalities. The male-to-female ratio was 1.2:1. The median age for mortality due to cancer was 63 years (65 years for males and 61 for females) [4].

No	Site	Freq	%
1	Trachea, Bronchus, Lung	362	12.9
2	Colorectal	335	11.9
3	Prostate	234	8.3
4	Bladder	226	8.0
5	Non-Hodgkin lymphoma	153	5.4
6	Leukemia	127	4.5
7	Stomach	91	3.2
8	Larynx	85	3.0
9	Kidney	82	2.9
10	Brain, Nervous system	82	2.9

Fig. 6.4 Top 10 cancers among males. Jordan 2016. (Jordan Cancer Registry) [4]. The 21st annual report of 2016 data. Copyright of this fig to Jordan cancer Registry, Report

No	Site	Freq	%
1	Breast	1263	39.7
2	Colorectal	308	9.7
3	Thyroid	202	6.3
4	Corpus Uteri	134	4.2
5	Non-Hodgkin lymphoma	111	3.5
6	Ovary	96	3.0
7	Trachea, Bronchus, Lung	86	2.7
8	Hodgkin disease	79	2.5
9	Brain, Nervous system	65	2.0
10	Stomach	58	1.8

Fig. 6.5 Top 10 cancers among females. Jordan 2016. (Jordan Cancer Registry) [4]. The 21st annual report of 2016 data. Copyright of this fig to Jordan cancer Registry, Report

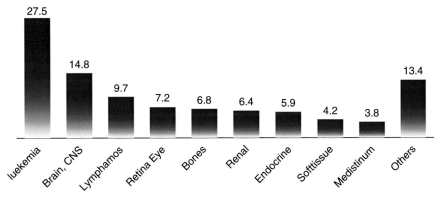

Fig. 6.6 Top 10 pediatric cancers among both genders. Jordan 2016 (Jordan Cancer Registry) [4]. The 21st annual report of 2016 data. Copyright of this fig to Jordan cancer Registry, Report

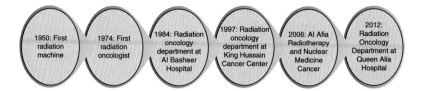

Fig. 6.7 Stage in development the milestones of radiation oncology in Jordan since 1950 [5]. Copyright to, History and Current State of Radiation Oncology Services and Practice in Jordan

Since the late 1950s, efforts have resulted in an ever-growing RT practice in Jordan. As a result, four cancer care facilities with cutting-edge technology has been successfully established as shown in Fig. 6.7 [5].

In 1967, the radiology department at the Ashrafeh hospital (AL Basheer Now) was expanded with the arrival of its first external beam radiotherapy machines that used gamma rays from cobalt-60 to treat cancer cells [5]. The MOH had no qualified radiation oncologists until 1974 when the International Atomic Energy Agency (IAEA) hired a Polish radiation oncologist to work at Al Basheer Hospital (Ashrafeh at that time). In 1987, the first resident joined the newly created radiation residency program.

The initiation and foundation of the King Hussein Cancer Center (KHCC) in 1997 was a major boost to the already growing radiation and oncology practice in Jordan. Currently, in Jordan, there are four Radiation Therapy Facilities, in the public sector (Ministry of Health) and the royal military services, private sector, and the KHCC (Non-Governmental Organizations NGOs) with a short new installment in the King Abdullah Hospital in the northern city, Irbid.

6.3   Healthcare System in Jordan

The healthcare system in the country is covered by different health sectors, public, military, private, and teaching hospitals as well as some NGOs and nonprofit health facilities. The whole spectrum of healthcare is available in Jordan, inequality, and inequity of those services to the vast public is one of the major obstacles and challenges faced by the health system sector that echoed on the population health.

6.4   Oncology Care in Jordan

Cancer care and treatment are provided in the different health sectors with diverse plans; in Jordan, the King Hussein Cancer Center (KHCC), a specialized cancer center with accreditation and moral reputation delivers a standard cancer treatment protocol.

Diagnosis and treatment of cancer are costly, though Jordanian citizens holding a national number are being treated in the Ministry of Health hospitals. Furthermore, references to other health facilities can be made including the King Hussein Cancer Center if service is needed. On government financial coverage, or cost exemptions granted by the royal court to the cancer patients as well as other diseases too. These dispensation canons can be applied to non-national in selected incidents.

6.5   Cancer Risk Factors

The major well-known risk factor is the consumption of the most incriminated cause i.e., tobacco smoking. Tobacco use, not only the cigarettes but also all different tobacco types and other forms like oriental tobacco narghile, shisha or cigars, and the electronic cigarettes recently among many others are risk factors for different cancers and other diseases too [6–8]. According to the Stepwise Survey conducted in 2019, Jordanian males' smokers are about 58–68% of the population, while in females it is 12–18% are smokers in the age group 18–69 years [9].

"The highest global smoking rates in Jordan have been blamed on tobacco manufacturers' interference by health officials, following an investigation by British newspaper The Guardian" [10, 11]. Obesity and overweight seem to be a public disorder among adult Jordanians, as it was revealed by the 2019 Stepwise figures, which showed more than 30% of the population is obese, while more than 60% are overweight [9].

Obesity, poor unhealthy diet, and physical inactivity create a major chronic disease burden including cancer in Jordan that is likely to increase substantially in the next coming years due to the westernization of the lifestyle and the unhealthy food and physical inactivity especially among the young population [12]. Alcohol consumption in Jordan is not alarming as three-step surveys 2004, 2007, and recently 2019 showed the drinking habit is less than 2% among the Jordanian population [13].

6.6   Cancer Screening Programs

Since the establishment of the Jordan Cancer Registry more than 20 years ago, breast cancer among females in Jordan ranks first and tops all registered cancers nationwide. Based on the national cancer registry epidemiological disseminated figures and data, national early diagnosis and screening strategies were in progress in the year 2006–2007.

The national program was started with the intention of screening goals. This was not achieved at that time and the program was modified to down-staging activities on the national level. "Jordan Breast Cancer Program" adopted three main lines of activities, expanding awareness between two main target groups, one in the public and female communities. The other target group is the medical staff increasing skills and raising awareness of the disease and its early diagnosis. The third activity is, improving the availability and standards of making mammograms with better qualities and qualified mammogram-readers [14].

The program is a success story and it has been going on for more than 10 years with good outcomes as a comprehensive service for the early detection and screening of breast cancer among both Jordanian and non-Jordanian women in Jordan. The screening is available in both selected primary and tertiary levels as well as two mobile units. Currently, a comprehensive report is being edited and prepared about the breast program; unfortunately, no statistical data from the program is released yet. While the data of breast cancer in the National Cancer Registry show some downstage and more cases are being discovered in early stages and little reduction in the late-stage numbers.

In Jordan, there is no established national screening program for cervical cancer. Nevertheless, there are scattered efforts of screening in the Ministry of Health, the screening is performed at the maternity clinics. As well as at the Jordan Association for Family planning (JAFP), and the private sector, limited opportunistic Pap smear screening activities are done. The screening services are not institutionalized yet, and no database is available. Still, no other screening programs are available. Plans have been pulled and brought to the table for the colorectal cancer screening program [15] as it is on the top of the list between both males and females' cancers in the country. Numerous local and national committees have been formed for such purposes and goals. The void and non-availability of endorsed NCCP besides the absence of financial support and funds backing such screening or other cancer activities make it hard to implement and carry on.

6.7   Cancer Prevention Programs

Disease prevention and control is not the task of the government alone, rather it is a collaboration of communities and society members in sharing, planning such activities, and adopting reliable prevention strategies and solutions [16]. For participation in such activities, some changes are required that includes the inclusion of programs geared toward various factors, such as socio-economic and behavioral patterns as well community and life alterations, in addition to environmental and appropriate legislative changes, especially if we knew that approximately 30–40% of cancers are preventable and can be reduced [17].

The Ministry of Health paid attention to creating a national plan to control cancer by preparing a comprehensive national plan with the participation of all medical and academic sectors in the Kingdom; a national committee was formed. Activities in the field of prevention and early detection of cancer with the aim of increasing awareness of the importance of early detection; urges citizens to get this service with the lowest costs, the least suffering, and the best guarantee of International standards according to the available capabilities.

The concept of prevention and healthy life starts from infancy and childhood. The national vaccine program covers the basic vaccines including the hepatitis B vaccine. The importance of early exercise and proper lifestyle with healthy nutrition, lower obesity figures, and the lack of physical activity along with many negative habits such as smoking. Smoke cessation program and law supporting smoke prohibition was passed banning smoking in public places with penalties and fines [18, 19]. Jordan was one of the first countries who joined the international community in this regard as well as the youth programs for stopping smoking. The Ministry of Health and the Jordan breast cancer program have joint activities regarding the awareness and prevention of breast cancer in Jordan. A drafted National Cancer Control Plan (NCCP) was written and prepared but unfortunately, it was not endorsed nor implemented in the country [20, 21].

6.8 Cancer Diagnosis

Cancer care and services in Jordan mainly focus on treatment, with less effort being put on other elements of the cancer continuum [22, 23]. Cancer care infrastructure and workforce are well available but with the inequity of such services. The major cancer treatment modalities (surgery, chemotherapy, and radiation) are generally available, and most services are focused on the capital, Amman. Most of the institutions offer multiple diagnostic and clinical specialties. However, across these institutions, variable gaps exist regarding the availability or sufficiency of equipment and staff in certain disciplines [22]. The King Hussein Cancer Center is the only specialized tertiary hospital that provides all treatment modalities and services for cancer care. With other functional nuclear medicine departments in Al Basheer Hospital (MOH), the Royal Medical Services (RMS), the teaching hospital of King Abdulla the founded in the northern part of the country, and some of the private sector in Amman. Other laboratories (private sector and the university) are present with the capacity of performing cytogenetic and molecular testing along with the genetic ones [24].

6.9 Treatment

The government bears the cost of treating Jordanian cancer patients. Cancer treatment is offered at no cost to all Jordanian citizens through public hospitals of the MOH, or any other referred facility if required and needed, but the services are not available in the MOH facilities. A full range of diagnosis and treatment is provided by other health sectors in the private and the military services as well. The King Hussein Cancer Center provides a specialized updated cancer care and treatment not only to the Jordanian citizens but to many from the neighboring and surrounding countries [23].

6.9.1 Medical Oncology

Jordan has several medical oncology facilities, which provide treatment of chemotherapy and stem cell transplant along with other oncological surgery services. The King Hussein Cancer Centre located in the capital city of Amman is a center of excellence with a regional reputation in the field. Nevertheless, not yet the robotic surgery. The stem cell transplantation is also done in the specific specialized center at the Jordan university hospital.

6.9.2 Radiation Therapy

Jordan has four sites or locations that provide radiation therapy and other spectra of cancer treatments. The country has eight linear accelerators with more than 130 registered radiation oncologists, who can provide services with other types of radiation being provided like Three-Dimensional Conformal Radiotherapy (3D-CRT)/ Intensity Modulated Radiation Therapy (IMRT)/Volumetric Modulated Arc Therapy (VMAT)/Stereotactic Radiosurgery (SRS)/Stereotactic Body Radiation Therapy (SBRT). The major centers that provide radiation oncology treatment are The King Hussein Cancer Center, Basheer Hospital, Al Afia Center.

6.9.3 Surgery

Understanding the challenges and beyond medical care, surgery services of high experience and with great proficiency for all types of cancers are available and provided to cancer patients in Jordan, and to many more out comers from outside the kingdom, whom they seek the treatment and cure for their diseases and illness. Some locations or centers have specialized and trained staff for such services with the proper settings and equipment. The other services like Brachytherapy and the Cyberknife and the Hyperthermic Intraperitoneal Chemotherapy (HIPEC) procedures are available in many locations and centers for oncological surgery while the robotic surgeries for cancer in Jordan are still not presented nor available currently.

6.9.4 Pediatric Oncology

Pediatric oncology has about 5.6% of the total cancers of the Jordanian population [4]. These cases are served and treated mainly in the KHCC center where comprehensive pediatric treatment and services are provided [13]. Other services are of limited numbers in some other locations in the private sector or the military services.

6.9.5   Survivorship Track

Surveillance of cancer survival by central analysis of population-based registry data to 5-year survival statistics can be calculated with the number of patients diagnosed with cancer still alive 5 years later after diagnosis. This data was obtained from the national Jordan Cancer Registry (JCR) and analyzed with Jordan cancer data. It was included in the international concord studies parts 2 and 3 as one of the participating countries in this international study of cancer survivals of different cancers [25].

6.9.6   Palliative Care Track

The palliative care initiative was launched in Jordan as the WHO demonstration project in 2003 to implement palliative care through training and education, changing policies related to opioids and drug availability. Palliative care is an approach that improves patients' and their families quality of life [26, 27].

There were improvements in the practice of palliative care. A national palliative care committee was formed with different stakeholders from different health and medical sectors in the kingdom. A national guideline was prepared and printed, a society for palliative care was established and courses in collaboration with local universities were founded and established. Certified nurses are graduating from university after 6 months of palliative training (study). Two international conferences were held in Amman, under the patronage of the Minister of Health. The legislation amendments were made regarding narcotics dispensing to the patients to facilitate prescription. The service of palliation is mainly provided at the KHCC and some private hospices. Recently home palliative care services have been made available with a trained team making home visits by qualified personnel [28].

6.10   Research and Education

The medical education and teaching programs in Jordan are considered the strongest in the region. Jordan had six advanced medical schools with a strong presence in the region. Some of these universities have postgraduate oncology programs, like master's and PhD degrees not for the physicians only but the nurses as well [29]. In addition, residency programs are available in almost all cancer-related specialties, including residency programs in radiation oncology and fellowship training programs in both pediatric and adult medical and surgical oncology, more recently in palliative care. In addition, many programs combined the training programs in radiology, cancer imaging, breast imaging, nuclear medicine, pathology, and anesthesia with those of many local hospitals or abroad. At KHCC, it introduces the opportunity for young pediatricians from Jordan and neighboring counties to specialize in pediatric hematology/oncology as this center is the first and only pediatric hematology/oncology training hub in Jordan [30, 31]. There are oncology fellowships to get the Jordanian board certificate.

Research is still limited due to many reasons, while the financial support and funds top the list of such obstacles. Many papers and descriptive types of research have been published in many peer-review magazines on the international levels. Many establishments of national and international collaborations programs in cancer research, of higher studies, at the University Science and Technology, and the University of Jordan as well as more studies and research and trials in collaboration with the King Hussein Cancer Center. Not to forget the activities and conferences managed by the Jordan Oncology Society, Jordanian Society of Pediatric Oncology, and the Jordan Cancer Society.

6.11 Cost-Effective Cancer Care

The new generation of treatments and available medications are quite expensive and are a huge burden to both the government and individuals. Increasing cancer prevalence rate, high new costly pharmaceuticals, physician's and facility's fees have all been added to the expenditure and therefore, it is raised in the cancer care issue. In Jordan, most of the cancer patients are treated at the expense of a third party, mainly the MOH or the royal court, which is a spot-on motive to have a very good and authentic cost-effective for such provided services to strengthen and improve as well as continue this benefit. However, most of the essential cancer drugs are available, and to some extent, the newly FDA-approved ones as well, but one of the biggest challenges in this country will be how to tackle the increasing cancer care cost, the increase in the utilization of expensive medications, radiation, chemo, etc. [32–35].

6.12 Challenges and Advantages

6.12.1 Medical Tourism in Jordan

Medical tourism in Jordan has seen an increase over the years, mainly due to the high level of services and the expertise provided by hospitals and the medical staff in the country. The International Medical Travel Journal (IMTJ) shows the increasing interest in medical tourism to Jordan and the healthcare provided in the country. Service quality, patient safety, levels of care, and experience to ensure that patient expectations are met and taken care of [22, 36].

Cancer treatment in Jordan is one of the main panels in the country, especially to the King Hussein Cancer Center "KHCC," one of the best comprehensive cancer centers in the region as well as many other clinics and specialized doctors in the private sector. Many patients seek services provided and the quality of the high standard and effective outcomes and results. Patients from the Gulf and Saudi Arabia, Yemen, Iraq, Syria, Libya, and many others are being treated in Jordan [26]. The high-quality standards in healthcare in Jordan vouched for by the numerous international and domestic accreditations that most hospitals in the country have earned. The healthcare facilities in Jordan ensure that visitors get only the best.

6.13 The Future of Cancer Care in Jordan

Over the past decade, cancer care in Jordan has witnessed a remarkable improvement through access to advanced diagnostics and therapeutic cancer care in the country, which focused on treatment, with less effort being employed on other elements of the cancer continuum. Cancer continues to be among the leading cause of morbidity, and mortality and the number of new cases are expected to rise, reaching levels that will challenge public and private healthcare systems and that may hinder access of patients to life-saving treatment.

Despite several initiatives, Jordan does not have a national cancer control plan, nor does organize cancer control, as promoted by international organizations such as the World Health Organization (WHO), International Agency for Research on Cancer (IARC), the Union for International Cancer Control (UICC), offers the best approach for healthcare systems to be more integrated, cost-effective, and efficient in preventing cancer. The cost of the recently introduced cancer drugs, sophisticated radiation therapy, and surgical techniques will create significant challenges for the current and future care providers. Scarcity in cancer care providers will be another challenge as Jordan experiences significant difficulties in attracting and retaining highly specialized Jordanian graduates.

This increase will constitute a challenging burden on healthcare systems in Jordan and many other neighboring countries. Planning is the key to managing the expected rise in the demand for cancer care, and this will require public health initiatives to guarantee access to quality cancer care [13, 16, 22, 23].

6.14 Conclusion

The healthcare system in Jordan is one of the best reputable and trustworthy prominent healthcare systems in the Middle East & North Africa (MENA) region, if not, it is globally well known. Wide-range oncology care is available in many public and private hospitals, healthcare facilities, and clinics. Twining with many western and well-known cancer and oncology facilities, patients and doctors have the advantage of such collaborations, in both directions.

Cancer treatment in Jordan is one of the main sites and country for the health tourism in the region and this can be reflected highly on the cost of the treatment to the visiting patients compared if they seek the services in the west or the USA, still delivering quality of high standard and effective results.

Jordan will be always open to all its Arab fellows, at the same time open for new and up-to-date innovations, cooperation, and collaboration with other scholars so the best available treatment can be presented to the patients.

Conflict of Interest Authors have no conflict of interest to declare.

References

1. Jorinfo_2019.pdf (dos.gov.jo)
2. Demographics of Jordan—Wikipedia.
3. Jordan Home (worldbank.org)
4. 05bd5575-f7e2-4943-8e66-2dd1510196cc.pdf (moh.gov.jo). https://wasel.moh.gov.jo/ Echobusv3.0/SystemAssets/05bd5575-f7e2-4943-8e66-2dd1510196cc.pdf.
5. Khader J, Al Mousa A, Al-Kayed S, Mahasneh H, Mubaidin R, Al Nassir N, Khatib S, Qasem A, Haddadin I, Elayan E, Al Khatib S. History and current state of radiation oncology services and practice in Jordan. https://www.ncbi.nlm.nih.gov/pmc/articles/PMC7328116/.
6. Narghile, water pipe smoking associated with earlier development of oral cancer. Asia Pac J Clin Oncol. 2014.
7. Kofahi MM, Haddad LG. Perceptions of lung cancer and smoking among college students in Jordan. 2005. sagepub.com
8. Water pipe smoking among bladder cancer patients: a cross sectional study of Lebanese and Jordanian Populations-HDJSC_6615832 1..8 (hindawi.com)
9. http://moh.gov.jo/Echobusv3.0/SystemAssets/aa28955c-cdef-4f8b-8b30-8f2f82ab3203.pdf
10. https://www.thelancet.com/journals/lanres/article/PIIS2213-2600(19)30077-3/fulltext
11. https://en.royanews.tv/news/21332/Highest-global-smoking-rates-in-Jordan-amid-concerns-of-big-tobacco-interference
12. https://www.liebertpub.com/doi/abs/10.1089/met.2007.0030
13. Cancer care for adolescents and young adults in Jordan. http://www.emro.who.int/emhj-volume-24-2018/volume-24-issue-7/cancer-care-for-adolescents-and-young-adults-in-jordan.html
14. Breast cancer screening and diagnosis guidelines. Amman 2008.
15. Dietary and lifestyle characteristics of colorectal cancer in Jordan: a case-control study. Asian Pac J Cancer Prev 2011;12
16. Health challenges and access to health care among Syrian refugees in Jordan. East Mediterr Health J 2018;24(7):680. Review.
17. The WHO site –Preventing cancer (who.int).
18. The Public Heath Law, passed in 2008/Three coffee shops closed for violating smoking ban I Jordan Times.
19. https://en.wikipedia.org/wiki/List_of_smoking_bans
20. https://www.almadenahnews.com/article/45784
21. http://www.jordanzad.com/print.php?id=15782
22. Cancer Care in Jordan. https://www.sciencedirect.com/science/article/pii/ S1658387615000230.
23. jordan_national_health_sector_strategy_2015-2019_pdf. https://extranet.who.int/country-planningcycles/sites/default/files/planning_cycle_repository/jordan/jordan_national_health_sector_strategy_2015-2019_.pdf.

24. The molecular genetics center at the Specialty Hospital is one of the best and most specialized academic molecular genetics labs in Jordan and in the Middle East.
25. Cancer survival: the CONCORD-2 study. https://www.thelancet.com/journals/lancet/article/PIIS0140-6736(15)61442-8/fulltext?rss%3Dyes=.
26. Jordan palliative care initiative: a WHO demonstration project. https://www.sciencedirect.com/science/article/pii/S0885392407001534
27. https://www.who.int/ncds/surveillance/steps/2007_Fact_sheet_Jordan.pdf?ua=1
28. https://www.khcc.jo/en/palliative-care
29. http://graduatedstudies.ju.edu.jo/Lists/OurPrograms/School_Master.aspx
30. Oncology medical training and practice. https://ascopubs.org/doi/full/10.1200/GO.20.00141
31. https://www.poemgroup.org/TrainingandActivities/TrainingSites/2/king-hussein-cancer-center
32. Fact Sheets.indd (moh.gov.jo) Jordan STEPS Survey 2019/. https://kaa.moh.gov.jo/Echobusv3.0/SystemAssets/256a175e-9de8-43a2-87a0-fc121aff76d4.pdf.
33. Cancer prevention and care. https://www.researchgate.net/publication/263712568_Cancer_Prevention_and_Care_a_National_Sample_from_Jordan
34. When is cancer care cost-effective? https://www.ncbi.nlm.nih.gov/pmc/articles/PMC2808348/
35. Importance of cost-effectiveness and value in cancer care and healthcare policy. J Surg Oncol. 2016 Sep;114(3):275–80.
36. Cancer Care Program (CCP) for Cancer Coverage | King Hussein Cancer Foundation (khcf.jo).
37. Jordan Population (2021) worldometers.info

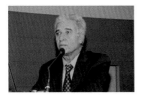

Sami Khatib is working as a senior Clinical Oncologist in Amman, Jordan. He graduated from Barcelona, Spain. He is the Secretary-General of the Arab Medical Association Against Cancer and the president of the Jordan Oncology Society. Khatib was deputy D.G. at King Hussein Cancer Center. He is a member of the regional and International Oncology Associations. He is the deputy Editor-in-Chief for The Pan Arab Journal of Oncology.

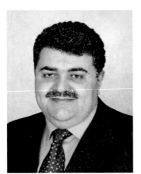

Omar Nimri is the Head of the Cancer Prevention Department/MOH, as well as the Director-PI, Jordan Cancer Registry. Nimri obtained his medical bachelor's degree from Pakistan and went on to obtain several higher degrees and diplomas, including Korean Acupuncture from Sri Lanka in 1991, Community medicine from Jordan in 2002, A two-year Comprehensive Postgraduate Training Program in Applied Epidemiology (FETP), Cancer Prevention and Control Diploma from the NIH; USA-2006. Cancer registration from IARC France in 2005/2007 and Cancer prevention and Etiology Diploma from the UM School of Public Health, University of Michigan, USA 2008. Master Public Health, Jordan University, 2017–2019.

Chapter 7
General Oncology Care in Kuwait

Ahmad Alhuraiji ⓘ**, Jinan Abdullah, Bader O. Almutairi, and Jasem Albarrak**

7.1 Kuwait Demographics

The State of Kuwait sits on the northeast corner of the Arabian Peninsula, sharing its borders with Saudi Arabia and Iraq. It is a part of West Asia. The total surface area of Kuwait is 17,818 km^2. Kuwait is a rapidly growing country; the current estimated population of 4.7 million has almost doubled over the last two decades [1]. Of those, one-third of the population is Kuwaiti nationals. Among Kuwaitis, there is a 1:1 ratio of male to female. However, in non-Kuwaitis, there is a 2.3:1 ratio of male to female. The median age among Kuwait's population is 29.3 years, and the country tends to have a younger population with fewer people above the age of 65 years (Fig. 7.1a, b) [2]. The life expectancy is 75.3 years.

Through a ministerial decree issued in 1984, Kuwait was divided into six health areas/regions, namely Capital, Hawalli, Ahmadi, Jahra, Farwania, and Al-Sabah. Each health region office supervises and manages at least one general hospital along with a few primary health centers and specialized clinics. The number of medical doctors increased from only 362 doctors in the country in 1962 to 3117 doctors in the governmental sector and 324 doctors in the private sector in 1998 and 7640 physicians in the governmental sector and 2149 physicians in the private sector in 2014 [3].

Kuwait has a petroleum-based economy; petroleum is the main export product of the country. The Kuwaiti dinar is the highest-valued unit of currency in the world with a high Gross Domestic Product (GDP) per capita as per a recent report from the World Bank [4], making it an attractive place for healthcare workers outside Kuwait.

A. Alhuraiji (✉)
Hematology Department, Kuwait Cancer Control Center, Kuwait, Kuwait
e-mail: aalhuraiji@moh.gov.kw

J. Abdullah · B. O. Almutairi · J. Albarrak
Medical Oncology Department, Kuwait Cancer Control Center, Kuwait, Kuwait
e-mail: jaalbarrak@moh.gov.kw

© The Author(s) 2022
H. O. Al-Shamsi et al. (eds.), *Cancer in the Arab World*,
https://doi.org/10.1007/978-981-16-7945-2_7

The first hospital for men was established in 1911, and the first hospital for women was established in 1919. In the 1950s, due to the increased oil revenues, free medical services were introduced to all Kuwaiti nationals. The expenditures on health ranked third in the national budget.

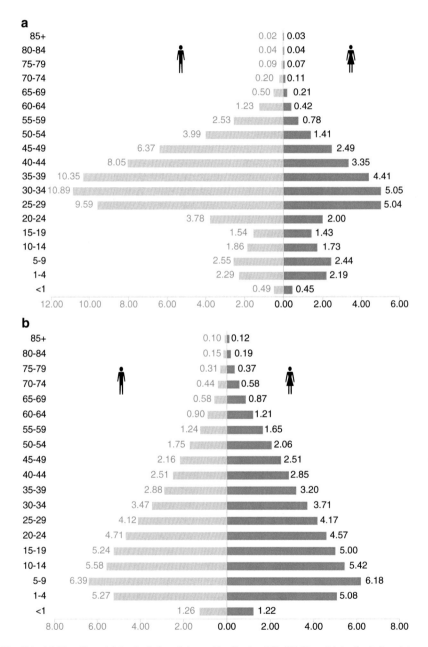

Fig. 7.1 (**a**) Non-Kuwaiti (male & female) age distribution [5]. (**b**) Kuwaiti (male & female) age distribution [5]

7.2   Cancer Statistics in Kuwait

Kuwait Cancer Control Center (KCCC) is the only cancer center in Kuwait, providing comprehensive care to oncology patients. Kuwait Cancer Registry (KCR) has, since 1971, systematically collected data of cancer cases occurring in Kuwait. It has a separate department at KCCC. Notification of cancer is compulsory through Ministerial decree 228/2014. The registry collects data from KCCC and other hospital notes, pathology reports and mortality reports from the health information system at the Ministry of Health (MOH). The cancer registry helps in defining the problem, monitoring the trends, prevention of cancer by identifying high-risk individuals, research, and education.

The cancer statistics have been stable over the last years, but there was a drop in 1990 that corresponds to the gulf war, which led to missed follow-up cases. Figure 7.2a, b shows the Age Standardized Incidence Rate (ASIR)/100,000 of females and males, respectively [5].

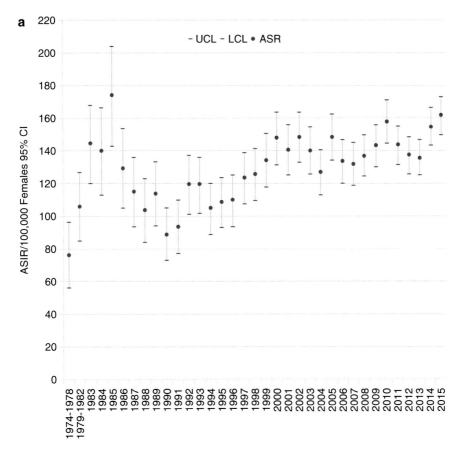

Fig. 7.2 (**a**) Age Standardized Incidence Rate (ASIR)/100,000 females [5]. (**b**) Age Standardized Incidence Rate (ASIR)/100,000 males [5]

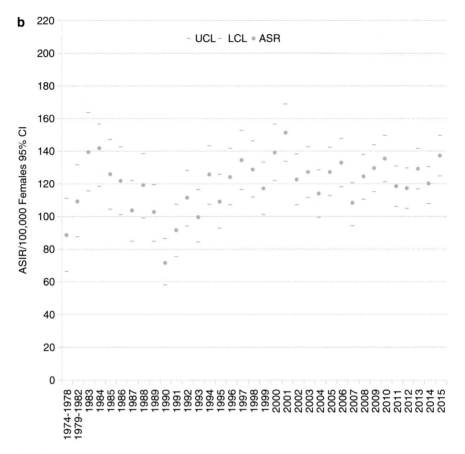

Fig. 7.2 (continued)

According to the most recent health statistics, cancer is recognized to be the second cause of death (21.7 per 100,000 population) in Kuwait, preceded only by cardiovascular diseases (58.6. per 100,000) [5]. There were 2700 new cases of cancer in Kuwait in 2015, of which 1319 cases occurred among Kuwaitis and 1381 among Non-Kuwaitis. The most common cancers among Kuwaiti and non-Kuwaiti males were colorectal followed by prostate cancers and among females were breast followed by thyroid cancer (Table 7.1).

Table 7.1 Top ten cancers among Kuwaiti population (2015) [5]

Males (N = 515)*			Females (N = 797)*		
Site	N (%)	ASIR**	Site	N (%)	ASIR**
Colorectum	72 (14.0)	20.2	Breast	325 (40.8)	66.6
Prostate	55 (10.7)	17.8	Thyroid	84 (10.5)	14.0
Lung	50 (9.7)	15.0	Colorectum	69 (8.7)	15.4
†NHL	39 (7.6)	8.9	Corpus uteri	54 (6.8)	12.2
Leukemia	39 (7.6)	7.4	NHL†	27 (3.4)	5.2
Pancreas	29 (5.6)	8.6	Leukemia	24 (3.0)	4.2
Bladder	25 (4.9)	7.3	Pancreas	23 (2.9)	5.1
Liver	24 (4.7)	6.8	Ovary	22 (2.8)	4.4
Kidney	21 (4.1)	5.5	Lung	18 (2.3)	3.7
Hodgkin's disease	21 (4.1)	3.1	Hodgkin's disease	17 (2.3)	2.7
Male (N = 678)			Females (N = 689)*		
Site	N (%)	ASIR**	Site	N (%)	ASIR**
Colorectum	90 (13.3)	10.5	Breast	286 (41.5)	50.0
Prostate	67 (9.9)	13.2	Thyroid	70 (10.3)	7.5
Leukemia	61 (9.0)	4.9	Colorectum	51 (7.4)	10.4
Bladder	51 (7.5)	7.4	Cervix uteri	31 (4.5)	2.9
Lung	48 (7.1)	5.4	Corpus uteri	30 (4.4)	6.2
NHL†	47 (6.9)	4.3	Ovary	26 (3.8)	4.7
Liver	33 (4.9)	3.2	Leukemia	22 (3.1)	4.4
Hodgkin's disease	30 (4.4)	2.1	NHL†	19 (2.8)	3.5
Thyroid	28 (4.1)	2.1	Lung	19 (2.8)	4.0
Brain and nervous system	22 (3.2)	1.6	Hodgkin's disease	17 (2.5)	2.2

*Number of all sites but non melanoma skin cancers (NMSC)
**ASIR = Age Standardized Incidence Rate/100,000
† = Non-Hodgkin lymphoma

The estimated cases per 100,000 population is 140–150 cases in Kuwait. Fig. 7.3a, b represent the situation in Kuwait in comparison to the international data and the Middle East and North Africa (MENA region) [5].

a

Esatimated cases per 100,000 population (ALL cancer sites except C44.)
all ages : both sexes

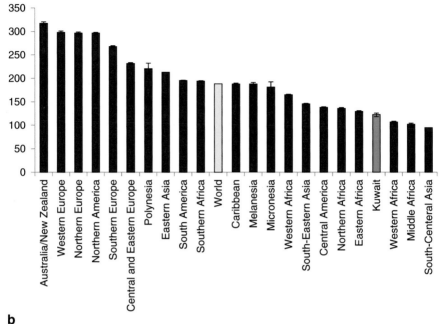

b

Esatimated cases per 100,000 population (ALL cancer sites except C44.)
all ages : both sexes

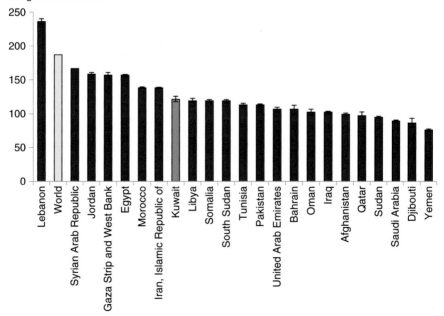

Fig. 7.3 (**a**) Age Standardized Incidence Rate (ASIR) in comparison to the international ASIR [5]. (**b**) Age Standardized Incidence Rate (ASIR) in comparison to the MENA region ASIR [5]

7.3 Cancer Risk Factors

The aim of this section is to describe the risk factors in Kuwait. It will thus be divided into two sections. First, we will state about ubiquitous cancer risk factors such as smoking and alcohol.

7.3.1 Part 1: Ubiquitous Risk Factors: Where Does Kuwait Stand?

Tobacco: According to Alzalabani [6], tobacco usage was as high as 40% in 2005 in Kuwait. In 2014, World Health Organization (WHO) data shows low figures of only 19% in 2014. It is not clear whether Hookah/shisha is included in Alzalabani et al's report. Either way, tobacco has been attributed to 16% of all cancer cases in the GCC countries, which includes Kuwait [6].

Alcohol: Alcohol is not a major cause of cancer in Kuwait. According to the WHO report 2014, almost 0.1% of the Kuwaiti population consumes alcohol. It is worth noting that drinking is stigmatized in Kuwait, and the actual figures may be higher than officially documented. As reported by WHO in 2018, the official recorded alcohol consumption in Kuwait in 2016 was almost zero. However, the alcohol-attributable fraction of cancer deaths is 10 per 100,000 people. Therefore, the official figures of alcohol consumption do not represent reality.

Infection: Vaccination against Hepatitis B virus (HBV) is mandatory in Kuwait for the prevention of HBV infection and ultimately Hepatocellular carcinoma (HCC). However, the HPV vaccine against cervical cancer is not obligatory in Kuwait as this disease is socially and ethically stigmatized. The second part of this section will go more into depth regarding risk factors for cervical cancer.

7.3.2 Part 2: Other Kuwait-Specific Risk Factors

Inactivity and Obesity: Obesity is common among the Kuwaiti population, and it seems to be a main reason for the higher incidence of cancer. The total number of motor vehicles in Kuwait has increased by 162% between 2005 and 2014 [7]. This has led to two things: a decrease in physical activity and an increase in air pollution. According to the World Health Organization report (WHO) 2014, 53% of the Kuwaiti population is considered inactive and 38% are obese [8]. This, along with the importation of the Western diet, can explain the rising cases of colorectal cancer. Elbasmi et al. have already shown similar results. In this study, a fivefold increase in colorectal cancer cases in Kuwait, between 2003 and 2007, was attributed to diet and lack of physical activity [9]. Decreased activity and obesity did not explain the rise in breast cancers. However, among nine retrospective registry data, only one showed an association between breast cancer and obesity, with an odds ratio of 2.29. Note that most included cases were premenopausal women who could have affected the results [10].

7.4   Cancer Screening Programs

Screening programs are evolving in Kuwait, and it is challenging to establish other screening programs for lung, prostate, and cervical cancers, which will reflect positively on preventing such serious illnesses.

In Kuwait, the public awareness of colorectal cancer and screening is higher than comparable countries [11], which can be attributed to the small community in Kuwait with early interchangeable knowledge and available access to information. The colorectal cancer screening program started in 2016, which adapted the recommendations of Northern American societies due to paucity of data and underutilization of the Kuwait Cancer Registry. Yet, the program helped in detecting early-stage cancers, according to a news report. However, the full impact of such screening programs is yet to be studied. On the other hand, The Kuwait National Mammography Screening Program (KNMSP), launched in 2014, provides annual screening mammograms for women between 40 and 69. In 2016, the KNMSP screened 4.2% of all Kuwaiti ladies eligible for screening, and the incidence of cancer was 1.2% of total screened ladies found to have breast cancer [12].

7.5   Cancer Prevention Programs

Prevention and early detection of cancer are still one of the most valuable tools in improving cancer outcomes. Nearly 30–50% of cancers are preventable and avoidable cancers [13], in addition to that, the predictions of a 75% increase in the global burden of newly diagnosed cancers and a 40% increase in the number of mortality related to cancer by year 2030 [14]. With such odds, early detection of cancer by well-implemented screening programs will play a major role in improving cancer care in the upcoming near future.

In Kuwait, the healthcare system provides a comprehensive vaccination program for all residents of Kuwait. It is mandatory to get vaccinated according to the MOH program, which includes the HBV vaccine, as mentioned earlier. There are some vaccines that are not mandatory, such as the Herpes Simplex Virus (HSV) vaccine, yet it is widely available in the private sector. It is understandable that the screening and prevention of cervical cancer by implementing a national screening and vaccination program will be a challenge in the coming years. Using social media with scientific advertisements will help the public to be convinced to participate actively in such programs.

Smoking is the leading preventable cause of cancer. According to The International Agency for Research on Cancer (IARC), smoking is linked to 20 cancer sites or subtypes. In the state of Kuwait, smoking is considered a serious health issue with around 25% prevalence among the young population in 2001, according to WHO, and it is expected to increase with the introduction of E-cigarettes and its popularity among the young population. Such a challenge was faced by multiple awareness campaigns from both the government and the civil society. On the same page, the Ministry of Health provides a free service for smokers who wish to quit smoking via smoking cessation clinics in MOH polyclinics throughout the country. The authorities believe stressing on such interventions by expanding the campaigns and enforcing laws to prevent smoking in public areas will help in fighting this hazardous habit.

7.6   Cancer Diagnosis

The state of Kuwait provides a high standard of healthcare to all residents of Kuwait. With easy access to seven general government hospitals that are equipped with state-of-the-art diagnostic facilities, not to mention more than the number of Sabah centers, specialized centers. Cancer diagnosis and treatment was and still one of the top priorities in Kuwait's Health system. Kuwait Cancer Control Center (KCCC) is one of the oldest specialized centers in the region. It was established in 1968, and since then, the center has been providing its services to Kuwait residents and nearby countries. With time, the center expanded to a multicenter compound that includes Sheikha Badria Alahmad Chemotherapy Center, Husain Makki Al Juma Center for Specialized Surgery, Faisal Sultan Center for Diagnosis and Radiation Therapy, Yacob Behbehani Center for Specialized Laboratories and Bone Marrow Transplantation and The Palliative Care Center. Since the establishment, it has the main center for treating all cancer patients in the state of Kuwait, along with one center for pediatric hematology and oncology patients (National Bank of Kuwait Specialized Hospital for Children).

In Kuwait, all the general hospitals are equipped with a diagnostic radiology department along with molecular imaging and nuclear medicine such as Positron Emission Tomography (PET) scans, which is also available in specialized centers like KCCC and Kuwait Center for Molecular Imaging (along with the chest hospital).

Moreover, all the general government hospitals have fully equipped laboratory services that conduct the needed investigations to help in diagnosing patients with access to reference laboratories such as Yacob Behbehani Center for Specialized Laboratories and Bone Marrow Transplantation, which is a part of KCCC. Since its opening in 2017, the center has played a crucial part in diagnosing and treating cancer by providing specialized laboratories for cytogenetics, Fluorescence in situ Hybridization (FISH), qualitative and quantitative Polymerase Chain Reaction (PCR) and more recently, Next Generation Sequencing (NGS) along with molecular testing. KCCC is now able to provide genetic testing and counseling clinics in parallel with Ghanima Ahmed Alghanim Center for Premature and genetic in the Alsabah health region, which provides genetic testing and counseling for non-oncological inherited diseases.

It is widely known that 'Interventional Radiology' plays an integral part in diagnosing oncological conditions. This service is available in all government hospitals under the umbrella of the Ministry of Health. The interventional radiology departments provide a wide range of diagnostic and therapeutic interventions, which help in diagnosing and treating oncological conditions and their complications.

With the rapidly progressing environment in the region, GCC countries have adapted long-term strategies to ensure the prosperity and development of their communities and countries. Kuwait launched its vision for 2030, which includes a massive expansion in the infrastructure of the healthcare system. This vision brought KCCC to an ambitious project intended to be the largest cancer center in the Middle East with more than 680 beds; dedicated to diagnosing and treating cancer in a state-of-the-art institute. For that purpose, this project will need well-trained staff. The Kuwait Institute for Medical Specialties (KIMS) established a 3-year fellowship program for medical oncology in 2014, where the fellow will be exposed and trained in the facilities of KCCC and the Ministry of Health. On the other hand, training abroad is one of the valuable opportunities for Kuwaiti physicians to gain experience and to explore the full spectrum of this rapidly growing medical subspecialty. The Kuwaiti fellows enrolled in multiple fellowship programs in Northern America, Europe, and nearby countries.

7.6.1 Specialized Laboratory Services

Fortunately, KCCC has access to in-house cytogenetic and molecular studies. The department can send for conventional cytogenetic, Fluorescence in Situ Hybridization (FISH) studies for hematological and solid tumors. The Next Generation Sequencing (NGS) tests use different panels for different disease entities. This helped in risk stratifying the cases in a more efficient way to deliver the best care to the patients. One of the advantages of having such services in-house is the rapid turnaround time for these tests, which most of the time is between 10 and 14 days. KCCC also has a flow cytometry machine which is used extensively in hematological malignancies using 8-color and 10-color machines.

7.7 Treatment

7.7.1 Medical Oncology

Sheikha Badriya Al Ahmad Al Jaber Al-Sabah Medical Oncology Center is a member of the Kuwait Cancer Control Center (KCCC), established in 2010. It accommodates the medical oncology department and its ancillary services. The medical oncology department contains 13 specialized medical oncologists and 19 registrars and senior registrars. Members function within tumor site-based treating units. Patient care provided includes but not limited to offering anti-cancer treatment, genetic counseling, survivorship programs and supportive care.

Medical oncology practice guidelines are updated frequently to incorporate high-quality evidence and advancements in patient care. Anti-cancer medical treatments offered include cytotoxic chemotherapy, hormonal therapy, targeted therapy, and immunotherapy. Treatment protocols are updated and accessed through the KCCC website: https://kuwaitcancercenter.net/. KCCC has established a Compassionate Drug Access Program through the affiliation and cooperation with charities and non-profit organizations. The Compassionate Drug Access Program aims to alleviate the financial concerns for few expatriate patients and present state-of-the-art cancer treatment options. Hundreds of patients enjoy the benefits of this program annually and it helps in organizing the efforts among all charities to maximize access to expensive modern cancer treatments.

7.7.1.1 Malignant Hematology and Bone Marrow Transplantation (BMT)

At KCCC, the department of hematology and stem cell transplantation has a very active service with dedicated units such as leukemia/myeloma, lymphoma, and Bone Marrow Transplant (BMT). It has an inpatient service of 40–50 beds along with 8-beds for BMT. The department has different academic activities on a weekly or monthly basis as well as other multidisciplinary meetings with other specialties. The academic activities and inpatient discussion rounds are being held every Tuesday morning. There are multiple daily clinics held at AM and PM.

BMT programs initiated in 2001, starting with autologous Stem Cell Transplantation (SCT) till 2011. More than 200 patients have had SCT at KCCC so far. The issue of donor availability and drug shortage are the two main obstacles for expanding the Bone Marrow Transplantation program [15].

7.7.2 Radiation Therapy

The radiotherapy department in KCCC has an intensity-modulated radiotherapy and brachytherapy. It encompasses an inpatient and an outpatient service. The department is divided into subunits according to the cancer type: head and neck, cervical and genito-urinary cancers, sarcomas, thoracic and brain, breast, and gastrointestinal (GIT). Gamma-knife surgery is present in Ibn Sina hospital, which is the center of excellence for neurology and neurosurgery in Kuwait. The radiotherapy department works with the medical and surgical department in decision-making. The three departments attend the tumor board review and multidisciplinary meetings together for decision-making.

7.7.3 Surgery

KCCC has the only dedicated surgical oncology department in the country. In addition, dedicated surgical units provide treatment at secondary hospitals as well. Subspecialty oncology units for Colorectal and Hepatobiliary cancer exist currently in Al-Amiri, Mubarak, and Jaber Hospitals. Surgeons from different sites collaborate in a multidisciplinary setting to execute their plans. Skillful Kuwaiti surgeons constitute most of the staff with extensive experience in minimally invasive procedures, breast oncoplastic procedures and multivisceral resections. Robotic surgery is available at two sites and is primarily utilized for urological malignancies. More recently, robotic surgery has been introduced for gastrointestinal cancer. A peritoneal carcinomatosis treatment program combined with Hyperthermic Intraperitoneal Chemotherapy (HIPEC) has started at Al-Amiri hospital.

7.7.4 Pediatric Oncology

Pediatric hematology/oncology unit was first established in 1976 within the department of pediatric in Alsabah hospital that was expanded in 1986 to a 24-bed capacity in the ward- dedicated only to treat inpatient and outpatient children with hematological and oncological disorders. In April 2000, the Kuwait's Ministry of Health established a dedicated specialized pediatric hematology/oncology center (NBK Children's hospital) in Sabah medical district, where all children up to the age of 16 years are referred from all over the country.

The center has a 24-hour emergency room, inpatient wards for children with benign and malignant hematological disorders as well as oncology care, outpatient clinic and a day care unit. The service for Stem Cell Transplantation was recently introduced in Kuwait for children, and the first Stem Cell Transplant was done for a child with neuroblastoma in Oct 2020.

7.7.5 Survivorship Track

Survivorship programs have been established for breast and colon cancer. There are dedicated clinics and staff that conduct the survivorship programs according to specific guidelines for active surveillance and management of post-treatment sequelae. Patients are screened for recurrences, counseled for secondary prevention, and assessed for their physical and mental well-being. Patients' material for the survivorship programs are published on the KCCC website: https://kuwaitcancercenter.net/.

7.7.6 Palliative Care Track

The Palliative Care Center is closely affiliated with KCCC. Their services span from symptom management to end of life care in a multidisciplinary setting. Patients with advanced cancers are strongly advised to receive joint care by oncologists and palliative care specialists at the beginning of their cancer journey.

Sheikha Badriya Al Ahmad Al Jaber Al-Sabah Medical Oncology Center has been accredited and designated center of integrated oncology and palliative care by the European Society of Medical Oncology since 2015.

7.8   Research and Education

Scientific and clinical research is a cornerstone in any healthcare system, and it plays a catalytic role in improving medical practice based on the best available evidence. In the case of Kuwait and cancer research, there is a long history of such new healthcare systems, with early publications back to the 70s, being considered the earliest publications in the region. Since then, clinicians and researchers in Kuwait have published hundreds of medical publications in clinical and preclinical fields. On the other hand, Kuwait has well-established scientific and academic institutes, i.e., Kuwait University (KU), Kuwait Foundation for the Advancement of Sciences (KFAS) and Kuwait Institute of Scientific Research (KISR), which were established in the late 1960s. Such institutes and scientific entities help in creating a progressive environment for researchers to help them in their scientific quest.

The Kuwait cancer registry started with the establishment of the Kuwait cancer center and it gave valuable information about the dynamics of cancer over more than 40 years. More recently, in September 2019, a malignant hematology registry was established to capture cases of leukemia, lymphoma, and myeloma prospectively with dedicated teams to different disease entities with the aim to look at our statistics, demographic distribution, assess our quality of care and assess our outcomes in different disease areas. We believe the utilization of such historical data will help us in understanding the changes in disease's nature and it might help in creating prediction models, which will be a useful tool for clinicians and researchers.

7.9   Challenges and Advantages

Recognizing the impact of cancer on public health and on society starts with addressing the problem and formulating a comprehensive future plan highlighting the current and upcoming challenges. According to WHO reports, cancer is one of the leading causes of death in people below the age of 70 worldwide [16]. In Kuwait, for example, breast cancer alone was the seventh cause of death in 2019, followed by colon cancer as the 10th most common cause [16]. With a rising concern regarding the increase in the incidence of particular cancers among young age populations, such as colon cancer [17], solidifies early detection and screening argument by expanding the national screening programs. On the other hand, the importance of cancer research in both clinical and preclinical phases is more crucial than ever before, and the investment in improving the research infrastructure should have a high priority. Nevertheless, constant updates and improvements in the established system, particularly in diagnostics and therapeutics aspects, are still of high importance and should not be overlooked as we expect an increase in demand for such interventions. One of the challenges we face in Kuwait is the paucity of practicing oncologists, hem-oncologists, Radiation oncologists and researchers, which will create a burden in the near future. Such rarity can be overcome by improving the established postgraduate training programs and by creating attractive chances for cancer researchers.

7.10   The Future of Cancer Care in Kuwait

The field of oncology is rapidly evolving across all the areas of diagnostic, therapeutic, and prognostic factors; furthermore, people are aging, which results in higher incidence and prevalence of cancer. Primarily, expanding the infrastructure through building a new cancer center with 618 beds capacity. Moreover, to increase the number of healthcare professionals at KCCC (physicians, nurses, technicians, and other important ancillary services). Lastly, building home health programs to facilitate patient care and treatment. One of the most important steps the country is facing is to move to a paperless work environment and have electronic medical records to optimize research, registries and capturing our data. Research is one of the core services that allow us to know our performance and improve the quality of care; this needs to be done in collaboration with Kuwait University, KFAS or KSIR.

7.11   Conclusion

Cancer care in Kuwait was established more than 50 years ago. It has been rapidly evolving with more advanced technology in the era of personalized medicine. Both infrastructure and healthcare professionals are increasing to keep up with these advances.

Contribution   AA, JA, BA and JA wrote and reviewed the manuscript.

Conflict of Interest   Authors have no conflict of interest to declare.

References

1. https://www.paci.gov.kw/stat/. Accessed on 10 Oct 2020.
2. http://stat.paci.gov.kw/englishreports/. Accessed on 10 Oct 2020.
3. Annual report of Kuwait Cancer Report, 2012.
4. https://data.worldbank.org/country/kuwait. Accessed on 28 Oct 2020.
5. Ministry of Health Report, Kuwait 2015.
6. Al-Zalabani AH. Cancer incidence attributable to tobacco smoking in GCC countries in 2018. Tob Induc Dis. 2020;18(18) https://doi.org/10.18332/tid/118722.
7. Al-Mutairi A, Smallbone A, Al-Salem SM, Roskilly AP. The first carbon atlas of the state of Kuwait. Energy. 2017;133:317–26.
8. https://www.who.int/cancer/country-profiles/kwt_en.pdf?ua=1. Accessed on 2 Nov 2020.

9. Elbasmi A, Al-Asfour A, Al-Nesf Y, Al-Awadi A. Cancer in Kuwait: magnitude of the problem. Gulf J Oncolog. 2010;8:7–14.
10. Lara Theresa Annette Tanner KLC. Correlation between breast cancer and lifestyle within the Gulf Cooperation Council countries: a systematic review. World J Clin Oncol. 2020;11(4):217–42.
11. Raed Saeed Saeed YYB, Alkhalifah KH, Ali LM. Knowledge and awareness of colorectal cancer among general public of Kuwait. Asian Pac J Cancer Prev. 2018;19(9):2455–60.
12. Victoria L, Mango HA-K, David Dershaw D, Ashkanani MH, Pennisi B, Turner P, Thornton C, Morris EA. Initiating a National Mammographic Screening Program: the Kuwait experience training with a US Cancer Center. J Am Coll Radiol. 2019;16(2):202–7.
13. https://www.who.int/cancer/prevention/en/. Accessed 28 Oct 2020.
14. Cancer epidemiology and prevention, Edition Chapter 8.
15. Al SH, Shemmari RA. Kuwait bone marrow transplantation activities. Hematol Oncol Stem Cell Ther. 2017;10(4):308–10.
16. World Health Organization (WHO). Global Health Estimates 2020: deaths by cause A, sex, by country and by region, 2000–2019. WHO; 2020. Accessed 11 Dec 2020. https://www.who.int/data/gho/data/themes/mortality-and-global-health-estimates/ghe-leading-causes-of-death.
17. Abualkhair WH, Zhou M, Ahnen D, Yu Q, Wu XC, Karlitz JJ. Trends in incidence of early-onset colorectal cancer in the United States among those approaching screening age. JAMA Netw Open. 2020;3(1):e1920407.

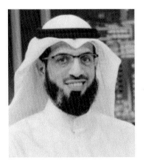

Ahmad Alhuraiji is a Hemato-Oncology consultant working in the department of hematology at the Kuwait Cancer Control Center. Dr. Alhuraiji has graduated from the Royal College of Surgeons in Ireland and is board certified in internal medicine and hematology from King Faisal Specialist hospital and research center in Riyadh, Saudi Arabia. He has been at the MD Anderson Cancer Center where he did a leukemia fellowship. He is a member of the Kuwait national amyloidosis program. He ranked no. 1 at the Saudi hematology fellowship program in 2015 and has the best abstract at the Pan Arab Hematology Congress 2017.

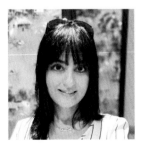

Jinan Abdullah is MBBS in medicine and surgery, Kuwait University. Diplôme d'études Supérieures d'oncologie médicale, université Sorbonne, Paris, France. She chose medical oncology because more work is needed to provide adequate treatment for this highly morbid and mortal disease. She believes that the Gulf needs its own research and guidelines as the population profile is different than that in the west. She is a strong supporter of euthanasia.

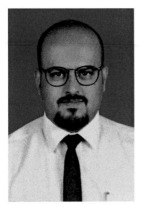

Bader O. Almutairi graduated from Jordan University of Science and Technology. He worked in the internal medicine department in Farwaniya hospital and joined the Kuwaiti board in internal medicine. He graduated in 2019. Currently, he is working in the Kuwait cancer control center as a clinical fellow in a medical oncology fellowship.

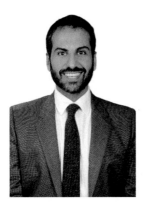

Jasem Albarrak is a consultant in internal medicine and medical oncology along with gastrointestinal oncology. Albarrak is the Deputy Director of the Kuwait Cancer Control Center. He is also the Chairman of the Department of Medical Oncology-Kuwait Cancer Control Center (2016–2021).

Chapter 8
General Oncology Care in Lebanon

Razan Mohty and Arafat Tfayli

8.1 Lebanon Demography

Lebanon is relatively a small country located on the eastern coast of the Mediterranean Sea. Its surface area is around 10.452 km² [1]. Lebanon was established in September 1920. The country is divided into governorates (Mohafazat), and each governorate is divided into districts (Caza) except Beirut and Akkar [1]. The eight governorates are Akkar, North Lebanon, Baalbek-Hermel, Beqaa, Mount Lebanon, Beirut, Nabatiyeh, and South Lebanon. These governorates are divided into 25 districts. The total Lebanese population in 2019 was around 4,546,618 people, excluding foreign residents and refugees. Among the Lebanese residents, 24.6% (1,118,468 people) are aged less than 15 years, 65.7% (2,987,128 people) are aged between 15 and 65 years, and 9.7% (441,022 people) are aged more than 65 years. 50.6% of the Lebanese population are females and 49.4% are males (Fig. 8.1) [2]. The life expectancy in Lebanon at birth is 79 years [3].

8.2 Cancer Statistics in Lebanon

The National Cancer Registry in Lebanon is managed by the ministry of public health (MOPH) and started in 2002. The overall incidence of cancer in Lebanon in 2020 is 253.5/100,000 in males and 262.2/100,000 in females [5, 6]. The number of new cases in 2020 is 11,589 with the most common cancers being Breast cancer 16.9%, Lung cancer 12.1%, Prostate cancer 8.9%, Colorectal cancer 7.8%, and

R. Mohty · A. Tfayli (✉)
Division of Hematology/Oncology, Department of Internal Medicine, American University of Beirut Medical Center, Beirut, Lebanon
e-mail: at35@aub.edu.lb

© The Author(s) 2022

H. O. Al-Shamsi et al. (eds.), *Cancer in the Arab World*,
https://doi.org/10.1007/978-981-16-7945-2_8

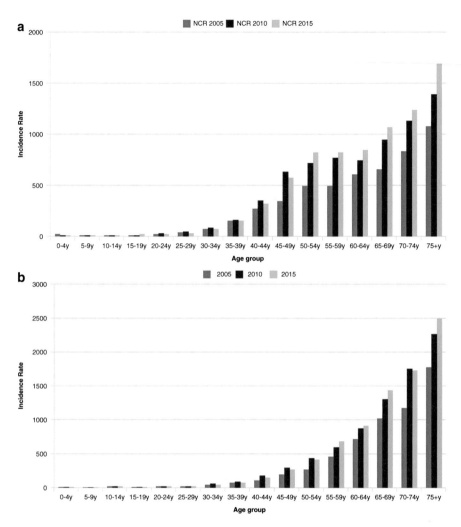

Fig. 8.1 Cancer Age-Specific Incidence Rate (100,000), Lebanon, 2005, 2010, 2015, (**a**) Females, (**b**) Males (Source: Republic of Lebanon—Ministry of Public Health—National Cancer Registry 2015) [4]

Bladder cancer 5.4%. The number of cancer deaths in 2020 is around 6438 [7, 8]. In 2016, cancer distribution according to age was as follows: 2.9% in patients age < 15, 39.1% in patients aged between 20 and 65 years, 46.8% in patients aged 65 years or older, and 11.3% in patients had missing age [9]. In 2019, cancer mortality represented 18.92% of hospital mortality in Lebanon. Hospital cancer deaths are distributed as follow lung cancer in 23.3% of the cases, breast 10.3%, colon 7%, pancreas 7%, leukemia 5.6%, liver and biliary ducts 5.2%, cancer of unknown primary 4.6%, bladder cancer 4.1%, neoplasm of the brain 3.9%, and prostate cancer 3.8% (Table 8.1) [2].

Table 8.1 Percentage (% of total) by primary site and age group (Source: Republic of Lebanon—Ministry of Public Health—National Cancer Registry 2016) [4]

Primary site	All ages	Age group 0–4y	5–9y	10–14y	15–19y	20–24y	25–29y	30–34y	35–39y	40–44y	45–49y	50–54y	55–59y	60–64y	65–69y	70–74y	75+y	Unsp.	ICD (10th)
Lip	0.0	0.0	0.0	0.0	0.0	0.0	0.0	0.0	0.0	0.0	0.0	0.0	0.0	0.0	0.0	0.0	0.0	0.0	C00
Tongue	0.2	0.0	0.0	0.0	0.0	0.0	0.0	0.0	0.0	0.0	0.0	0.0	0.0	0.0	0.0	0.0	0.1	0.0	C01–C02
Mouth	0.2	0.0	0.0	0.0	0.0	0.0	0.0	0.0	0.0	0.0	0.0	0.0	0.0	0.0	0.0	0.0	0.0	0.0	C03–C06
Salivary glands	0.2	0.0	0.0	0.0	0.0	0.0	0.0	0.0	0.0	0.0	0.0	0.0	0.0	0.0	0.0	0.0	0.0	0.0	C07–C08
Tonsil	0.0	0.0	0.0	0.0	0.0	0.0	0.0	0.0	0.0	0.0	0.0	0.0	0.0	0.0	0.0	0.0	0.0	0.0	C09
Other oropharynx	0.0	0.0	0.0	0.0	0.0	0.0	0.0	0.0	0.0	0.0	0.0	0.0	0.0	0.0	0.0	0.0	0.0	0.0	C10
Nasopharynx	0.1	0.0	0.0	0.0	0.0	0.0	0.0	0.0	0.0	0.0	0.0	0.0	0.0	0.0	0.0	0.0	0.0	0.0	C11
Hypopharynx	0.0	0.0	0.0	0.0	0.0	0.0	0.0	0.0	0.0	0.0	0.0	0.0	0.0	0.0	0.0	0.0	0.0	0.0	C12–C13
Pharynx unsp.	0.0	0.0	0.0	0.0	0.0	0.0	0.0	0.0	0.0	0.0	0.0	0.0	0.0	0.0	0.0	0.0	0.0	0.0	C14
Oesophagus	0.3	0.0	0.0	0.0	0.0	0.0	0.0	0.0	0.0	0.0	0.0	0.0	0.0	0.0	0.0	0.1	0.1	0.0	C15
Stomach	2.0	0.0	0.0	0.0	0.0	0.0	0.0	0.0	0.1	0.1	0.2	0.2	0.2	0.2	0.2	0.2	0.3	0.2	C16
Small intestine	0.2	0.0	0.0	0.0	0.0	0.0	0.0	0.0	0.0	0.0	0.0	0.0	0.0	0.0	0.0	0.1	0.1	0.0	C17
Colon	6.0	0.0	0.0	0.0	0.0	0.0	0.0	0.1	0.1	0.2	0.3	0.5	0.5	0.5	0.5	0.6	1.5	1.1	C18
Rectum	1.7	0.0	0.0	0.0	0.0	0.0	0.0	0.0	0.0	0.1	0.1	0.2	0.2	0.3	0.1	0.2	0.1	0.3	C19–C20
Anus	0.2	0.0	0.0	0.0	0.0	0.0	0.0	0.0	0.0	0.0	0.0	0.0	0.0	0.0	0.0	0.0	0.1	0.0	C21
Liver	0.9	0.0	0.0	0.0	0.0	0.0	0.0	0.0	0.0	0.0	0.0	0.0	0.1	0.2	0.1	0.1	0.3	0.1	C22
Gallbladder etc.	0.6	0.0	0.0	0.0	0.0	0.0	0.0	0.0	0.0	0.0	0.0	0.1	0.1	0.1	0.0	0.1	0.1	0.1	C23–C24
Pancreas	1.5	0.0	0.0	0.0	0.0	0.0	0.0	0.0	0.0	0.0	0.1	0.0	0.2	0.2	0.3	0.2	0.3	0.2	C25
Nose & sinuses & etc.	0.1	0.0	0.0	0.0	0.0	0.0	0.0	0.0	0.0	0.0	0.0	0.0	0.0	0.0	0.0	0.0	0.0	0.0	C30–C31

continued

Table 8.1 (Continued)

Primary site	All ages	0–4y	5–9y	10–14y	15–19y	20–24y	25–29y	30–34y	35–39y	40–44y	45–49y	50–54y	55–59y	60–64y	65–69y	70–74y	75+y	Unsp.	ICD (10th)
Larynx	0.6	0.0	0.0	0.0	0.0	0.0	0.0	0.0	0.0	0.0	0.1	0.0	0.1	0.1	0.1	0.1	0.0	0.1	C32
Trachea bronchus & lung	5.9	0.0	0.0	0.0	0.0	0.0	0.0	0.0	0.0	0.1	0.4	0.6	0.8	0.9	0.8	0.7	0.9	0.7	C33–C34
Other thoracic organs	0.3	0.0	0.0	0.0	0.0	0.0	0.0	0.0	0.0	0.0	0.1	0.0	0.0	0.0	0.0	0.0	0.0	0.0	C37–C38
Bone	0.5	0.0	0.0	0.1	0.1	0.0	0.0	0.0	0.0	0.0	0.0	0.0	0.0	0.0	0.0	0.0	0.0	0.0	C40–C41
Melanoma of skin	0.6	0.0	0.0	0.0	0.0	0.0	0.0	0.0	0.0	0.0	0.0	0.1	0.0	0.0	0.1	0.1	0.1	0.1	C43
Other skin	5.4	0.0	0.0	0.0	0.0	0.0	0.0	0.1	0.0	0.1	0.1	0.4	0.3	0.4	0.4	0.5	1.7	1.2	C44[a]
Mesothelioma	0.1	0.0	0.0	0.0	0.0	0.0	0.0	0.0	0.0	0.0	0.0	0.0	0.0	0.0	0.0	0.0	0.2	0.2	C45
Kaposi sarcoma	0.0	0.0	0.0	0.0	0.0	0.0	0.0	0.0	0.0	0.0	0.0	0.0	0.0	0.0	0.0	0.0	0.0	0.0	C46
Connective & soft tissue	0.8	0.0	0.0	0.0	0.0	0.0	0.0	0.0	0.0	0.1	0.0	0.1	0.1	0.1	0.1	0.1	0.1	0.1	C47; C49
Breast	36.2	0.0	0.0	0.0	0.0	0.1	0.4	1.0	1.8	3.4	4.1	4.9	4.5	3.6	2.9	2.1	2.9	4.3	C50
Vulva	0.7	0.0	0.0	0.0	0.0	0.0	0.0	0.0	0.0	0.0	0.0	0.0	0.0	0.1	0.1	0.1	0.2	0.2	C51
Vagina	0.1	0.0	0.0	0.0	0.0	0.0	0.0	0.0	0.0	0.0	0.0	0.0	0.0	0.0	0.0	0.0	0.0	0.0	C52
Cervix uteri	1.7	0.0	0.0	0.0	0.0	0.0	0.0	0.0	0.1	0.2	0.3	0.2	0.2	0.1	0.1	0.1	0.1	0.4	C53
Corpus uteri	3.5	0.0	0.0	0.0	0.0	0.0	0.0	0.0	0.1	0.1	0.2	0.4	0.4	0.6	0.6	0.3	0.4	0.4	C54
Uterus unsp.	0.7	0.0	0.0	0.0	0.0	0.0	0.0	0.0	0.0	0.1	0.1	0.1	0.1	0.0	0.1	0.0	0.1	0.1	C55
Ovary	3.1	0.0	0.0	0.0	0.0	0.1	0.0	0.0	0.0	0.1	0.4	0.6	0.4	0.3	0.3	0.2	0.3	0.4	C56
Other female genital	0.4	0.0	0.0	0.0	0.0	0.0	0.0	0.0	0.0	0.0	0.4	0.0	0.0	0.1	0.1	0.0	0.0	0.1	C57
Placenta	0.0	0.0	0.0	0.0	0.0	0.0	0.0	0.0	0.0	0.0	0.0	0.0	0.0	0.0	0.0	0.0	0.0	0.0	C58
Kidney	1.1	0.0	0.0	0.0	0.0	0.0	0.0	0.0	0.0	0.0	0.0	0.1	0.2	0.2	0.1	0.1	0.2	0.1	C64
Renal pelvis	0.0	0.0	0.0	0.0	0.0	0.0	0.0	0.0	0.0	0.0	0.0	0.0	0.0	0.0	0.0	0.0	0.0	0.0	C65
Ureter	0.1	0.0	0.0	0.0	0.0	0.0	0.0	0.0	0.0	0.0	0.0	0.0	0.0	0.0	0.1	0.0	0.0	0.1	C66

Primary site	All ages	Age group																Unsp.	ICD (10th)
		0–4y	5–9y	10–14y	15–19y	20–24y	25–29y	30–34y	35–39y	40–44y	45–49y	50–54y	55–59y	60–64y	65–69y	70–74y	75+y		
Bladder	2.2	0.0	0.0	0.0	0.0	0.0	0.0	0.0	0.0	0.0	0.1	0.1	0.2	0.4	0.3	0.3	0.4	0.4	C67
Other urinary organs	0.0	0.0	0.0	0.0	0.0	0.0	0.0	0.0	0.0	0.0	0.0	0.0	0.0	0.0	0.0	0.0	0.0	0.0	C68
Eye	0.1	0.0	0.0	0.0	0.0	0.0	0.0	0.0	0.0	0.0	0.0	0.0	0.0	0.0	0.0	0.0	0.0	0.0	C69
Brain & nervous system	1.4	0.1	0.0	0.0	0.0	0.0	0.1	0.1	0.1	0.1	0.1	0.2	0.1	0.1	0.1	0.1	0.1	0.1	C70–C72
Thyroid	4.2	0.0	0.0	0.0	0.0	0.1	0.2	0.4	0.5	0.5	0.5	0.3	0.3	0.3	0.2	0.1	0.2	0.7	C73
Adrenal gland	0.1	0.0	0.0	0.0	0.0	0.0	0.0	0.0	0.0	0.0	0.0	0.0	0.0	0.0	0.0	0.0	0.0	0.0	C74
Other endocrine	0.0	0.0	0.0	0.0	0.0	0.0	0.0	0.0	0.0	0.0	0.0	0.0	0.0	0.0	0.0	0.0	0.0	0.0	C75
Hodgkin disease	1.6	0.0	0.0	0.1	0.2	0.2	0.3	0.2	0.1	0.1	0.1	0.0	0.1	0.1	0.0	0.0	0.1	0.1	C81
Non-Hodgkin lymphoma	4.2	0.0	0.0	0.0	0.1	0.1	0.1	0.1	0.2	0.1	0.4	0.4	0.4	0.5	0.4	0.3	0.6	0.3	C82–C85; C96
Immuno-proliferative dis.	0.0	0.0	0.0	0.0	0.0	0.0	0.0	0.0	0.0	0.0	0.0	0.0	0.0	0.0	0.0	0.0	0.0	0.0	C88
Multiple myeloma	1.3	0.0	0.0	0.0	0.0	0.0	0.0	0.0	0.0	0.0	0.1	0.1	0.2	0.2	0.1	0.2	0.3	0.0	C90
Lymphoid leukemia	1.5	0.2	0.1	0.0	0.0	0.0	0.0	0.0	0.0	0.0	0.0	0.0	0.1	0.1	0.1	0.1	0.4	0.0	C91
Myeloid leukemia	1.1	0.0	0.0	0.0	0.0	0.0	0.0	0.0	0.0	0.1	0.1	0.1	0.1	0.1	0.1	0.1	0.2	0.0	C92–C94
Leukemia unsp.	0.3	0.0	0.0	0.0	0.0	0.0	0.0	0.0	0.0	0.0	0.0	0.0	0.0	0.0	0.0	0.0	0.0	0.0	C95
Other & Unspecified	4.1	0.1	0.0	0.0	0.0	0.1	0.0	0.1	0.1	0.1	0.2	0.3	0.4	0.4	0.4	0.4	0.6	0.8	OTHER
All sites, total	*100.0*	*0.6*	*0.3*	*0.5*	*0.8*	*0.9*	*1.4*	*2.7*	*3.6*	*5.9*	*8.3*	*10.7*	*10.7*	*10.6*	*9.2*	*7.8*	*13.2*	*12.8*	*All*
All sites but C44	*94.6*	*0.6*	*0.3*	*0.5*	*0.8*	*0.9*	*1.4*	*2.6*	*3.6*	*5.8*	*8.1*	*10.3*	*10.4*	*10.1*	*8.8*	*7.3*	*11.5*	*11.6*	*Not C44*

aC44 refers to non melanoma skin cancer

8.3 Healthcare System in Lebanon

Lebanon has one of the most developed healthcare systems in the Middle East and North Africa (MENA) region through excellent hospital infrastructure, availability of novel equipment, and world-renowned physicians and healthcare professionals. The 2018 Health Care Access and Quality ranked Lebanon in the 33rd rank worldwide being the first in the MENA area [10]. Most of the university hospitals in Lebanon require healthcare professionals to do advanced training in most developed countries. This prerequisite is a source of diversity and excellence in patient care and allows collaboration with worldwide peers in the fields. Despite all difficulties, economic and political instability, the healthcare system continues to grow and improve showing remarkable resilience. According to the World Health Organization (WHO) estimates, Lebanon spent 10.7% of its Gross Domestic Products (GDP) on health in 2000 dropping to 6.4% in 2018 through a successful targeted strategy mainly in the field of investment in technology [10, 11].

The Lebanese healthcare system is based on a collaboration between the public and private sectors. In 2019, the numbers of private and public hospitals in Lebanon were 118 and 28, respectively. Furthermore, the Lebanese MOPH established an accreditation system to assure the best quality of care through strict rules, regulations, and continuous updates of standards [10].

In 2014, the MOPH founded Universal Health Coverage as part of the Lebanese National Health Strategy. This universal coverage is established by filling the gaps in cost coverage. In fact, almost half of the Lebanese population is covered by the National Social Security Fund (NSSF) which is an autonomous public organization established in 1963 to provide health coverage to most of the Lebanese residents working in the private sector [12]. Furthermore, Lebanese are covered by other governmental organizations including the army, civil servants cooperative, internal security forces, general security forces, state security forces, mutual funds, or private insurances. The MOPH serves the rest of the Lebanese population non-adherent to any of the listed organizations. This strategy made treatment accessible to almost all Lebanese patients [13].

8.4 Oncology Care in Lebanon

Cancer incidence has been steadily increasing in Lebanon challenging the healthcare system. The MOPH established the national cancer database in 2002. The most recent estimate of cancer cases in 2020 is around 11,589 new cases compared to 7200 new cases in 2004 [8]. Cancer care is provided mainly in university hospitals including the Naef Basil Cancer Institute at the American University of Beirut Medical Center (AUBMC) established in 1995, Hotel Dieu de France, the Lebanese American University Medical Center Rizk Hospital, Mount Lebanon Hospital, Clemenceau Medical Center, and other cancer centers. Outside university hospitals, medical oncology services are also provided in peripheral hospitals and private clinics. Since 1999, the MOPH has provided free provision of cancer drugs to cancer patients who do not have any other financial coverage accounting for around half of the Lebanese population. This major step in cancer care provided equity in healthcare access to all Lebanese cancer patients. In a report by the MOPH, the average cost of cancer care increased steadily between 2008 and 2013 reaching $52 million in 2016. The average drug cost by patient was around $8400 in 2016. This increase was insignificantly affected by the MOPH strategy of providing access to novel immunotherapy and targeted therapy [14].

8.5   Cancer Risk Factors

In 2017, globally, around 30–50% of cancer can be prevented by modifying or avoiding risk factors including smoking, obesity, alcohol use, unsafe sex practice, infections like hepatitis B (HBV), hepatitis C (HCV), and Human Papilloma Virus (HPV), and exposure to ultraviolet light or ionizing radiation. Tobacco smoking is prevalent in Lebanon mainly in the young adult population. 38% of Lebanese people smoke cigarettes [15]. Alcohol consumption is also high among Lebanese, being 39.8%. 73.4% of the Lebanese people eat a non-healthy diet, meaning eating less than 5 servings of fruit and/or vegetables and 61% have a decreased physical activity and do not reach WHO recommendations on physical activity for health. In 2018, a total of 253 cases of HBV and a total of 103 HCV were reported [15, 16].

8.6   Cancer Screening Programs

Several cancer screening programs are established in Lebanon aiming for early detection of disease. Lebanon follows the international guidelines of cancer screening including the American Society of Clinical Oncology (ASCO) and the European Society of Medical Oncology (ESMO) guidelines for screening. The breast cancer screening program was established in 2002 by the Lebanese breast cancer foundation educating young women on early breast cancer detection through annual breast cancer awareness campaigns targeting all populations in addition to several other campaigns throughout the year [17]. The Lebanese breast cancer foundation also helps in establishing national screening guidelines for breast cancer prevention and recommends yearly mammography starting at the age of 40 [18]. In addition to breast cancer, colon cancer, and HBV, lung cancer screening is advocated in Lebanon using an annual low-dose CT scan of the chest but remains with very limited applicability. Women are encouraged to do cervical cancer by PAP smear screening through a national campaign for the prevention of cervical cancer [19].

8.7   Cancer Prevention Programs

The MOPH and Lebanese cancer societies established cancer prevention and control programs that play an important role in raising awareness through educating the general population about cancer prevention, screening, counseling, and cancer research [17]. The MOPH developed national guidelines in collaboration with the Lebanese order of physicians, the Lebanese society of medical oncology, and the Lebanese society of gastroenterology for the prevention of colon cancer through colonoscopy [20]. Furthermore, the HBV vaccination program for newborns started in 1998 aiming to screen and vaccinate high-risk populations for the prevention of hepatocellular carcinoma among other morbidities due to HBV. Moreover, the National Tobacco Control Program of the MOPH established a smoking cessation program to spread awareness about this disease. Also, the Tobacco Control Law (174/2011) was introduced in August 2011 for Tobacco Control and Regulation of Tobacco Products' Manufacturing, Packaging, and Advertising that forbid smoking in indoor, at workplaces, and in public transportation [21]. The HPV prevention vaccine is supported for the prevention of cervical cancer. However, a population-based vaccination program for cervical cancer is still not established [19].

8.8   Cancer Diagnosis

8.8.1   Imaging

According to the 2014 National Cancer Registry (NCR) data, 110 Computerized Tomography (CT) scans and 41 Magnetic Resonance Imaging (MRI) machines are available in Lebanon. The numbers of these diagnostic modalities are increasing and higher in 2020. PET-CT scan availability is high in Lebanon in relation to the population number having more than 2.2 machines per million people. Based on the latest 2020 national data from the Lebanese society of nuclear radiology and the MOPH, 16 physicians with nuclear medicine training are available, in addition to 50 technologists and 6 radiochemistry specialists for cyclotron units. Regarding the equipment, Lebanon has 24 Single Photon Emission Computed Tomography (SPECT), 3 SPECT-CT, and 18 Positron Emission Tomography (PET)-CT (unpublished data from the Lebanese society of nuclear medicine). In 2021, there are 2 cyclotrons, one mini and one big cyclotron with extra-large targets. These cyclotrons produce ^{18}F, ^{11}C, and ^{68}G as radioactive materials. In addition, ^{18}F-fluorodeoxyglucose (FDG), $^{18}FNaF$, ^{18}F-DOPA, ^{13}N ammonia, ^{11}C-methionine (MET), ^{68}Ga-DOTA-TOC, and ^{68}Ga-PSMA are all available radiotracer materials. Furthermore, advanced theragnostic agents including 131-iodine, lutecium DOTATE, lutecium PSMA, and actinium PSMA are also used. Additionally, radio-embolization of liver lesions using Yttrium is used for the treatment of primary or metastatic liver masses (unpublished data from the Lebanese society of nuclear medicine). Those procedures are only available in private university hospitals.

8.8.2 Laboratory

Advances in laboratory testing revolutionized the management of malignant disorders through better characterization and classification of the disease. According to the 2020 WHO cancer country profile, the 2005 number of medical and pathology lab scientists per 10,000 cancer patients was 309.4 [7].

8.8.3 Cytogenetics and Medical Genetics

Novel cytogenetics techniques are present in Lebanon and mainly in big centers and university hospitals. Tertiary centers in Lebanon are national referral centers for peripheral blood, bone marrow, amniotic fluid, skin and lymph node karyotyping, and cytogenetic analysis for both constitutional and non-constitutional disorders. These tertiary centers are equipped with metaphase and image-capture platforms as well as highly trained and dedicated staff with many years of technical and analytical expertise. They also provide Sanger Sequencing and Fluorescent in Situ Hybridization (FISH) for numerous disorders including CLL, multiple myeloma, CML, and solid tumors.

8.8.4 Molecular Diagnostics

Big molecular laboratory centers in Lebanon are national and regional referral centers for Molecular Microbiology, Histocompatibility (HLA), and Molecular Pathology. They utilize a wide range of molecular techniques from conventional Polymerase Chain Reaction (PCR) to Reverse Transcription (RT)-PCR, and quantitative PCR for diagnosis and residual disease monitoring like testing for FLT3, NPM1, JAK2, CALR, BCR-ABLbcr-abl International Scale, and common and major translocations for both Acute Myeloid Leukemia (AML) and Acute Lymphoblastic Leukemia (ALL) in addition to solid tumors like sarcomas. Quantitative real-time PCR is utilized to follow all patients on treatment and the tests cover a large panel of infectious organisms as well as important genes adopted for targeted therapy including EGFR, KRAS, and BRAF like in colon cancer. State-of-the-art liquid biopsy testing is also available in big centers and has been introduced to assist in cases requiring frequent monitoring as well as for patients where a re-biopsy is not an option. The molecular lab at the AUBMC, affiliated with the

American Association for Molecular Pathology (AMP) and its Director, is currently the Chairman of the AMP International Affairs Committee (2021) is particularly equipped with Next-Generation Sequencing platforms, that are currently utilized for targeted gene panels for Leukemias, solid tumors, and immunoglobulin variable heavy chain gene (IGVH) Somatic Hypermutation assessment in Chronic Lymphocytic Leukemia (CLL). Next-Generation Sequencing (NGS) is available at AUBMC and is now done for myeloid hematologic diseases. Other NGS panels will also be available for solid tumors.

8.9 Treatment

8.9.1 Medical Oncology

Oncology treatment in Lebanon is provided by doctors specialized in malignant hematology, medical oncology, or hematology/oncology. The Lebanese physicians are very well-trained oncologists who did advanced training outside the country including Europe (mainly France, Belgium, the United Kingdom, and Germany) and the United States of America. In university hospitals, hematology/oncology is divided into subspecialties according to organs. This specialized treatment is important to refine the quality of care. All Lebanese oncologists are registered in the Lebanese Order of Physicians (LOP). In 2021, there are around 173 adult Lebanese hematology/oncology physicians including 21 physicians who are registered at the LOP but are currently practicing outside Lebanon (Data from the LOP).

8.9.2 Radiation Therapy

Radiation oncology is a well-developed medical specialty in Lebanon, attracting patients from different parts of the region for its state-of-the-art equipment and well-renowned physicians. The radiation oncology department at the AUBMC, for example, provides treatment for an average of 900 new patients per year (unpublished data from the AUBMC). There are 12 radiation oncology centers in Lebanon, and practically all of them are part of a larger medical center or hospital. Traditional 2D/3D conformal radiation therapy as well as Intensity Modulated Radiation Therapy (IMRT) are available in most of the centers in the country, whereas High-dose-rate brachytherapy, Stereotactic Radiosurgery (SRS), Stereotactic Body Radiation Therapy (SBRT) and modern Image-Guided Radiotherapy (IGRT) techniques are only available in few centers all located in Beirut. Through well-developed physician training and skills, in addition to modern machinery and technology, patients benefit from improved oncologic outcomes with reduced radiation toxicity. Radiation therapy is covered by third-party payers for eligible patients, including insurance and the National Social Security Fund (NSSF) etc. If the patients have no healthcare coverage, the Ministry of Public Health (MOPH) provides financial coverage at a few governmental hospitals. Finally, there is still a shortage in the number of available radiation oncologists in the country, whose total number remains less than 30 in 2021. Many radiation oncologists have clinics in at least two radiation therapy facilities to be able to cope with the patient load.

8.9.3 Surgery

Advanced cancer surgery is provided in big hospitals, mainly university hospitals, by surgeons specialized in surgical oncology, which is organ specific. Robotic surgery is provided in highly specialized centers. Hyperthermic Intraperitoneal Chemotherapy (HIPEC) is also provided mainly for gynecologic and gastrointestinal malignancies.

8.9.4 Pediatric Oncology

Based on the 2015 NCR of the MOPH, the most common cancers in the pediatric Lebanese population are hematologic malignancies with 29% for leukemias and 19% for lymphomas, followed by Central Nervous System malignancies (10.4%), followed by malignant epithelial tumors and melanoma (8.5%), soft tissues sarcomas (8.3%), malignant bone tumors (7.2%), neuroblastoma (4.8%), germ cell tumors (3.9%) and others more rare tumors like renal and hepatic tumors (Table 8.2) [22]. There are around 10 pediatric cancer treatment centers in Lebanon with 30 pediatric hematology/oncology physicians. As part of the Lebanese Pediatric Society, a group of pediatric hematologists and oncologists was founded in 2001, aiming to standardize pediatric oncology treatment across the different treatment centers in Lebanon. Furthermore, palliative pediatric care started in 1990 to address patient quality of care mainly for patients with non-curative diseases [23]. Among children's cancer centers the Children's Cancer Center for Lebanon (CCCL) was the first to be established in 2002 at the AUBMC and affiliated with St Jude Children's Research Hospital being a tertiary care center and receiving referrals from Lebanon and the region. Later many other centers were founded. The following are examples of hospitals comprising pediatric oncology units (list being not exhaustive): the pediatric oncology unit at Geitawi hospital, Saint-George hospital, Hotel-Dieu de France, Rafic Hariri University Hospital, Rizk Hospital, and many others. Most pediatric cancer patients do not pay out-of-pocket bills. A big amount of the treatment bill is covered by third-party payers (NSSF, MOPH, and others) and the rest of the bill is covered by Non-Governmental Organizations (NGOs). In fact, the yearly needed budget for a single tertiary center is around $15 million USD [24].

Table 8.2 Reported pediatric cases (% of total) by main ICCC-3 group and age group (Source: Republic of Lebanon—Ministry of Public Health—National Cancer Registry 2015) [4]

ICCC main groups	0–4 years	5–9 years	10–14 years	15–19 years	0–19 years
I. Leukemia & myeloproliferative & myclodysplastic dis	11.3	8.8	3.5	5.5	29.1
II. Lymphomas & recitucloendothelial neoplasms	1.4	4.2	5.1	9.2	19.9
III. CNS & miscellaneous intracranial & intraspinal neo	2.8	3.0	2.5	2.1	10.4
IV. Neuroblastoma & other peripheral nervous cell tumor	3.9	0.7	0.2	0.0	4.8
V. Retinoblastoma	1.2	0.7	0.0	0.0	1.8
VI. Renal rumors	1.6	0.9	0.2	0.2	3.0
VII. Hepatic rumors	0.2	0.0	0.0	0.0	0.2
VIII. Malignant bone tumors	0.7	0.7	3.2	2.5	7.2
IX. Soft tissue & other extraosseous sarcomas	2.1	1.8	1.6	2.8	8.3
X. Germ cell & trophoblastic & neoplasms of gonads	0.7	0.5	0.5	2.3	3.9
XI. Other malignant epithelial neo. & malignant melanomas	0.7	0.7	1.6	5.5	8.5
XII. Other & unspecified malignant neoplasms	0.5	1.2	0.2	0.9	2.8
All sites	**27.0**	**23.1**	**18.7**	**31.2**	**100.0**

ICCC-3 International Classification for Childhood Cancer, 3rd

8.9.5 Survivorship Track

Patients are followed based on international guidelines. Most survivor patients get involved in cancer societies to spread awareness about the disease through campaigns in addition to sharing their experience and supporting other cancer patients.

8.9.6 Palliative Care Track

In June 2013, the MOPH recognized Palliative Care (PC) as a specialty which was as important as it is to establish PC as an independent specialty, it is not enough by itself to quickly move the specialty forward. The palliative care track in Lebanon is still continuously developing. The National Committee for Pain Control and Palliative Care (NCPCPC) was established in May 2011, under the Ministry of Public Health (MOPH) with the main objective to work toward the development of palliative care. Well-established hospital-based and outpatient clinic palliative care programs and services are still very limited due to many factors related mainly to financial and personnel-related challenges. Home care palliative care services (Home Hospice) are provided through Non-Governmental Organizations (NGOs) mainly in the Beirut area occasionally extending beyond Beirut but rarely covering rural areas. Their main goals are to provide home-based patient care and 24 h home consultation services to minimize patient suffering(s) and support family members/caregivers taking care of terminal patients, but also, they participate in spreading knowledge about palliative care among healthcare providers and the public. Although establishing PC as a specialty, conducting national awareness campaigns about the importance of this specialty, and establishing (though limited) hospital and home-based PC services, have helped this specialty find its way through the healthcare system and the general population; however, many challenges lie ahead that will hinder further progress which is highly needed. Third-party payers are still not clearly covering these services whether at home or in the hospitals, thus increasing the financial burden on families and patients as they pay from out-of-pocket. Moreover, these challenges may hinder the establishment of PC fellowship programs for physicians and palliative care specialty education for nurses; an endeavor greatly needed as the health care system needs increase. Addressing challenges at a population health system level requires national efforts. National standards that regulate palliative care services are currently under development which will help in improving those services and request financial coverage for patients.

8.10 Research and Education

Lebanon has the biggest and most renowned higher education system in the MENA region. The first medical school in the Middle East was established in Beirut in 1867 by an evangelical missionary named the American University of Beirut (AUB). In 1875, a second medical school was established by the Jesuit missionary at the University of Saint Joseph (USJ). In 1983, a public medical school was established as part of the Lebanese University. Later, four additional medical schools were founded as part of the following universities: Beirut Arab University, Saint-Esprit University of Kaslik, University of Balamand, and the Lebanese American University. All the mentioned medical schools have a hematology/oncology training program [25]. There are two radiation oncology programs in Lebanon at the AUBMC and USJ.

Lebanon is well known for its focus on research compared to other countries in the MENA region. It comprises one of the highest research per physicians or scientists. Almost all medical schools in Lebanon integrate research modules as mandatory fields during medical studies which help early integration of doctors in the research field. In addition to retrospective studies, clinical trials, translation research, and basic science research are also well developed leading to publications in high-impact factor journals. Clinical trials are either multi-institutional within Lebanese institutions, regional or international. Those researches are concentrated within academic centers and regulated by the Institutional Review Board.

8.11   Cost-Effective Cancer Care

The burden of cancer cost is increasing due to several factors including the aging of the population, increasing cancer cases, increasing diagnoses, and treatment costs. In addition, national economic load and explosions causing damage to hospitals and cancer centers increased the financial burden. Novel diagnostic techniques are more costly, increasing the financial weight on MOPH, third-party payers, and patients.

In 2010, WHO recognized Lebanon for its effective strategy in decreasing its health cost from GDP by mainly decreasing out-of-pocket payments. This was possible through a series of reforms by the MOPH. Part of the reform was improving the public health sector including hospitals and laboratories. This decreased the cost spent in private hospitals mainly for the low-income population. Also, MOPH was able to negotiate with the private hospitals for the cost of services. Furthermore, the use of approved generic drugs lowers health care costs. Regulating the use of medical technology was also one of the important components of this reform. This reform led to a decrease in percentage of GDP from 12.4% to 8.4% and a decrease in out-of-pocket from 60% to 44% [26].

8.12   Challenges and Advantages

8.12.1   Facilities Providing Cancer Care

Cancer care is provided mainly by private hospitals, primarily academic hospitals, and to a lesser extent by public hospitals. Lebanon currently has around 29 public hospitals and 128 accredited private hospitals. Oncology care is delivered in big academic hospitals in addition to small peripheral hospitals and private clinics.

Lebanon is leading in the treatment of oncologic diseases in general and malignant hematologic diseases. It includes one of the biggest transplant activities in the MENA region. The Hematopoietic Stem Cell Transplant activity reached 897 transplants between 2012 and 2016 with 303 (33.8%) allogeneic transplants and 594 (66.2%) autologous transplants [27]. Autologous stem cell transplantation is provided at four centers including the AUBMC, Makassed General Hospital (MGH), Middle East Institute of Health (MEIH), and Mount Lebanon hospital (MLH). Centers for allogeneic stem cell transplantation are three, the AUBMC, MGH, and MEIH. The bone marrow transplantation program at the AUBMC was founded in July 2004. It has been accredited by the joint accreditation committee ISCT-European Blood and Bone Marrow Transplantation (EBMT) (JACIE) since 2016. In addition, a cellular therapy program is under development that will provide patients horizons for novel and effective therapies [27].

8.12.2 Treatment Availability

Most of the treatments are available in Lebanon, including immunotherapy, chemotherapy, and novel target therapies. Many patients also get access to newly approved drugs through compassionate use programs. National cancer treatment guidelines were developed by the MOPH to standardize national cancer treatment and organize cancer drug provision to patients [28].

8.13 The Future of Cancer Care in Lebanon

In summary, Lebanon includes tertiary cancer centers that represent national and regional referral centers. Worldwide renowned physicians and healthcare professionals are key players in cancer treatment in Lebanon. Almost all cancer treatments are available in Lebanon which is crucial for continuous improvement of patient care.

Despite development in governmental health care services, Lebanese people still have a negative perception of those services. Implementing more standardized national cancer treatment guidelines developed through experts in the field is crucial. Cancer centers in public hospitals should be developed and healthcare workers at these centers, primarily nurses, should get specialized training in oncology services. This will encourage patients, mainly those with low income, to seek care in affordable public hospitals.

After the conflict in Syria, numerous Syrian refugees moved to Lebanon increasing the Lebanese total population by around 30%. This influx of refugees increased the burden on the Lebanese government and notably on the healthcare system. However, despite all constraints, the healthcare system showed significant resilience with its continued ability to provide acceptable healthcare and most importantly providing cancer drug coverage. This economically deprived population with absent financial coverage by third-party payers is in urgent need to enable access to healthcare, similar to the Lebanese population. The United Nations High Commissioner of Refugees (UNHCR) and NGOs help refugees by covering those vulnerable patients offering them a decent level of care [29]. However, as of 2014, the UNHCR decreased the percentage of in-hospital coverage from 85% to 75%, limiting access to a big number of refugees who are not able to pay 25% of the bill out of pocket.

The advancement of molecular techniques increased our ability to detect targetable mutations. Targeted therapy and immunotherapy are rapidly emerging, replacing conventional chemotherapy in many types of cancer. The drawback of these drugs is their availability, accessibility, and affordability especially in middle-income countries like Lebanon. In addition, given the current economic crisis in Lebanon, the MOPH and third-party payers might not be able to afford novel expensive treatment jeopardizing patient care. Moreover, due to the current economic situation, many healthcare workers immigrated outside Lebanon putting healthcare again in a stressful situation. These difficulties might render advanced expensive treatments accessible only for high-income individuals leading to inequity in cancer care.

Enhancing research in the country will be an asset to improve patient care. Developing national clinical trials and involving Lebanese patients in regional and international clinical trials will enrich our healthcare and benefit our patients.

Our wishes as physicians are to build a health care system resilient enough to face economic, political, and natural constraints minimizing the burden of these constraints on patients. Continuous review and constant update of local treatment guidelines, improvement of health care coverage system to ensure a universal coverage of cancer patients in Lebanon, building a health care strategic plan considering these constraints, continuous update of cancer epidemiology and mortality data to build health care strategy based to national statistics are important steps to build this resilient health care system.

8.14 Conclusion

In conclusion, Lebanon, a relatively small country, comprises the most advanced and well-reputed cancer care and well-renowned physicians. Despite economic constraints, it remains one of the most developed countries in terms of healthcare and notably cancer treatment. Strategies to overcome difficulties affecting the healthcare system are needed.

Conflict of Interest Authors have no conflict of interest to declare.

Acknowledgments We would like to thank the following doctors for their help in providing resources and information: Dr. Jean El-Cheikh, Dr. Antoine Finianos, Dr. Alain Abi Ghanem, Dr. Mohamad Haidar, Dr. Rami Mahfouz, Dr. Raya Saab, and Dr. Bassem Youssef from the American University of Beirut Medical Center.

References

1. The republic of Lebanon [Internet]. 2013. Available from: http://www.cas.gov.lb/index.php/about-lebanon-en.
2. Statistics 2019 [Internet]. Ministry of Public Health. 2019 [cited November 22, 2020]. Available from: http://www.moph.gov.lb/en/DynamicPages/index/8/327.
3. The World Bank Data—Lebanon [Internet] 2019. Available from: https://data.worldbank.org/indicator/SP.DYN.IMRT.IN?locations=LB.
4. Health MoP. National Cancer Registry. Available from: https://www.moph.gov.lb/en/Pages/8/19526/national-cancer-registry.
5. National Cancer Registry: Incidence rate per 100,000 by primary site & age group [Internet]. Lebanese Ministry of Public Health. 2016 [cited November 22, 2020].

6. National Cancer Registry: Frequency (nb) of incident cases by primary site & age group [Internet]. Lebanese Ministry of Public Health. 2016 [cited November 22, 2020].

7. Cancer Country Profile 2020 [Internet]. World health organization. 2020 [cited November 22, 2020]. Available from: https://www.who.int/cancer/country-profiles/LBN_2020.pdf?ua=1.

8. Organization WH. Lebanon fact sheet: https://gco.iarc.fr/today/data/factsheets/populations/422-lebanon-fact-sheets.pdf; 2020 [.

9. National Cancer Registry: Percentages (% of total) by primary site & age group [Internet]. Lebanese Ministry of Public Health. 2016 [cited November 22, 2020].

10. Access GBDH, Quality C. Measuring performance on the healthcare access and quality index for 195 countries and territories and selected subnational locations: a systematic analysis from the global burden of disease study 2016. Lancet. 2018;391(10136):2236–71.

11. Lerberghe WV, Mechbal A, Kronfol N. The collaborative governance of Lebanon's health sector. 2018. Available from: https://www.moph.gov.lb/userfiles/files/Programs%26Projects/PSO/The-Collaborative-Governance-of-Lebanons-Health-Sector.pdf.

12. Ibrahim MD, Daneshvar S. Efficiency analysis of healthcare system in Lebanon using modified data envelopment analysis. J Healthc Eng. 2018;2018:2060138.

13. Ammar W. Universal health coverage: bridging the gaps. Available from: https://www.moph.gov.lb/en/view/1287/universal-health-coverage-bridging-the-gaps.

14. Elias F, Bou-Orm IR, Adib SM, Gebran S, Gebran A, Ammar W. Cost of oncology drugs in the middle-eastern country of Lebanon: an update (2014-2016). J Glob Oncol. 2018;4:1–7.

15. Mansour Z, Said R, Dbaibo H, Mrad P, Torossian L, Rady A, et al. Non-communicable diseases in Lebanon: results from World Health Organization STEPS survey 2017. Public Health. 2020;187:120–6.

16. Notifiable communicable diseases: reported cases by time [Internet]. Republic of Lebanon Ministry of Public Health. 2018 [cited November 22, 2020].

17. Lebanese breast cancer foundation: awareness 2020. Available from: http://www.lbcfoundation.org/FactsAndFigures.aspx.

18. Adib SM, El Saghir NS, Ammar W. Guidelines for breast cancer screening in Lebanon Public Health Communication. J Med Liban. 2009;57(2):72–4.

19. Bahr S, Bzieh R, El Hayek GY, Adib S. Cost-benefit analysis of a projected national human papilloma virus vaccination programme in Lebanon. East Mediterr Health J. 2019;25(10):715–21.

20. National Guidelines for Cancer Colorectal Early Detection In: Health RoLMop, editor. 2019.

21. aub.edu.lb. Smoking cessation support 2018. Available from: https://www.aub.edu.lb/tobaccofree/Pages/Smoking-Cessation-Support.aspx.

22. Health LMoP. Table pediatric B: reported cases (%/total) by main ICCC-3 group and age group. MOPH. 2017. Available from: https://www.moph.gov.lb/userfiles/files/Esu_data/Esu_ncr/PB2015.HTM.

23. Noun P, Djambas-Khayat C. Current status of pediatric hematology/oncology and palliative care in Lebanon: a physician's perspective. J Pediatr Hematol Oncol. 2012;34(Suppl 1):S26–7.

24. Lebanon CsCCo. Cost & Budget 2020. Available from: https://cccl.org.lb/p/16/Cost-Budget.

25. Nemr E, Meskawi M, Nemr R, Yazigi A. Undergraduate medical education in Lebanon. Med Teach. 2012;34(11):879–82.

26. Health Strategic Plan [Internet]. Ministry of Public Health. 2016. Available from: https://www.moph.gov.lb/en/Pages/9/1269/strategic-plans.

27. Bazarbachi A, Zahreddine A, Massoud R, El Cheikh J, Hanna C, Nasr F, et al. Trends in hematopoietic stem cell transplant activity in Lebanon. Hematol Oncol Stem Cell Ther. 2017;10(4):315–20.

28. UNDP_cancerbook [Internet]. 2009. Available from: https://www.moph.gov.lb/userfiles/files/Quality%26Safety/NationalGuidelines/UNDP_cancerbook.pdf.

29. Ammar W, Kdouh O, Hammoud R, Hamadeh R, Harb H, Ammar Z, et al. Health system resilience: Lebanon and the Syrian refugee crisis. J Glob Health. 2016;6(2):020704.

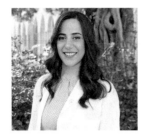

Razan Mohty, MD, is currently a blood and marrow transplantation and cellular therapy fellow at Mayo Clinic Florida. She completed her hematology and oncology fellowship in June 2021 at the American University of Beirut Medical Center, Lebanon. She graduated from the Lebanese University medical school in June 2015, where she completed 3 years of internal medicine residency training. She is currently an active member of the European Blood and Marrow Transplantation Society (EBMT) trainee committee and served as an EBMT young ambassador in 2018. She also serves as a reviewer for several international journals, including the British Journal of Hematology, European Journal of Hematology, Bone Marrow Transplantation, and Transplantation and Cellular Therapy. Dr. Mohty's research interest is blood and marrow transplantation and cellular therapy focusing on preventing and treating associated complications on which she authored several articles.

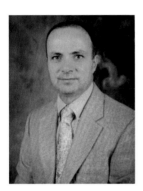

Arafat Tfayli is a Professor of Clinical Medicine at the American University of Beirut Medical Center in Beirut, Lebanon. He received his medical degree from the American University of Beirut in 1995 and completed his Internal Medicine training at the State University of New York at the Stony Brook University Hospital and his Hematology/Oncology training at the Lombardi Cancer Center, Georgetown University. He is a fellow of the Royal College of Physicians. He is also the Director of research at the Naek K Basile Cancer Institute, AUB.

Chapter 9
General Oncology Care in Libya

Adel Attia, Ismail Siala, and Fathi Azribi

9.1 Libya Demographics

Libya is in the north of the African continent and its total land area is about 1.76 million km^2 [1]. The country was declared as an independent state on 24th December 1951. Tripoli is the capital of Libya and is in the Northern west while Benghazi is the second largest city and is in the Northern east. Libya depends on oil as the main source of income, and it has the 10th largest proven oil reserves in the world.

In 2020, the population of Libya was estimated to be 6.93 million [2]. Based on the 2006 Libyan Census, the estimated growth rate in the period from 1995 to 2006 was 1.8%. Almost 42% of the population are 19 years or younger and 4.2% are 65 years or older. The median age in Libya is 28.8 years and about 78.2% of population is urban [3].

9.2 Cancer Statistics in Libya

Benghazi Cancer Registry (BCR) is the first population-based cancer registry in Libya. It was established in 2002 in collaboration with Modena Cancer Registry and the National Center for Epidemiology of the Italian National Institute of Health [5]. The main office of BCR is currently present in Benghazi Medical Center. The results of BCR were published in volume X of Cancer Incidence in Five Continents (2014), which is one of the publications of International Association of Cancer

A. Attia
Benghazi Cancer Centre, University of Benghazi, Benghazi, Libya

I. Siala
Tripoli Cancer Centre, Tripoli University, Tripoli, Libya

F. Azribi (✉)
Division Chief, Tawam Hospital, Abu Dhabi, United Arab Emirates
e-mail: fazribi@seha.ae

© The Author(s) 2022
H. O. Al-Shamsi et al. (eds.), *Cancer in the Arab World*,
https://doi.org/10.1007/978-981-16-7945-2_9

Registries (IACR) [4]. It is also published in other international journals [5]. It covers a population of 1.58 million people in the eastern part of Libya as per 2006 census (28% of Libyan population). Other hospital-based registry reports were published from cancer centers in Sabratha and Misrata and non-published data from Tripoli Oncology Departments. These hospital-based data are consistent with the population-based cancer registry of Benghazi.

The data of a total of 3396 new cancer cases were diagnosed in Eastern Libya during the calendar period from 2003 to 2005 (Table 9.1) [4]. The Age-Standardized

Table 9.1 Benghazi Cancer Registry Data [4]. Used with permission from International Agency for Research on Cancer (IARC/WHO)

*Libya, Benghazi (2003-2005)

	Male						Female						
SITE	No. cases	Freq. (%)	Crude rate (per 100,000)	ASR world	Cum. rates 0-64 (%)	0-74	No. cases	Freq. (%)	Crude rate (per 100,000)	ASR world	Cum. rates 0-64 (%)	0-74	ICD-10
Lip	2	0.1	0.1	0.2	0.01	0.01	1	0.1	0.0	0.1	0.00	0.03	C00
Tongue	5	0.3	0.2	0.4	0.03	0.06	3	0.2	0.1	0.2	0.01	0.01	C01-02
Mouth	8	0.5	0.3	0.7	0.03	0.09	9	0.6	0.4	0.8	0.08	0.10	C03-06
Salivary glands	3	0.2	0.1	0.2	0.02	0.02	5	0.3	0.2	0.3	0.03	0.03	C07-08
Tonsil	2	0.1	0.1	0.2	0.02	0.02	0	0.0	0.0	0.0	0.00	0.00	C09
Other oropharynx	0	0.0	0.0	0.0	0.00	0.00	1	0.1	0.0	0.1	0.00	0.01	C10
Nasopharynx	42	2.4	1.8	2.8	0.21	0.31	25	1.6	1.1	1.4	1.10	0.16	C11
Hypopharynx	2	0.1	0.1	0.2	0.00	0.00	1	0.1	0.0	0.0	0.00	0.00	C12-13
Pharynx. unspecified	1	0.1	0.0	0.1	0.01	0.01	2	0.1	0.1	0.2	0.02	0.02	C14
Oesophagus	18	1.8	0.8	1.6	0.08	0.23	3	0.2	0.1	0.2	0.01	0.01	C15
Stomach	62	3.6	2.6	4.9	0.26	0.59	37	2.3	1.6	3.0	0.15	0.41	C16
Small intestine	3	0.2	0.1	0.3	0.01	0.04	4	0.3	0.2	0.3	0.02	0.02	C17
Colon	111	6.4	4.6	8.8	0.51	1.10	126	8.0	5.6	9.0	0.53	1.06	C18
Rectum	64	3.7	2.7	5.0	0.29	0.66	48	3.0	2.1	3.3	0.24	0.39	C19-20
Anus	5	0.3	0.2	0.3	0.02	0.02	3	0.2	0.1	0.2	0.02	0.02	C21
Liver	58	3.3	2.4	4.9	0.19	0.66	44	2.8	1.9	3.7	0.18	0.48	C22
Gallbladder etc.	17	1.0	0.7	1.3	0.10	0.13	42	2.7	1.9	3.2	0.19	0.30	C23-24
Pancreas	64	3.7	2.7	5.4	0.26	0.67	37	2.3	1.6	2.9	0.17	0.29	C25
Nose, sinuses etc.	5	0.3	0.2	0.4	0.02	0.06	1	0.1	0.0	0.1	0.01	0.01	C30-31
Larynx	66	3.8	2.8	5.5	0.33	0.63	8	0.5	0.4	0.7	0.05	0.09	C32
Trachea, bronchus and lung	326	18.7	13.7	27.8	1.34	3.67	37	2.3	1.6	3.1	0.18	0.40	C33-34
Other thoracic organs	1	0.1	0.0	0.0	0.00	0.00	3	0.2	0.1	0.2	0.01	0.03	C37-38
Bone	12	0.7	0.5	0.4	0.02	0.02	16	1.0	0.7	0.8	0.05	0.07	C40-41
Melanoma of skin	4	0.2	0.2	0.2	0.02	0.02	5	0.3	0.2	0.3	0.04	0.04	C43
Other skin	47		2.0	3.8	0.11	0.44	26		1.1	2.1	0.08	0.24	C44
Mesothelioma	3	0.2	0.1	0.3	0.01	0.03	0	0.0	0.0	0.0	0.00	0.00	C45
Kaposi sarcoma	6	0.3	0.3	0.5	0.02	0.07	1	0.1	0.0	0.1	0.01	0.01	C46
Connective and soft tissue	41	2.4	1.7	2.4	0.14	0.24	38	2.4	1.7	2.3	0.15	0.23	C47-C49
Breast	6	0.3	0.3	0.5	0.03	0.08	364	23.0	16.0	22.9	1.82	2.46	C50
Vulva							5	0.3	0.2	0.4	0.01	0.04	C51
Vagina							3	0.2	0.1	0.2	0.02	0.02	C52
Cervix uteri							62	3.9	2.7	4.5	0.26	0.48	C53
Corpus uteri							7	0.4	0.3	0.6	0.02	0.10	C54
Uterus unspecified							98	6.2	4.3	8.3	0.62	1.08	C55
Ovary							75	4.7	3.3	4.7	0.33	0.49	C56
Other female genital organs							0	0.0	0.0	0.0	0.00	0.00	C57
Placenta							0	0.0	0.0	0.0	0.00	0.00	C58
Penis	0	0.0	0.0	0.0	0.00	0.00							C60
Prostate	162	9.3	6.8	14.7	0.29	1.74							C61
Testis	10	0.6	0.4	0.6	0.05	0.05							C62
Other male genital organs	0	0.0	0.0	0.0	0.00	0.00							C63
Kidney	51	2.9	2.1	3.9	0.20	0.40	27	1.7	1.2	2.0	0.12	0.22	C64
Renal pelvis	2	0.1	0.1	0.1	0.01	0.01	0	0.0	0.0	0.0	0.00	0.00	C65
Useter	0	0.0	0.0	0.0	0.00	0.00	1	0.1	0.0	0.1	0.00	0.00	C66
Bladder	174	10.0	7.3	14.9	0.64	1.74	26	1.6	1.1	2.3	0.10	0.36	C67
Other urinary organs	1	0.1	0.0	0.1	0.00	0.03	0	0.0	0.0	0.0	0.00	0.00	C68
Eye	4	0.2	0.2	0.2	0.01	0.01	6	0.4	0.3	0.3	0.01	0.04	C69
Brain, nervous system	87	5.0	3.6	5.2	0.38	0.62	50	3.2	2.2	3.0	0.16	0.32	C70-72
Thyroid	13	0.7	0.5	0.8	0.06	0.07	64	4.0	2.8	3.8	0.25	0.37	C73
Adrenal gland	3	0.2	0.1	0.1	0.01	0.01	4	0.3	0.2	0.2	0.01	0.02	C74
Other endoceine	0	0.0	0.0	0.0	0.00	0.00	2	0.1	0.1	0.1	0.01	0.01	C75
Hodgkin lymphoma	38	2.2	1.6	1.6	0.11	0.11	44	2.8	1.9	1.8	0.13	0.15	C81
Non-Hodgkin lymphoma	88	5.1	3.7	5.8	0.31	0.70	67	4.2	3.0	4.3	0.26	0.45	C82-85,C96
Immunoproliferative diseases	0	0.0	0.0	0.0	0.00	0.00	0	0.0	0.0	0.0	0.00	0.00	C88
Multiple myeloms	18	1.0	0.8	1.6	0.08	0.19	16	1.0	0.7	1.2	0.08	0.14	C90
Lymphoid leukaemia	27	1.6	1.1	1.4	0.06	0.08	24	1.5	1.1	1.2	0.05	0.10	C91
Myeloid leukaemia	43	2.5	1.8	2.7	0.15	0.30	48	3.0	2.1	2.9	0.19	0.31	C92-94
Leukaemia unspecified	10	0.6	0.4	0.7	0.06	0.09	15	0.9	0.7	0.7	0.06	0.06	C95
Myeloproliferative disorders	8	0.5	0.3	0.5	0.05	0.11	11	0.7	0.5	0.9	0.05	0.11	MPD
Myelodysplastic syndromes	3	0.2	0.1	0.1	0.01	0.01	0	0.0	0.0	0.0	0.00	0.00	MDS
Other and unspecified	60	3.5	2.5	4.7	0.23	0.53	65	4.1	2.9	4.9	0.22	0.54	O&U
All sites	1786		74.8	138.5	6.78	16.62	1640		71.0	110.0	7.21	12.32	C00-96
All sites except C44	1739	100.0	72.8	134.6	6.67	16.19	1584	100.0	69.8	107.9	7.13	12.08	C00-96 exc. C44

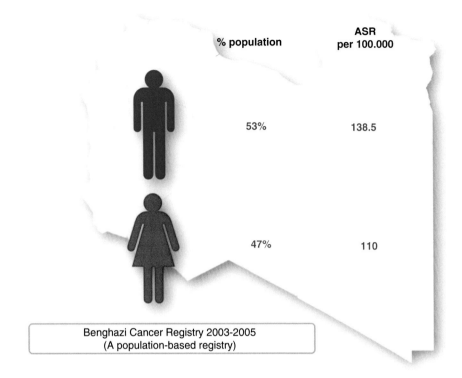

% population

**ASR
per 100.000**

53%   138.5

47%   110

Benghazi Cancer Registry 2003-2005
(A population-based registry)

Fig. 9.1 ASR for all cancer sites, BCR 2003–2005 [4]

Rate (ASR) was 138.5 and 110 per 100,000 for men and women, respectively (Fig. 9.1) [4]. There was a slight male excess (53% of all cancer cases). The incidence of disease was found to increase with age, presenting a median age at diagnosis of 61 years for males and 50 years for females.

Among men, cancers of lung (18.7%), colorectum (10.1%), bladder (10.0%), prostate (9.3%), and Non-Hodgkin lymphoma (5.1%) represented the most frequently reported malignancies, whereas the five most diagnosed types of cancer among women were breast (23.0%), colorectum (11.0%), uterus (unspecified) (6.2%), leukemias (5.5%), and ovary (4.7%) (Fig. 9.2) [4].

The most lethal cancers in both sexes combined were lung cancer showing a 5-year Relative Survival (RS) of 2.3%, followed by liver cancer with a 5-year RS of 2.4%, and stomach cancer with a 5-year RS of 3.3%. Thyroid, breast, and colorectal cancers were associated with a best prognosis showing a 5-year RS of 64.9%, 56%, and 29.5%, respectively [5].

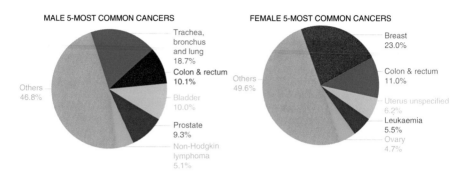

Fig. 9.2 Five most common cancers in both sexes, BCR 2003–2005 [4]

9.3 Healthcare System in Libya

The unstable political situation had adversely affected the provision of healthcare in the country. Still the services are free but suffer disruptions of continuity of care, which has resulted from drug and diagnostic reagents unavailability. These issues are more clearly reflected on patients suffering from chronic diseases including cancer.

Health care delivery in Libya is organized into three levels of care: primary, secondary, and tertiary. The primary health care level includes the services delivered in primary health care units and polyclinics. The secondary care level is formed of hospitals either general hospitals or rural hospitals and the tertiary level includes the university hospitals and the specialty-oriented hospitals and centers such as the cardiac, eye, oncology, diabetes, trauma, chest, and psychiatric hospitals. Cancer is the second leading cause of death in Libya after cardiovascular diseases (The Report on the causes of death in Libya, data analysis of causes of death in the years 2016–2017; Health Information Center, Ministry of Health—Libya, 2019) [19].

9.4 Oncology Care in Libya

Specialist cancer care in Libya started in the late 1970s in both Tripoli and Benghazi. It started as hematology and oncology clinics as part of the general medical and pediatric departments. In Tripoli, the adult oncology service was based at the Department of Medicine of Tripoli Central Hospital, while the pediatric oncology/hematology services were based at Aljala Children's hospital. In Benghazi, Howari hospital was the first hospital to deliver comprehensive cancer care in the eastern part of Libya.

The first cobalt radiotherapy machine was operated in Tripoli Central Hospital in the 1980s. In 1994, in Sabratha—80 km west to Tripoli—a new cancer center was established. In 1995, a radiotherapy center was established in Benghazi. In 1996, the new 1200 beds Tripoli Medical Center was opened; it contained a 78-beds department for medical oncology and hematology, a 39-beds department of pediatric oncology that moved from the old unit in Aljala Children's Hospital. In 1998, a Medical Oncology unit at Al-Jamhoriya Hospital in Benghazi was established; in the same year the second radiotherapy department was launched at Tripoli Medical Center with a cobalt machine first and now it has two linear accelerators and a brachytherapy service. In 2005, a medical oncology service was launched in Misrata initially as a branch of Sabratha Cancer Center, then in 2007, it became Misrata Cancer Centre. Figure 9.3 shows the development of oncology in Libya.

In 2016, a new medical oncology service was launched in Sebha in collaboration with Sabratha Cancer Centre. In 2017, new medical oncology units were opened in Tobruk, Albayda, Ajdabiya, Sirt, and Zintan. In 2018, radiotherapy services were launched in Misrata Cancer Center and in January 2021, the radiotherapy services in Sabratha were launched.

Recently, a decree to establish Tripoli Cancer Center was signed to organize and modernize cancer care in the Tripoli area, where almost a third of the Libyan

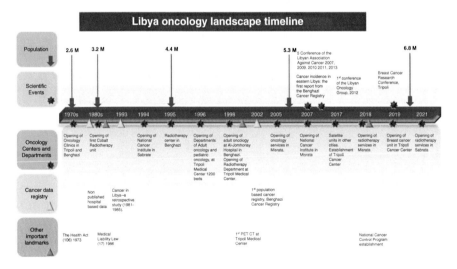

Fig. 9.3 Development of Oncology in Libya [4, 5]

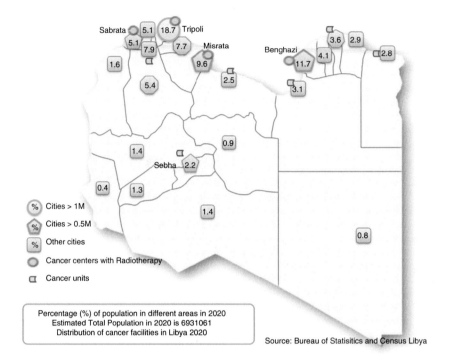

Fig. 9.4 Distribution of current cancer services in Libya [2]. Source: Bureau of Statistics and Census Libya

population live. It has already started with a dedicated Breast Cancer unit, opened in July 2019. It provides diagnostic and therapeutic services to breast cancer patients. This expansion of services allowed cancer patients to access facilities closer to their residential areas (Fig. 9.4).

A Bone Marrow Transplant (BMT) unit was established at Sabratha Cancer Center in collaboration with an Italian team that unfortunately stopped because of the political conflict. As mentioned earlier, the whole cost of oncology care of all Libyan citizens is fully funded by the government either locally or abroad, in case there is a need to refer patients for treatment abroad.

Private oncology care, particularly medical and surgical oncology has emerged and started providing their services, the cost is covered as out-of-pocket or through insurance and on some occasions, it is covered by the government, when there is a huge pressure on the public hospitals, particularly during COVID-19 Crisis.

9.5 Cancer Risk Factors

Cigarette smoking is an important modifiable risk factor for cancer in Libya. In a study published in 2014 on random samples from different Libyan cities (33,739 males and 33,527 females) about cigarette smoking, 15.5% were smokers and the highest age interval of smoking was 40–49 years. Cigarette smoking is more common in males (23.9%) than females (1.7%) [9]. The second risk factor is childhood obesity, a study showed that 30% of the children are obese, males are more affected, with the highest percentage is in Tripoli and the lowest in Sabha [10]. In Libya, STEPS Survey 2009 (WHO) showed 30.5% of the population studied were obese (BMI ≥30, males 21.4%, females 40.1%) [10]. Physical inactivity is another well recognized risk factor, in Libya STEPS Survey 2009 (WHO) showed that 43.9% of adults have low levels of activity (defined as <600 MET-minutes per week) [10].

Hepatitis B and C infections are risk factors for Hepatocellular Carcinoma (HCC). In a study published in 2000, the prevalence of hepatitis B in healthcare workers was 4% [11]. In a more recent study published in 2001, the prevalence of HBV surface antigen (HBsAg) and anti-HCV was 2.2% and 1.3%, respectively, among the general population [12]. Although the studies were different in design, a drop in hepatitis B prevalence was observed. This is possibly due to the introduction of hepatitis B vaccination. HPV infections are related to cervical cancer and oral cancer. In a study published in 2019, the overall prevalence of the most common oncogenic HPV types was 4.5% [13].

Dietary habits are also important risk factors for cancer in Libya. Libya STEPS Survey 2009 (WHO) showed that 97.4% of adults eat less than five servings of fruits/vegetables per day [10]. The BRCA mutation is an important risk factor for breast and ovarian cancers. In a systematic review and meta-analysis study published in 2019, the pool estimate of BRCA mutations among women with hereditary breast and ovarian cancer in the Arab countries was 20% [14].

9.6 Cancer Screening Programs

Unfortunately, patients diagnosed with cancer in Libya are still present in later stages [6, 7]. Hence, awareness of the need for early diagnosis is required, especially those cancers whose screening has proved effective. The breast and colon are among the common cancers in Libya. They constitute almost 21% of cases in both sexes.

Screening activities are not based on well-structured government led programs; it is an initiative of Non-Governmental Organizations (NGOs) in collaboration with the health sector. Awareness campaigns about the importance of early detection of breast cancer started in 2008 by a group of active Libyan doctors in both Benghazi and Tripoli through regular and organized visits to girl schools, women's groups in governmental and private institutes, and through local media and Internet. This effort helped to change some attitudes and beliefs in our community towards breast cancer and increased the awareness of the benefits of its early detection. Since 2011, every October, breast cancer screening campaigns have become a regular event. Breast cancer screening units were established at many of the primary healthcare facilities that accept women for screening and early detection in major cities.

The first early detection units for breast cancer in both Tripoli and Benghazi were opened in 2017 in Alkesh polyclinic-Benghazi, later moved to Benghazi Medical Center, Al-Badri and Triq Al-Matar polyclinics-Tripoli and thereafter, many other clinics opened in other cities. This initiative was highly successful and unexpectedly the units received a large number of women. The early detection clinics work in coordination with multidisciplinary teams of pathology, surgery, oncology, radiotherapy, and radiology departments, to agree on the appropriate management recommendation for these screened women. The early detection units provide screening and diagnostic mammography, ultrasound scan for ladies, who are before the age of screening mammogram and breast diagnostic intervention (FNAC & Tru-cut biopsy).

In one series reported from Benghazi, the breast cancer detection rate was around 20%. Interestingly, almost more than a third of these cases were at an advanced stage [8]. An awareness campaign for cervical cancer was launched in many cities of Libya in January 2020, the campaign of 2021 used the digital platform.

9.7 Cancer Prevention Programs

Smoking is officially banned in public places and to sell it to underage by the law (206) issued in the year 2009. This law also bans tobacco advertisements and enforces tobacco factories to put a warning label on the cigarette packets.

Hepatitis B vaccination programs were started in Libya in the late 1980s and were incorporated in the National Immunization Program in 2001. Libya reported the highest estimate of vaccination in African countries [15]. In 2003–2005, Benghazi cancer registry, hepatocellular carcinoma constituted only 3% of all cancers [4]. This could be explained by the effective vaccination program.

Interestingly, the incidence of cervical cancer in 2004 was one of the lowest in the world. This is most likely due to lower incidence of extramarital relations and the protective role of male circumcision [16]. In anticipation of changes in cancer incidence and social changes, the HPV vaccination was introduced in Libya in 2013 and targeted young females only. It is not yet included in the compulsory vaccination list.

9.8 Cancer Diagnosis

9.8.1 Imaging

Ultrasound, Computed Tomography (CT), and Magnetic Resonance Imaging (MRI) scans are available in all hospitals taking care of cancer patients. Positron Emission Tomography (PET/CT) scan is available at Tripoli University Hospital. Nuclear medicine departments services like bone isotope scan and a multigated acquisition (MUGA) scan are available in some hospitals. Interventional radiology services such as CT-guided lung biopsy and US-guided liver biopsy are available at the major hospitals.

9.8.2 Laboratory

There are six pathology laboratories in the governmental hospitals, one in Sabratha, Misrata, Benghazi and three in Tripoli. However, many private pathology laboratories are delivering their services in various cities. Pathology laboratories are performing routine pathological examination as well as immunohistochemical studies.

Some of the biomarker testing such as RAS in colorectal cancer is done in two of the governmental laboratories, i.e. Sabratha and Misrata. EGFR, ALK, ROS1, and BRAF for lung cancer testing are done in a private laboratory. Currently, PD-L1 testing is sponsored by pharmaceutical companies. Other molecular testing like the BCR-ABL gene testing is performed in Tripoli. Flow cytometry is also available in some of these laboratories. Cytogenetics is referred abroad through few governmental and private laboratories. The tests for hereditary breast and ovarian cancer (BRCA1 & 2) can also be referred and sent abroad through hospital arrangements.

9.9 Treatment

9.9.1 Medical Oncology

Medical oncology and radiation oncology are separate specialties in Libya, while hemato-oncology is a separate specialty in some centers and covered with medical oncology in others. Almost all oncologists are Libyans, and the majority received their postgraduate training locally. For more details about the training, please refer to the education section. Medical oncology and hematology specialists (Adult and Children) are estimated to be around 57 (0.82 per 100.000 population), and the radiation oncologists are estimated to be around 14 (0.2 per 100.000 population). The number of specialists in oncology remains less compared to North America [17].

9.9.1.1 Advanced Treatments

U.S. Food and Drug Administration (FDA) and/or European Medicines Agency (EMA) approved innovative medications including immunotherapy and targeted treatments. These are offered to the patients in Libya through different governmental hospitals. However, political instability adversely affected the timely budgeting, processing, and importing of essential drugs. Furthermore, frequent closure of airports and ports added to the delay of arrival of medicines and other supplies.

9.9.1.2 Bone Marrow Transplantation

Bone Marrow Transplantation (BMT) unit was established in Sabratha in 2003, it contained two laminar flow rooms and was operated in collaboration with Hematology Division, San Martino's Hospital, Genova, Italy. Then it was operated with visiting doctors from Egypt. It is currently non-operational due to the current situation in the country. A new Bone Marrow Transplant unit is under construction in Misrata that is expected to be in service in 2022.

9.9.2 Radiation Therapy

There are 6 radiation oncology units in Libya, 1 in Sabratha (1 Linac, brachytherapy), 1 in Misrata (2 Linac, brachytherapy), 2 units in Tripoli (1 with cobalt, the other has 1 cobalt, 2 Linac and brachytherapy), 2 units in Benghazi each with 1 Linac. The nuclear medicine departments are in Tripoli, Benghazi, Misrata, and Sabratha. PET CT service is available only in Tripoli. Due to the current political instability and shortage of essential operational substances, some of these units are out of service.

9.9.3 Surgery

The dedicated surgical oncology departments are available at Sabratha and Misrata cancer centers. They perform routine oncological surgery for most of the sites. In Tripoli and Benghazi, oncological surgery is performed by surgical departments in the Major Hospitals. Advanced surgical techniques like laparoscopic surgery are available, but robotic surgery has not been introduced yet. The occasional patients, who are deemed appropriate for the Hyperthermic Intraperitoneal Chemotherapy (HIPEC) procedure, are referred abroad.

9.9.4 Pediatric Oncology

Childhood cancer represents 4% of all malignant cancers reported in Benghazi Cancer Registry data [18]. Three hematology and oncology units for pediatrics are in pediatric hospital-Benghazi, Tripoli University Hospital, and Misrata Cancer Center. They are busy units and serve the whole country.

9.9.5 Survivorship Track

Formal survivorship clinics do not exist and patients who have completed their active treatment will continue their surveillance and follow-up at the medical oncology clinics. This includes patients who had their treatment at these clinics as well as those who did not have systemic therapy. Some patients may prefer to be followed-up in the private sector. For patients who were treated abroad, follow-up at the hospital would be more convenient to them.

9.9.6 Palliative Care Track

The palliative care for advanced cancer patients is very important especially that we still see a high proportion of patients in the advanced stage. The care of these patients is not limited to oncology units but also in medical or surgical departments. There are pain clinics that are primarily run by anesthesia specialists in collaboration with oncologists. Unfortunately, there is a significant shortage of this essential service across the country and the National Cancer Control Program is trying to address this issue.

9.10 Research and Education

9.10.1 Research

Most of internationally published oncology research in Libya is limited to epidemiological studies, case reports, and single center experiences. There is no infrastructure and necessary personnel to conduct phase 1, 2, or 3 clinical trials, especially in the current difficult times of the country.

9.10.2 Education and Training

Oncology is incorporated into the curricula of the main medical schools in Libya. Post graduate training is conducted under the umbrella of the Libyan Board of Medical Specialties, which was established in 1994. Medical oncology and hematology training are incorporated into the General Medical Training Program, while radiation oncology, pathology, and diagnostic radiology have their separate training programs. Diploma degrees in medical oncology and pediatric oncology were started in 2020, offered by private academies and recognized by the Ministry of Health.

9.11   Cost-Effective Cancer Care

The increasing cost of cancer care is a global issue faced by all societies around the world. The need for more sophisticated and high technology diagnostic procedures, high cost of the new antineoplastic agents such as immunotherapies and targeted therapies, the advances in cancer treatment resulted in long survival of increasing number of patients who may require expensive maintenance therapy for many years, the complexity of care needs large multidisciplinary team to address the needs of cancer patients. All these factors inevitably lead to soaring costs of cancer care.

Although the diagnostic workup and treatment of cancer are primarily covered by the government, which constitutes a large portion of the health care budget. However, in the current circumstances of the country that led to supply interruptions, patients may have to bear some of the cost of their treatment.

In Libya, one of the well-established strategies for cost saving is the bulk purchasing of drugs from the pharmaceutical industry rather than individual hospital purchasing. Furthermore, there is an increased awareness among the oncology community and policy makers of the high cost of cancer care. In the heart of cost saving approaches there is an emphasis on considering the use of biosimilars in cancer treatment as a proven strategy already adopted by many other countries.

Attempts to regulate the use of advanced imaging modalities such as PET/CT scan, MRI or CT scans have been implemented to decrease the cost of imaging that cancer patients often need. Further attempts to reduce the cost of cancer care is to invest more in early detection, which is a well-established way of reducing the cost through having more patients diagnosed earlier and avoiding the usually higher cost of advanced-stage care. In recent years, there are regular campaigns to increase the awareness of the importance of the early diagnosis of cancer and opening of clinics of early detection across several cities in the country. Currently, many Libyan patients are seeking treatment abroad and naturally this is more expensive than local treatment. Therefore, there are many efforts to reduce the number of patients traveling abroad by investing in making more specialized cancer care available and more readily accessible by opening more specialist oncology units in different cities across the country.

9.12   Challenges and Advantages

9.12.1   Medical Tourism in Libya

Cancer patients constitute the highest percentage of Libyan patients treated abroad; most of them in the neighboring countries. Treatment abroad is supported by the government. A specialized committee oversees the whole procedures of treatment abroad including the eligibility of patients.

On the other hand, because of the location and climate of Libya, it is a potential place for medical tourism from neighboring countries. This seems to be feasible soon because of the striving private health care sector in Libya once political stability is achieved.

9.13   The Future of Cancer Care in Libya

Although healthcare in general and cancer care in particular are facing considerable challenges currently due to political and economic instability of the country as well as COVID-19 crisis. However, there are ambitious plans and strategies to transform cancer care in Libya in the coming years.

- *The National Cancer Control Program:* The program was launched in 2019. It is a governance body that is responsible for putting the cancer control plans, supervising the population-based cancer registry, setting the standards of the cancer care, updating the essential cancer medicine list on a regular basis, organizing the training programs and supervising the NGO activities directed towards cancer awareness and early detection.
- *Cancer Registry*: In a meeting with WHO and International Agency for Research on Cancer (IARC) late in 2016, agreed to start a population-based cancer registry both in Tripoli and Benghazi regions and to improve hospital-based cancer registry in other regions.
- *National Cancer Screening Programs:* In collaboration with other stakeholders, the National Cancer Control Program is planning to start two or more pilot projects for breast cancer screening.
- *Strategic Cancer Areas:* The National Cancer Control Program recommended to divide the country into five strategic cancer areas, each having a comprehensive cancer center and satellite units. This initiative will improve access of patients in remote areas to effective cancer care and will ensure equity in health care delivery across the country.
- *Sustainable Supply of Essential Cancer Medicines:* To explore different options of securing continuous supply of cancer medicines, for example, signing long-term contracts with the major pharmaceutical companies to guarantee continuous supply.
- *Bone Marrow Transplant:* It is one of the essential services that are unfortunately currently unavailable, and there is a big effort to resume the service in Sabratha and to open new transplant units in other centers.
- *Palliative Care*: This area is still not well developed in Libya and there is a bad need for introducing the service in the cancer centers. Training specialists in the field and building enough capacity are among the priorities of the government.
- *Private Sector:* It is striving and complements the public service, regulations and support for the private sector is necessary to augment cancer care based on international standards.

9.14   Conclusion

The cancer incidence rate is rising worldwide, and Libya is not an exception. The complexity of care, the soaring cost, high expectations of patients and their families are global challenges. The situation in Libya is further complicated by fragility of the healthcare system, the large size of the country with long distances between cities and towns, and lack of national programs. Despite all these challenges, the oncology services in Libya are covering a wide range of population and providing decent oncology care. The establishment of The National Cancer Control Program will certainly help to improve the cancer care in Libya and overcome these challenges in the coming years.

Conflict of Interest   Authors have no conflict of interest to declare.

References

1. https://www.worldatlas.com/articles/which-are-the-10-largest-countries-of-africa-by-size.html.
2. Bureau of Statistics and Census Libya. 2020. www.bsc.ly.
3. www.worldometers.info/world-population/libya-population.
4. Forman D, Bray F, et al. Cancer incidence in five continents volume X, Benghazi, Libya; 2014. p. 130–1.
5. El Mistiri M, Salati M, Marcheselli L, Attia A, Habil S, Alhomri F, Spika D, Allemani C, Federico M. Cancer incidence, mortality, and survival in Eastern Libya: updated report from the Benghazi Cancer Registry. Ann Epidemiol. 2015;25:564–8.
6. Ermiah E, Abdalla F, Buhmeida A, et al. Diagnosis delay in Libyan female breast cancer. BMC Res Notes. 2012;5:452. https://doi.org/10.1186/1756-0500-5-452.
7. Boder JE, Elmabrouk Abdalla FB, Elfageih MA, Abusaa A, Buhmeida A, Collan Y. Breast cancer patients in Libya: comparison with European and central African patients. Oncol Lett. 2011;2:323–30. https://doi.org/10.3892/ol.2011.245.
8. Alzwae A. Early breast cancer screening unit report. 2020.
9. Zidan A, Muhammad A. Bureau of statistics and census-Libya. National Libyan Survey of Family Health, main report. 2014. p. 15–6.
10. WHO STEPS chronic disease risk factor surveillance, www.who.int/chp/steps.
11. Daw MA, Siala IM, Warfalli MM, Muftah MI. Seroepidemiology of hepatitis B virus markers among hospital health care workers. Analysis of certain potential risk factors. Saudi Med J. 2000;21(12):1157–60.
12. Elzouki A-N, Smeo M-N, Sammud M, Elahmer O, Daw M, Furarah A, Abudher A, Mohamed MK. Prevalence of hepatitis B and C virus infections and their related risk factors in Libya: a National Seroepidemiological Survey. East Mediterr Health J. 2013;19(7):589–99.
13. Hani A, Lubna A, Ahmed E, Omar E, Abdulla B. Prevalence of high-risk human papillomavirus types 16 and 18 among Libyan women in Tripoli Libya. Libyan J Med Sci. 2019;3(4):125–30.
14. Abdulrashid K. BMC Cancer. 2019;19(1):256. https://doi.org/10.1186/s12885-019-5463-1.
15. Auta A, Adewuyi EO, Kureh GT, Onoviran N, Adeloye D. Hepatitis B vaccination coverage among health-care workers in Africa: a systematic review and meta-analysis. Vaccine. 2018;36(32):4851–60.
16. Bruni L, Albero G, Serrano B, Mena M, Gómez D, Muñoz J, Bosch FX, de Sanjosé S. ICO/IARC Information Centre on HPV and Cancer (HPV Information Centre). Human papillomavirus and related diseases in Libya. Summary Report 17 June 2019.

17. American Society of Clinical Oncology. The State of Cancer Care in America, 2017: a report by the American Society of Clinical Oncology. J Oncol Pract. 2017;13(4):e353–94.
18. El Mistiri M, et al. Cancer incidence in eastern Libya: the first report from the Benghazi Cancer Registry, 2003. Int J Cancer. 2007;120(2):392–7. https://doi.org/10.1002/ijc.22273.
19. https://seha.ly/en/wp-content/uploads/2020/02/Death-Certification-report_FINAL2020.pdf.

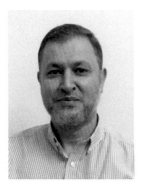

Adel A. Attia is a consultant physician and a medical oncologist at Benghazi Medical Center and an Assistant Professor of Medicine at the University of Benghazi. In addition to taking care of cancer patients and teaching medical students, he is also the director of the Benghazi Cancer Registry. His researches related to cancer incidence in Libya were published in Annals of oncology, Annals of epidemiology, and the WHO book titled *Cancer Incidence in Five Continents Volume X* (2014). Adel has recently finished the WHO course of improving the quality of cancer screening (train the trainer) and has become one of the WHO collaborators.

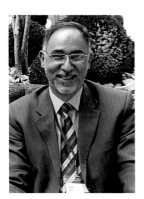

Ismail Siala, CABIM, FRCP, is a consultant of Medical Oncology, Founder and Director General of Tripoli Cancer Center, and a consultant at the Department of Medical Oncology and Hematology of Tripoli University Hospital as well as an Assistant Professor of Medicine at the University of Tripoli. He graduated from Tripoli University and completed his Arab Board Training and Certification in 1996 and became a fellow of the Royal College of Physicians of the UK-London in 2009. He joined the Division of Medical Oncology of The European Institute of Oncology, Milan-Italy as a visiting fellow for six months. His main interest is in breast, prostate, and gastro-intestinal malignancies, with experience in the set-up of chemotherapy units and treatment with chemotherapy, hormonal therapy and biological treatment, medical training and education.

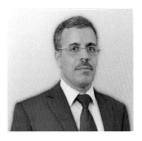

Fathi Azribi, FRCP (UK), CCT (Medical Oncology), is a consultant Medical Oncologist and Chief of the Medical Oncology Division at Tawam Hospital. He graduated from Tripoli University, Libya, then completed specialty training in Oncology in the UK and obtained a Certificate of Completion of Training in Medical Oncology in October 2009. His main interest is in thoracic, breast, gynecological, and gastro-intestinal malignancies, with expertise in treatment with chemotherapy, immunotherapy, hormonal, and targeted therapy. He published several papers and abstracts in peer-reviewed journals. He is also the Program Director of the medical oncology fellowship program at Tawam Hospital.

Chapter 10
General Oncology Care in Mauritania

Selma Mohamed Brahim, Ekhtelebenina Zein, Ahmed Houmeida, and Ahmedou Tolba (iD)

10.1 Mauritania Demographics

The Islamic Republic of Mauritania (RIM) is situated in northwestern Africa, bordering the Atlantic Ocean, and located between Senegal and Mali in the south, Algeria and Morocco in the north. It belongs to both the Sahel and the Maghreb regions. Apart from the coastal region, the climate is often hot and windy with an annual rainfall ranging from 150 mm (5.9 in) in the north to about 600 mm (23.6 in) in the South. The total area of the country is 1,030,000 km^2 formed mainly of vast arid plains except the Senegal River valley where most of the country's agricultural production is harvested. Livestock is raised primarily in the south east. Mineral's export, produced in the north, is dominated by iron but includes copper, gold, gypsum, oil, and steel [1, 2].

The country is organized in thirteen regions or "wilaya" all depending on the central interior ministry. A former French colony, Mauritania became independent in 1960. Estimated then at 850,384 inhabitants, now the total population counts 4,649,658 people according to UN data with a male to female ratio of 1.03.03 for residents aged 0–24 years and a growth rate of 2.72% [3]. The urban population represents 56.9% with about 5000 migrants. Arabic is the official language with the

S. Mohamed Brahim
Université de Nouakchott Al-Asriya, Nouakchott, Mauritania

E. Zein
Pediatric Oncologist, Centre National d'Oncologie (CNO), Nouakchott, Mauritania

A. Houmeida
Laboratoire de biomarqueurs dans la population Mauritanienne, Faculté de Sciences et Techniques, Université de Nouakchott Al Asriya, Nouakchott, Mauritania

A. Tolba (✉)
Radiation Oncologist, Unit Scientific Research, and Higher Education, Centre National d'Oncologie (CNO), Nouakchott, Mauritania

© The Author(s) 2022
H. O. Al-Shamsi et al. (eds.), *Cancer in the Arab World*,
https://doi.org/10.1007/978-981-16-7945-2_10

French spoken as a foreign language and four ethnic minority languages Wolof, Pulaar, Soninke, and Bambara. The Gross Domestic Product (GDP) was worth 7.59 billion US dollars in 2019 [4, 5].

10.2   Cancer Statistics in Mauritania

Two studies carried out, respectively, between (2000–2009) on 3305 patients and (2009–2020) on 10,437 patients showed that breast cancer (BC) was the most common cancer in the screened population (16.19% and 7.2%, respectively) (Figs. 10.1 and 10.2) [6, 7]. Deaths from cancer and communicable diseases represent, respectively, 5% and 59% of the total loss toll. Data from the registry of the Center National d'oncologie (CNO) also revealed an increase in cancer incidence rate since 2009 with a median age of 55 years at diagnosis. Table 10.1 shows the distribution by

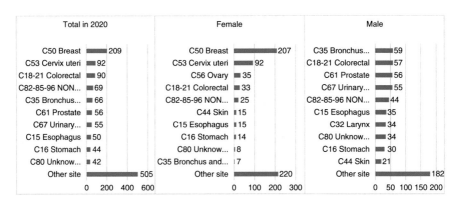

Fig. 10.1 Incidence of common cancers in Mauritania in 2020 [6]

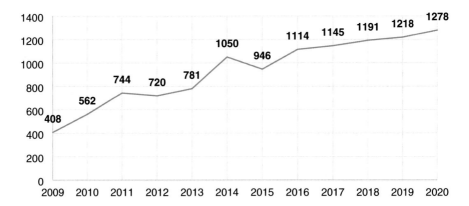

Fig. 10.2 Evolution of cancer incidence in Mauritania for the period of 2009–2020 [6]

Table 10.1 Description of cases by site, male, and female [8]

Total (n = 3305) Site	n	(%)	Âge moyen	Tranche d'âge	Hommes (n = 1403) Site	n	(%)	Âge moyen	Tranche d'âge	Femmes (n = 1902) Site	n	(%)	Âge moyen	Tranche d'âge
Sein	495	15.0	51	20-75	Peau	218	15.5	62	10-95	Sein	485	25.5	47	20-75
Col uterin	344	10.4	49	24-89	Prostate	203	14.5	71	30-92	Col uterin	344	18.1	49	24-89
Peau	332	10.0	59	2-96	Lymphomes	151	10.8	46	6-74	Peau	114	6.0	55	2-96
Lymphomes	213	6.4	42	6-90	Colorectal	92	6.6	49	3-86	Ovaire	114	6.0	45	8-90
Prostate	203	6.1	71	30-92	Œsophage	87	6.2	54	16-70	Corps uterin (endomètre+myomètre)	104	5.5		25-75
Colorectal	173	5.2	50	3-86	Estomac	75	5.3	56	28-83	Thyroïde	83	4.4	44	16-86
Œsophage	165	5.0	50	16-75	Vessie	62	4.4	52	18-84	Colorectal	81	4.3	50	20-86
Estomac	118	3.6	55	20-83	Poumon	57	4.1	59	25-89	Œsophage	78	4.1	46	20-75
Ovaire	114	3.4	45	8-90	Tissu mou	53	3.8	35	3-75	Lymphomes	62	3.3	37	12-90
Thyroïde	104	3.1	45	16-86	Cavité buccale	47	3.3	54	22-85	Estomac	43	2.3	54	20-80
Corps uterin (endomètre/myomètre)	104	3.1		25-75	Pharynx (hypo+pharynx+oro)	40	2.9		13-76	Cavité buccale	41	2.2	51	13-80
Tissu mou	90	2.7	39	1-82	Œil	40	2.9	52	2-85	Tissu mou	37	1.9	44	1-82
Cavité buccale	88	2.7	53	13-85	Langue	37	2.6	51	11-75	Rein	37	1.9	44	1-77
Vessie	82	2.5	54	18-84	Os	29	2.1	36	6-75	Vulve	36	1.9	57	3-82
Pharynx (hypo+pharynx+oro)	70	2.1		13-76	Nasopharynx (cavum+naso+sinus)	27	1.9		17-80	Pharynx (hypo+pharynx+oro)	30	1.6		20-75
Poumon	67	2.0	59	25-89	Rein	26	1.9	44	1-70	Langue	23	1.2	51	21-70
Rein	63	1.9	44	1-77	Thyroïde	21	1.5	46	18-70	Vésicule biliaire	22	1.2	57	41-70
Langue	60	1.8	51	11-75	Amygdale	21	1.5	54	30-70	Vessie	20	1.1	55	40-73
Œil	58	1.8	46	2-85	Glandes salivaires	17	1.2	58	45-75	Os	20	1.1	39	12-80
Os	49	1.5	37	6-80	Anus	14	1.0	52	23-73	Œil	18	0.9	41	2-70
Nasopharynx (cavum+naso+sinus)	40	1.2		18-75	Grêle	11	0.8	44	13-70	Nasopharynx (cavum+sinus)	13	0.7		17-75
Larynx	36	1.1	53	13-76	Larynx	10	0.7	54	3-82	Glandes salivaires	12	0.6	55	24-80
Vulve	36	1.1	57	3-82	Testicule	8	0.6	40	21-80	Amygdale	11	0.6	51	32-65
Amygdale	32	1.0	53	30-70	Système nerveux central	7	0.5	32	3-65	Vagin	11	0.6	43	25-67
Glandes salivaires	29	0.9	56	24-80	Lèvre	6	0.4	53	29-82	Poumon	10	0.5	60	45-80
Vésicule biliaire	25	0.8	63	41-75	Mandibule	4	0.3	54	23-70	Grêle	10	0.5	38	4-66
Grêle	21	0.6	41	4-70	Pancréas	4	0.3	43	40-65	Utérus	8	0.4	42	23-70
Anus	20	0.6	51	23-75	Vésicule biliaire	3	0.2	69	56-75	Larynx	6	0.3	50	30-75
Système nerveux central	13	0.4	41	3-68	Foie	3	0.2	50	38-65	Anus	6	0.3	50	18-75
Vagin	11	0.3	43	25-67						Système nerveux central	6	0.3	51	39-68
Lèvre	9	0.3	52	29-82						Cliteris	5	0.3	59	40-75
Testicule	8	0.2	40	21-80						Mandibule	4	0.2	40	36-48
Mandibule	8	0.2	47	23-70						Lèvre	3	0.2	50	40-60
Utérus	8	0.2	42	23-70						Pancréas	3	0.2	55	50-60
Pancréas	7	0.2	49	40-65						Foie	2	0.1	51	50-52
Foie	5	0.2	51	38-65										
Cliteris	5	0.2	59	40-75										

cancer type in the global cohort and in both genders (men: 1403 cases, 42% and women: 1902 cases, 58%), the mean age at detection and age group affected [8]. Overall, breast (15%) followed by cervical (10.4%) and skin (10%) cancers are the most common cancers in our population. This same order was found in women with, respectively, (25.5%), (18.1%), and (6%). In men, skin cancer (15.5%), prostate cancer (14.5%), and lymphomas (10.8%) were the most prevalent. Although the average age at diagnosis varied with cancer type, most cancer patients were 40–50 years old except, understandably, prostate cancer where the mean age was above 70 years [8–10].

10.3   Healthcare System in Mauritania

The healthcare service is organized in central hospitals in Nouakchott, the capital city, and regional hospitals in the 13 regions of the country supported by few dispensaries, maternal and child care centers in the less populated urban and rural zones (Table 10.2). Private health clinics also exist. All these facilities remain suffering from a lack of equipment, supplies, and well-trained staff. The state insurance covers 500,000 people and less than 1% of residents have a private health cover. Government health expenditure per person is estimated at 22 USD against 29 USD out-of-pocket spending [11]. There are about 15 physicians per 100,000 inhabitants [12]. Communicable, maternal, prenatal, and nutrition associated diseases represent 53% of the population total deaths. Infant mortality is 60.42 deaths/1000 live births. Life expectancy at birth is 67 years for females and 63 years for male [11, 12].

Table 10.2   Main hospitals offering care in Mauritania

Location	Hospital name: *specialized activity*
Nouakchott	– Centre Hospitalier National (CHN): *Multicare hospital* – Centre Hospitalier Amitié: *Multicare hospital* – Centre Hospitalier Cheikh ZAYED: *Multicare hospital* – Centre Hospitalier Militaire: *Multicare hospital* – Centre Hospitalier Mère et Enfant (CHME): gynecology and pediatric care – Centre National d'oncology (CNO): Oncology care – Centre National de Cardiologie (CNC): cardiovascular care – Centre National des spécialités (CNS): head and neck care – Centre National d'Hépatovirologie (INHV): gastroenterology and hepatology care
Nouadhibou	Centre Hospitalier de Nouadhibou: *Multicare hospital*
Hodh Echarghi	Centre Hospitalier de Néma: *Multicare hospital*
Hodh El Gharbi	Centre Hospitalier d'Aioun: *Multicare hospital*
Assaba	Centre Hospitalier de Kiffa: *Multicare hospital*
Gorgol	Centre Hospitalier de Kaedi: *Multicare hospital*
Brakna	Centre Hospitalier d'Aleg: *Multicare hospital*
Trarza	Centre Hospitalier de Rosso: *Multicare hospital*
Adrar	Centre Hospitalier d'Atar: *Multicare hospital*
Tagant	Centre Hospitalier de Tidjikja: *Multicare hospital*
Guididimagha	Centre Hospitalier de Sélibaby: *Multicare hospital*
Tiris Zemmour	Centre Hospitalier de Zouératt: *Multicare hospital*
Inchiri	Centre Hospitalier d'Akjoujt: *Multicare hospital*

10.4   Oncology Care in Mauritania

Overall, there are 22 main hospitals in Mauritania (9 in Nouakchott and 13 in the remaining regions of the country). Five of these hospitals are providing specialized care (Table 10.2). Of these hospitals, Centre National Oncology (CNO) is the main cancer care center. Oncology activity in Mauritania began only in 1990 at the internal medicine department of Nouakchott Central Hospital. Most patients were then transferred abroad for treatment until the creation of the Centre National Oncology (CNO) in 2008 (Fig. 10.3). Before the inauguration of the first radiotherapy accelerator in 2010, the only service provided to cancer patients by the CNO was medical oncology [13].

Currently, the CNO, an autonomous public institution, is the single institution in charge of cancer care in the country. There is no private cancer care in the country. The mission of CNO includes:

- Offering and supervising cancer treatments. The CNO works with the anatomy and pathology departments of the various central and regional hospitals for cancer diagnosis.
- Following-up treated patients.
- Ensuring the full and free care of all nationals for radio-chemotherapy.
- Coordination of patients' evacuations abroad. This action is currently limited to bone marrow transplants and severe leukemias. Costs of all oncology care are largely covered by the state. People with relatively higher income seek treatment abroad at their expense.
- The CNO undertakes and assists in campaigns to fight and raise awareness against the possible causes of cancer.
- The CNO also provides statistics on cancer types and cancer patients in Mauritania.

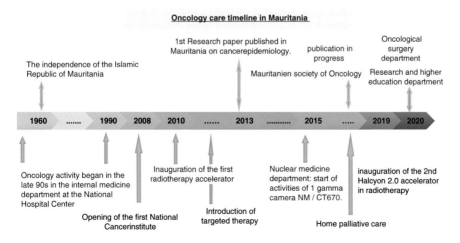

Fig. 10.3 Development of oncology in Mauritania [6]

10.5 Cancer Risk Factors

According to the Global Youth Tobacco Surveillance (*GYTS*) surveys conducted in Mauritania in 2000, 2006, and 2009, the prevalence of tobacco use is steadily increasing among adolescents aged 13–15 years. It was 41%, 59%, and 68%, respectively. Among adults (16–64 years), a study carried out by *STEP-Wise* NGO in 2006 showed a prevalence of 32% in men and 4.9% in women, respectively. Traditional tobacco called *Meneiyge*is very accessible and preferably used by rural aged women [14, 15].

Although female obesity is slightly decreasing, it is estimated that about 60% of Mauritanian women have a Body Mass Index (BMI) over 25 and therefore considered overweight [16–18]. The high rate of consanguinity and endogamy in the Mauritanian population (about 40–60%) particularly in some ethnic groups of sub-Saharan African origin (*Sonikés*) is also a risk factor for cancer and other disease with genetic trait such as heart diseases, hypertension, hearing deficit, and diabetes mellitus known to be more frequent in consanguineous marriages [19, 20].

Lifestyles such as high red meat consumption by many people in Mauritania particularly in the south may also contribute to various cancers like bowel (colorectal) cancer [21]. Hepatitis B (prevalence: 14%) and other infectious illnesses such as diarrhea, malaria, and tuberculosis remain endemic in the country [22, 23].

10.6 Cancer Screening Programs

There are no nationwide cancer screening programs in Mauritania because of funding priorities and lack of skilled healthcare workers to perform efficient screening plans. However, many promotional activities to raise public awareness on cancer risks (mainly smoking and obesity) are frequently undertaken by the state and Non-Governmental Organizations (NGOs) across the country such as "pink October," a nationwide campaign organized every October to raise awareness on cervical and breast cancer and promote early diagnosis of these cancers. Screening mammograms are available in the country. The cost of the service is either covered by the state for patients with national insurance or by NGO for those with no medical insurance. For insured besides, irregular screening actions are also launched on the most common cancers like breast, cervical, and lung cancers. Counseling services remain scarce. The plans to introduce state screening programs and national registry for cancer are underway [24].

10.7 Cancer Prevention Programs

Few steps have been taken to prevent cancer in the country. For instance, a total ban on use of plastic bags has been effective since 2014 as a measure in the fight to reduce carcinogen items in consumers' lifestyle although there is no clear evidence that people can get cancer from using plastic bags. High taxation on tobacco has been implemented. TV sketches on the risks of child and women obesity are regularly launched by the Ministry of Social Affairs [23]. Due to the high prevalence of hepatitis B in the country, vaccination against Virus of all newborn babies has been added since 2010 to the national program of child vaccination which already include (*programme Elargie de Vaccination (PEV)*). The screening for hepatitis B and the vaccine are also advised and freely available for all health workers but not yet mandatory. Vaccination for Human papillomavirus (HBV) is also recommended for girls when 12 years old [25].

10.8 Cancer Diagnosis

Evaluation of cancer in the country uses mainly patient history, physical examination, and basic laboratory testing such as tumor markers. Access to more reliable diagnostic tools such as imaging (X-ray), endoscopic exams, tumor biopsies is still limited and available only in few hospitals of the capital city such as the Institut National d'Hépatovirologie (INHV), Cheikh ZAYED hospital, and the Centre Hospitalier National (CHN). Advanced imaging facilities, Computed Tomography Scan (CT scan), and Mammograms are available in the CNO, at few public hospitals and some private clinics.

The main department of histopathology, located in the CNO, is supported by secondary services both in Nouakchott's hospitals and in few private clinics. There is only one Nuclear Medicine Department, created at the CNO in June 2015 [26]. An Immunohistochemistry laboratory and oncogenetic unit (for genetic testing) have been recently added to the CNO diagnostic and follow-up facilities.

10.9 Treatment

10.9.1 Medical Oncology

The CNO is the major fully competent facility for cancer treatment in the country. The medical staff currently (2020) available consists of three medical oncologists and two hematologists all men, two pediatric oncologists both women, 10 nurses and technicians (4 women and 6 men). The CNO also uses clinical help from other medical departments based in different hospitals of Nouakchott like surgery, ophthalmology, etc. Oncologists in CNO are all former General Practitioners (GP) who then received their training in oncology largely abroad.

Cancer drugs, chemotherapy, and targeted therapy such as Trastuzumab/Pertuzumab for breast cancer, Rituximab for B lymphomas, and Bevacizumab used in broader applications like malignant solid tumors are only available in the

CNO. Treatments are free at the CNO for indigent patients and offered at much reduced cost for patients with state insurance. Two private clinics *Sahel and twvigh* provide conventional chemotherapy for patients with insurance or self-pay.

Conventional-dose chemotherapy and targeted therapy are accessible only at the CNO. However, high dose chemotherapy, Bone Marrow Transplant (BMT), and immunotherapy are not yet available at the center due to their high cost, the associated equipment, and isolation rooms. Efforts are currently undertaken to introduce these therapies in the CNO [13].

10.9.2   Radiation Therapy

The single radiotherapy Linear Accelerator (LINAC) in the country, using Intensity-Volumetric Modulated Arc Therapy (VMAT), Modulated Radiation Therapy (IMRT), and 3D Conformal Radiation Therapy, is based at the CNO. It is operated by a Radiation therapist. The appropriate treatment volume and dosage prescribed to the patients by the radiation oncologist is then followed by the medical physicist and the dosimeters [27]. The radiotherapy staff currently (2020) available consists of four radiation oncologists and six physicists all men trained in Turkey, Morocco, and France.

10.9.3   Surgery

An oncological surgery has recently been set in the CNO. However, most organs and pieces removal procedures are still carried out within the surgery departments of the main hospitals of Nouakchott (Table 10.2) as part of their daily actions. There is no robotic or Hyperthermic Intraperitoneal Chemotherapy (HIPEC) surgery.

10.9.4   Pediatric Oncology

There is only one fully specialized pediatric oncology unit in the CNO since 2011. All hospitals refer young patients once diagnosed with cancer in their pediatric services to the CNO. The service is run by pediatric oncologists, all women and two juniors. It also includes two junior pediatric oncologists and four pediatric oncology nurses performing an integrated role of childhood cancer care and family support. Overall, 151 patients have been referred and followed at the CNO between 2017 and 2019 [6].

10.9.5 Survivorship Track

Data on cancer survival remain inaccurate in Mauritania as many patients do not complete their treatment or do not come back for checkup after completion of treatment. This group is termed "lost patients" by the CNO due to lack of possibility of tracking such patients. However, efforts are undertaken to minimize this loss and set an updated register of patient outcomes in the center. For instance, recent data have shown that 26% of women diagnosed with breast cancer in 2018 have died giving a 2–3-year survival rate 64% [6].

10.9.6 Palliative Care Track

Palliative care was successfully integrated in Mauritania in 2015. The country has about 50 nurses and a dozen of doctors specialized in medical care for people living with serious illnesses, mainly those with terminal cancers. Their task includes, besides improving the quality of life and outcome for patients of advanced diseases, the moral and spiritual support for stressed families, mainly those looking after their patients at home. There are no wards or hospice dedicated for palliative care in the country. However, in the plan for 2021, the CNO has approved a Department of Palliative Care to start in the first quarter of the year. Few Non-Governmental Organizations (NGO) charities such as *Cairdeas Medical* are also active in this field [28–30].

10.10 Research and Education

Oncology teaching program is part of the medical studies at the Faculty of Medicine but specialization in cancer practice remains largely carried out abroad. A program in oncology nursing is offered to nurses freshly joining the CNO but no national diploma in oncology nursing is yet available. Staff training in oncology remains very limited in local hospitals. They are provided mainly through exchange programs largely funded by the International Atomic Energy Agency (IAEA) allowing local staff to go for observation and skills learning in North African and European states.

Basic research on cancer is almost nonexistent. Few studies on the epidemiology of cancers such as breast and colorectal cancers in the Mauritanian population have been published [31–33]. A joint epidemiological study on breast cancer is underway between a team of the CNO and groups from the *institut Pasteur of Tunis* (Tunisia) and the *institut Pasteur of Casablanca* (Morocco). A Next Generation Sequencing (NGS) study aimed to identify gene mutations in a cohort of 135 breast cancer Mauritanian patients, being carried out by the oncogenetic unit of the CNO. The finding of this study may be useful in adapting standard treatment protocols to local patients if specific mutations were identified. There is a society of medical oncology.

10.11   Cost-Effective Cancer Care

Statistics are showing that cancer is rapidly being a public health problem in Mauritania. Due to the state's limited infrastructure in the field and patient low income, cancers are often diagnosed at an advanced stage. As in most African states, the high cost of oncological care and the scarcity of medical oncologists (pathologists, radiation oncologists, and other healthcare workers) are key factors in the poor prognosis and low survival rate. Patients with private insurance or sufficient income often seek treatment in countries such as Turkey, Tunisia, Morocco, and western countries [6].

10.12   Challenges and Advantages

Numerous factors are still decreasing the chance of good prognosis and the probability of recovery from cancer in the country. Among these different challenges in the fight against cancer we may cite, for instance:

- Absence of nationwide screening programs.
- Cost of the infrastructure needed for an advanced and adapted care. As a result, most cancers are identified at a late stage. Access to immunohistochemistry to quickly assess cancer proliferation is still very difficult. Drugs targeting specific cancer cells are often not available.
- Shortage of skilled oncology staff as training or recruiting specialized doctors and nurses is expensive for the state.
- Migration of trained workers seeking better opportunities offered in western countries.

However, the current stability of the political climate, the high percentage of a young population combined with the increasing awareness and priority given to education and health in the state economy programs are relatively reassuring on a better prospect of disease care in Mauritania.

10.13   The Future of Cancer Care in Mauritania

The government has recently implemented a new national policy making the cancer entirely supported by the state for needy patients and at reduced price to individuals with state insurance. To ease the burden on the CNO, being the only cancer care facility in the country, regional secondary oncology centers providing basic care before referring to the CNO are to be planned. Advanced equipment for treatments like radiotherapy, imaging, etc., should also be purchased. Another key element needed is the training of skilled cancer workers: specialized physicians and nurses.

10.14   Conclusion

As in most third world countries, lack of prioritization in funding, shortage of infrastructure, and qualified oncology workers remain a barrier for efficient care of cancer patients. Training programs in demanding specialized fields such as nursing and medical oncology ought to be developed. A national program for palliative care needs to be implemented. Efforts are made by the government to overcome these obstacles through more financial support and training through regional and international collaboration.

Conflict of Interest   Authors have no conflict of interest to declare.

References

1. https://www.diplomatie.gouv.fr/fr/dossiers-pays/mauritanie/presentation-de-la-mauritanie/. Accessed 1 Dec 2020.
2. https://www.tresor.economie.gouv.fr/Pays/MR/mauritanie-presentation-generale. Accessed 1 Dec 2020.
3. https://worldpopulationreview.com/countries/mauritania-population. Accessed 1 Dec 2020.
4. https://www.who.int/countries/mrt/fr/. Accessed 1 Dec 2020.
5. https://tradingeconomics.commauritania/gdp. Accessed 1 Dec 2020.
6. Centre National d'Oncologie CNO. Registry in 2020.
7. https://gco.iarc.fr/today/data/factsheets/populations/478-mauritania-fact-sheets.pdf. Accessed 1 Dec 2020.
8. Baba ND. Cancer in Mauritania: results of 10 years from the hospital register in Nouakchott. Pan Afr Med J. 2013;14:149. https://www.ncbi.nlm.nih.gov/pmc/articles/PMC3683519/
9. Torre LA. Global cancer statistics, 2012. CA Cancer J Clin. 2015;65(2):87–108. https://doi.org/10.3322/caac.21262.
10. Waleed M Sweileh, Sa'ed H Zyoud, Samah W Al-Jabi, Ansam F Sawalha, Contribution of Arab countries to breast cancer research: comparison with non-Arab Middle Eastern countries, BMC Womens Health 15, Article number: 25 (2015).
11. https://www.prb.org/wp-content/uploads/2020/06/Mauritanie-Plan-National-de-Developpement-Sanitaire-2017-2020.pdf. Accessed 1 Dec 2020.
12. http://www.africanchildforum.org/clr/policy%20per%20country/mauritania   /mauritania_health_2012-2020_fr.pdf. Accessed 1 Dec 2020.
13. https://www.t2s.ma/centre-doncologie-de-nouakchott/. Accessed 1 Dec 2020.
14. https://www.afro.who.int/sites/default/files/2017-09/Mauritania_report_card_0.pdf. Accessed 1 Dec 2020.
15. https://www.sante.gov.mr/?wpfb_dl=5. Accessed 1 Dec 2020.
16. Ba ML. Obesity in Mauritania: epidemiologic aspects. Tunis Med. 2000;78(11):671–6.
17. Manyanga T, El-Sayed H, TeyeDoku D, Randall JR. The prevalence of underweight, overweight, obesity and associated risk factors among school-going adolescents in seven African countries. BMC Public Health. 2014;14., Article number: 887
18. Hammami A, Elgazzeh M, Chalbi N, Mansour BA. Endogamy and consanguinity in Mauritania. Tunis Med. 2005;83(1):38–42.
19. Hammami A, Chalbi N, Ben Abdallah M, Elgazzeh M. Effects of consanguinity and social factors on mortality and fertility in Mauritania. Tunis Med. 2005;83(4):221–6.
20. Ferro-luzzi GA. Minist. Sanita, Serv. Nutriz., Rome the dietary and nutritional situation in Mauritania. Quadernidella; Nutrizione 1964;24:245–66.

21. Raad II. Challenge of hepatitis C in Egypt and hepatitis B in Mauritania. World J Hepatol. 2018;10(9):549–57. https://doi.org/10.4254/wjh.v10.i9.549.
22. Rui WZ, Baïdy BL, N'Diaye M. Hepatitis B virus infection in the school milieu of Kiffa and Selibaby, Mauritania. Bull Soc Pathol Exot. 1998;91(3):247–8.
23. https://screening.iarc.fr/doc/MfM_French_final.pdf. Accessed 1 Dec 2020.
24. Louie KS, De Sanjose S, Mayaud P. Epidemiology and prevention of human papillomavirus and cervical cancer in sub-Saharan Africa: a comprehensive review. Trop Med Int Health. 2009;14(10):1287–302. https://doi.org/10.1111/j.1365-3156.2009.02372.x.
25. Yusuf O. Soigner le cancer plus près de chez soi: la Mauritanie ouvre son premier centre de médecine nucléaire, IAEA Bulletin – mars 2015. https://www.iaea.org/sites/default/files/56105810607_fr.pdf. Accessed 1 Dec 2020.
26. https://www.iaea.org/search/google/Mauritanie%20radiation. Accessed 1 Dec 2020.
27. https://hospicecare.com/what-we-do/publications/newsletter/2016/02/featured-article/. Accessed 1 Dec 2020.
28. Dion Smyth M. Politics and palliative care. Int J Palliat Nurs 2016. https://doi.org/10.12968/ijpn.2016.22.11.570
29. Fearon D. Perceptions of palliative care in a lower middle-income Muslim country: a qualitative study of health care professionals, bereaved families and communities. Palliat Med. 2018; https://doi.org/10.1177/0269216318816275.
30. Baba ND. Cancer of the oral cavity in three brothers of the whole blood in Mauritania. Pan Afr Med J. 2016;25:156. https://doi.org/10.11604/pamj.2016.25.156.10377. Collection 2016
31. Sarr A, et al. Colorectal cancers in Mauritania: clinical aspects and treatment. Open J Intern Med. 6(4) https://doi.org/10.4236/ojim.2016.64019. https://www.scirp.org/journal/paperinformation.aspx?paperid=72878
32. Fearon D. Life journeys with advanced breast cancer in Mauritania: a mixed methods case study. 2020. https://doi.org/10.17635/lancaster/thesis/1013
33. Dey D. Understanding global challenges in Africa, Europe, Latin America, and Asia and proposing strategies for improvement. Rheum Dis Clin North Am. 2021;47(1):119–32. https://doi.org/10.1016/j.rdc.2020.09.009.

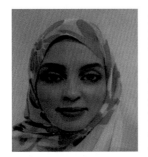

Selma Mohamed Brahim has obtained her baccalaureate in Natural Sciences and her BSc in Molecular Biology and Physiology from Alasriya University/Mauritania in 2016. After a master's in biology and Health Sciences at HASSEN II University/Morocco, she is now carrying out a Ph.D. in molecular biology on breast cancer mutation profile in Mauritania as part of a collaboration project between the research unit on biomarkers in the Mauritanian population/Alasriya University and the Onco-Virology Laboratory of Pasteur Institute/Morocco. She works at the Center National oncology, and she coordinates at unit Research. Thanks to numerous training programs home and abroad she developed a strong skill set in biomedical, molecular oncogenetics.

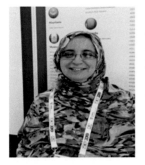

Ekhtelebenina Zein is the Director of the National Oncology Center, a reference structure for cancer care in Mauritania. She has been a pediatrician since 2003, holder of a pediatric oncology IUD from Med v University of Rabat and Paris Sud in 2015. Dr. Zein has been teaching at the Nouakchott Faculty of Medicine since 2010. Moreover, she is a member of the GFAOP group. She is involved in the development of pediatric oncology.

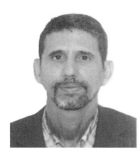

Ahmed Houmeida   holds a Ph.D. in muscle motility from Paul Sabatier University and a HDR (habilitation à diriger la recherche) from Louis Pasteur University (France). After nearly a decade of postdoctoral research at Bristol (School of Veterinary Medicine), then Leeds (School of Biomedical Sciences) Universities (UK) and Eastern Virginia Medical School (US), he returned to his home country to join the University of Nouakchott/Mauritania where he has taught biochemistry and immunology since 1998. He pursued his interest in research to create his own group aimed at introducing recent molecular techniques in profiling gene mutations associated to diseases with potential genetic components in the Mauritanian population. Numerous publications have come out of these investigations,which included hemoglobin Human molecular disorders.

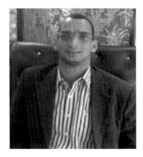

Ahmedou Tolba, MD, completed his medical studies at Sousse University, Tunisia in 2008. He had his training in Radiation Oncology at Mohammed V University, Morocco in 2013. Tolba has worked as a Radiation Oncologist at the Center National d'oncologie, Mauritania, since 2014. He has participated in many national and international fellowships and courses in radiation oncology, brachytherapy, and palliative care. Tolba has been actively involved in medical education and palliative care. He has been the chief of the research and Radiation oncology.

Chapter 11
General Oncology Care in Morocco

Saber Boutayeb and Mohammed Anass Majbar

11.1 Morocco Demographics

Morocco is a North African country. The current population of Morocco is estimated to be 37 million based on the projection of the United Nations data [1, 2]. Most of the local population lives in the Atlantic at the Mediterranean coastline. Casablanca is the biggest city with more than 7 million population. The other major cities are Marrakech, Rabat, Fez, and Tangier. The urban population represents around 60% of the entire population. The median age in the Moroccan population is young. Around 25% of the population is aged under 14 years [1]. The economy of Morocco is considered liberal and is the fifth largest African economy. The major Moroccan resources are represented by phosphate, tourism, agriculture, and car manufacturing. The Gross Domestic Product was evaluated at 118 USD billion dollars [3].

11.2 Cancer Statistics in Morocco

Morocco is currently in an epidemiological transition called, "double burden ", with the coexistence of infectious and chronic diseases. The two population-based registries are available in Morocco: Casablanca and Rabat [4, 5]. The registry of Casablanca covers more than 10% of the country's population (around 12%) and is used to

S. Boutayeb (✉)
Medical Oncology Department, National Institute of Oncology, University Mohammed V in Rabat, Rabat, Morocco
e-mail: saber.boutayeb@um5s.net.ma

M. A. Majbar
Surgical Oncology Department, National Institute of Oncology, University Mohammed V in Rabat, Rabat, Morocco
e-mail: anass.majbar@um5s.net.ma

© The Author(s) 2022   163
H. O. Al-Shamsi et al. (eds.), *Cancer in the Arab World*,
https://doi.org/10.1007/978-981-16-7945-2_11

Table 11.1 Top five cancers in Morocco between 2008 and 2012 according to the register of Casablanca [4]

Men cancers	Percentage	Women cancers	Percentage (%)
Lung	23%	Breast	35.6
Prostate	12.6%	Cervix	11.2
Colorectum	7.9%	Thyroid	8.6
Bladder	6%	Colorectum	5.9
Lymphoma	6%	Ovary	4

extrapolate the cancer incidence in Morocco [4]. These two registries provided descriptive information such as cancer type, histology, age, gender, and stage. To date, survival data is not provided by these registries. Table 11.1 shows the top five cancers in Morocco between 2008 and 2012 according to the registry of Casablanca [4].

The most frequent cancers in men are lung, prostate, bladder, colorectum, and lymphoma. Lung cancer represents 20.8% of all cancers in Men. Among them, the overall frequency of the EGFR mutation is 21%. Mutations were mainly detected in exon 19 (69%), followed by exon 21 (21%) and exon 20 (7%) [4, 6, 7]. Whereas, for women, the most frequent are breast, cervix cancer, colorectum, thyroid, and ovary [4, 5, 8]. Breast cancer is the leading cancer among females (36% of cancers in women) with an age-standardized incidence rate of 40.8 per 100,000. The median age at diagnosis is 49.5 years [9]. According to a large study conducted in Casablanca, the most common molecular phenotype was Luminal A (41.4%) Luminal B, HER2 and triple negatives occurred in 10.4%, 6.3%, and 11.2% [8].

11.3 Cancer Risk Factors

11.3.1 Tobacco

The prevalence in the general population is 18% in adults and 9% in youths. According to WHO, the mortality attributable to tobacco smoking is 8%. In 2008, the smoking prevalence among the Moroccan population was 16% (30% for males and 1% for females) [11–13]. Passive smoking is also high: 32% are exposed in their closed family circles and 60% are exposed in public places [13]. The anti-tobacco law was adopted in 1996 and Morocco signed the WHO Framework Convention on Tobacco Control in 2004 [10]. However, this legislation is poorly implemented, and the Moroccan population has generally not respected these laws.

11.3.2 Alcohol

In Morocco, alcohol is available in restaurants, bars, and hotels. However, drinking in public is strictly prohibited. The office of International Studies and Research on alcoholic beverages and spirits evaluated the Moroccans' alcohol consumption to nearly 120 liters annually. According to the WHO global status reports on alcohol and health, 95% of the population reported abstaining from alcohol [10, 13].

11.3.3 Obesity

The prevalence of obesity is increasing in the Moroccan population according to data on measured heights and weights. In 1984, 4.1% of the adult population was obese, and the prevalence increased to 13.3% in 2000 [12, 13].

11.3.4 Other Risk Factors

The relevance of BRCA1/2 mutations in the Moroccan population was not studied.
    Morocco is one of the low to intermediate endemic areas for hepatitis B virus (HBV) infection. However, no reports have been published on Occult HBV infection [10].

11.4 Cancer Screening Programs

The first Moroccan cancer plan (2010–2019) has given the priority to breast and cervix cancers [10, 13, 14]. For breast cancer, the program is based on clinical breast examination. In case of clinical abnormalities, patients are referred to the provincial diagnostic centers for digital mammography, breast ultrasound, and biopsy. The target age of the early detection program was 45–69 years. But in 2016, the age of initiation was lowered to 40 years [10]. For cervical cancers, the population-based screening program is based on visual inspection with acetic acid [10]. But in the private sector, the population with health insurance has a large access to mammography, cervical smear, colonoscopy, and prostate-specific antigen dosing.
    The Ministry of Health and the Lalla Salma Foundation organize annual campaigns called October Rose dedicated to breast cancer screening. Screening by mammography is widely available in all regions. The other cancers do not benefit from regular screening campaigns [10].

11.5 Cancer Prevention Programs

Cancer prevention policies are mentioned in the Moroccan cancer plan. However, so far cancer prevention actions are rare. The Moroccan Health Authorities and The Lalla Salma Foundation launches regular mass media campaigns to promote healthy lifestyles. For tobacco-induced cancers, a specific program exists focusing on promoting the tobacco-free area in the companies, universities, and high schools. For cervical cancer, the Ministry of Health planned to introduce the HPV vaccination in 2021. Concerning HBV vaccination is free as part of the National Vaccination Program [10].

11.6   Cancer Diagnosis

The diagnostic imaging infrastructure in the public sector includes 75 mammography machines, 56 CT scanners, eight MRI machines, one PET scanner, and seven nuclear medicine services. Endoscopy, bronchoscopy, and cystoscopy are in general available in all the regional public health centers. There are 31 pathology laboratories in the public sector but not all provide the complete panel of immunohisto-chemistry. Immunohistochemistry is in general more available in university hospitals and in private sectors [13, 14]. Biomolecular testings such as EGFR, ALK, HER, and BRAF are available in the main cancer centers [10].

11.7   Treatment

Cancer treatment is based on four primary disciplines: Surgical oncology, Radiation oncology, Medical oncology, and Palliative care. The cancer health care system (2020) in Morocco includes

- 11 Public Hospitals (6 university clinics), the major ones are the Institut National d'Oncologie (Rabat) and Mohammed VI Cancer Center in Casablanca
- 16 Private centers

The healthcare system is characterized by inequity medical insurance that covers only 40% of the population. A medical assistance plan called RAMED was launched in 2012 by the Moroccan authorities for the benefit of the low-income population with an aim of giving them free access to all health care services provided by public hospitals. Those patients who are not eligible for RAMED and not covered by health insurances need to pay for healthcare in public centers.

11.7.1   Medical Oncology

The medical oncologist specializes in diagnosing and treating cancer using chemotherapy, hormonal therapy, biological therapy, and targeted therapy. Moreover, the physician may coordinate treatment given by other specialists and give supportive care.

In Morocco, Medical Oncology (MO) is a relatively new specialty. Medical Oncology was recognized as a separate specialty by the Ministry of Health in 1994. However, the creation of the first chair of medical oncology at the University of Rabat was done in 2000. In 2020, overall, 150 medical oncologists are working in Morocco (mainly with a mixed training in Morocco and France or Belgium) [15]. The classical chemotherapies, hormonal therapies, and the first generation of monoclonal antibodies, i.e., Trastuzumab, Rituximab, Bevacizumab, Cetuximab, etc., are widely available for the entire population. Two immunotherapies are available in Morocco: Pembrolizumab and Atezolizumab, though their reimbursement is still conflictual. The access to immunotherapy is accorded based on an individual's assessment for each candidate patient by the National Health Insurance Agency.

Hyperthermic Intraperitoneal Chemotherapy (HIPEC) was first performed in 2014 and is now available at one public center (National Institute of Oncology in Rabat) and two private clinics in Rabat and Casablanca [21]. Stem Cells Transplantation (both autologous and allogeneic) are available in the main cities (Rabat, Casablanca, Fes, and Marrakech).

11.7.2 Radiation Therapy

The radiotherapy infrastructure and human resources available in public health services include 17 linear accelerators (LINAC), 3 brachytherapy units, 9 treatment planning systems, 9 CT simulators. In the private sector, linear accelerators with VMAT or IMRT techniques are available in Casablanca, Rabat, Kenitra, Marrakech, Tangier, Meknes, Fez, and Oujda. Radiosurgery has started with a gamma knife in Rabat. But nowadays, Stereotactic Body Radiation Therapy (SBRT) is operational in major cities [13].

11.7.3 Surgery

Morocco has made significant progress in the surgical treatment of cancer in the past 30 years. In the 1980s, oncological surgery was performed almost exclusively in two university hospitals in Rabat and Casablanca. In 1985, the National Institute of Oncology was created in Rabat, the first center dedicated to the treatment of cancers in the country. It included the first department specializing in Surgical Oncology, which treated gynecological, digestive, urological, ENT, and Soft tissue cancers. From the mid-1990s, four new university hospital centers were created in Fez, Marrakech, Oujda, and Tangiers. It helped to train more surgeons capable of performing surgical oncology in more areas in the country. In 2018, it was estimated that major oncological surgeries such as breast or colonic resections, could be performed in 35 public centers [16]. In addition, two departments specializing in gyneco-mammary oncological surgery were opened in Casablanca and Rabat, and another specializing in digestive oncological surgery was opened in Rabat. The surgical offer in the private sector has also grown over the past 20 years, with two private university hospitals in Rabat and Casablanca and at least 16 private oncology clinics, mainly in major cities, with more private university hospitals and oncology clinics are under preparation. Advanced surgical techniques and technologies have been introduced in Morocco in the last 20 years. Advanced minimally invasive techniques are now routinely performed for colorectal, liver, gynecologic, thoracic, and urologic cancers [17–20]. The first surgical robot was acquired by the university hospital in Fez in 2019.

There are also ongoing liver transplantation programs in university hospitals in Morocco. The first case of successful liver transplantation performed by a Moroccan team was reported in 2016 [21]. There is an ongoing program for living donor liver transplantation for liver cancers at the National Institute in Rabat.

11.7.4   Pediatric Oncology

Nearly 1000 new cases per year of pediatric cancer are diagnosed in Morocco. Among them, the incidence of leukemia is estimated to be 100 new cases per year [22]. Pediatric cancer patients are mostly managed by public hospitals. The pediatric cancer units exist in university hospitals [23]. Since 2019, the Moroccan Health Ministry has been considering pediatric cancer management as a priority.

11.7.5   Survivorship Track

Data about cancer survival is scarce, and only a few published studies reported survival outcomes of cancer patients. Most of the published data concern breast and rectal cancers. For breast cancer, Mouh et al. compared outcomes between triple-negative and non-triple-negative patients in Rabat. Three years disease-free survival rates for the local disease were 76% and 83%, respectively [24]. Slaoui et al. compared survival outcomes between young and aged patients in Rabat. The 5-year disease-free Survival of patients with local disease was 64.6% in young women and 71.5% in older women with breast cancer (p = 0.04) [25]. Finally, the 5-year survival rate of patients with Breast cancer treated at the National Institute of Oncology in Rabat in 2009 was 81.5% [13].

For rectal cancer, Souadka et al. reported in 2015 the survival data for patients who had abdominoperineal resections for low rectal adenocarcinoma at the National Institute of Oncology in Rabat. The 5-year overall survival and disease-free survival rate were 74.6% and 60.3% respectively. Local and distant recurrences occurred respectively in 10 (6.8%) and 29 (20%) patients [26]. In 2019, the same team reported survival after surgery for mid and low rectal cancers. The overall survival rate after 1 year, 2 years, and 3 years are 94%, 89.1%, and 82.8%, respectively. Predictive factors of impaired survival were high age and advanced T stage [27].

11.7.6   Palliative Care Track

The first national plan against cancer identified several issues in access to palliative care in Morocco [10]:

- Insufficient training of healthcare workers in the palliative care field
- Lack of human resources

- Absence of terminal palliative care
- Insufficient follow-up of the patients after return to the home

In 2013, Morocco changed the law concerning the distribution of morphine by increasing the number of days' prescription for opioid analgesic (7–15 days) [24]. However, till now, palliative care activities are rudimentary. Only the city of Casablanca has developed a regional network for palliative and terminal care with the possibility of home care by a mobile team. According to a national survey published by Ettahri et al in 2017, the number of palliative care units in Morocco was only three with a total of 48 beds [28].

11.8 Research and Education

11.8.1 Research

Research in oncology is mainly performed in universities and university hospitals in Morocco. A step forward was made in 2014, by the creation of The Institute for Research in Oncology (IRC), with the goal of promoting and coordinating the national research efforts in oncology. Since its creation, IRC has funded more than 40 research projects and created a network for researchers in oncology called "IRC Research Associates" with a mission to facilitate collaboration and coordination between researchers in oncology in Morocco. More recently, IRC launched the ambitious "Moroccan Oncology Big data" project, a multidisciplinary initiative that includes the creation of the first national biobank, OMICS in oncology research and a digital pathology research platform. Despite these initiatives, oncology research in Morocco is still fragmented, uncoordinated with lower scientific production compared to other countries in the Arab world [30]. Few Phase II trials were published by Moroccan teams. There is no local phase III trial conducted in Morocco, however, the main cancer centers had already participated in international trials.

11.8.2 Education

Undergraduate medical education in Morocco starts after passing a competitive exam. Five public and two private faculties of medicine are offering basic and postgraduate medical education in Morocco. Undergraduate medical education in morocco is organized as follows [29]:

1. 1st cycle is for 2 years and consists of pre-clinical sciences
2. 2nd cycle: 3 years of clinical sciences
3. Sixth year: externship full time at the hospital.
4. Seventh year: internship
5. Thesis

Access to medical specialty training (also called residency) in oncology is possible for:

- Medical oncology (Rabat, Casablanca, Marrakech, Fes, Oujda and Tanger)
- Radiotherapy (Rabat, Casablanca, Marrakech, Fes, Oujda and Tanger)

None of the Moroccan faculties offers direct training in surgical oncology. They provide General surgery certification.

The access to residency training is done in two ways [29]:

- Through Internship Exam: Students who have successfully completed their 5th year and all training should sit for the Internship Exam and complete a 2-year internship at the University Hospital after which they are called residents. They are given priority in choosing the specialty.
- Through the Residency exam: Doctor of medicine after graduation can pass residency entrance exam and can start his/her medical residency training.

The duration of Morocco medical residency training varies from 4 to 5 years (4 years for medical specialties and biology, 5 years for surgical specialties and internal medicine).

11.9 Cost-Effective Cancer Care

The pharmaco-economy is not well developed in Morocco. Despite the existence of a medical society for health technology assessment, published articles in this field are rare.

11.10 Challenges and Advantages

Many achievements in cancer diagnosis and treatment in Morocco were achieved during the past 20 years. The country has improved its infrastructure from primary to tertiary care, allowing a wider part of the population to access specialized cancer care and successful screening programs for breast and cervix cancers were launched. The major achievement was the strong commitment of the Moroccan government to ensure the implementation of the National Plan for Cancer Prevention and Control 2010–2019; an ambitious plan covering all the aspects of cancer care from prevention, diagnosis, treatment, and management. With the collaboration of non-profit organizations such as the Lalla Salma Foundation for Cancer Prevention and Treatment, donors, and international organizations such as the World Health Organization and the International Agency for Research on Cancer, the International Atomic Energy Agency, and the United Nations Population Fund, Morocco ensured a strong political and financial support of the Plan during the past 10 years [13]. Figure 11.1 shows the evolution of the number of public cancer centers from 2004 to 2020.

However, there are still many challenges ahead that need to be addressed. First, cancer patients are still mainly diagnosed at late stages. Early screening programs for breast and cervix cancers should be enhanced to increase population access.

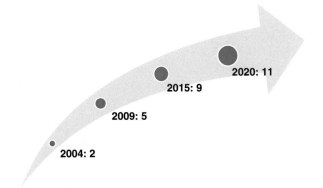

Fig. 11.1 The evolution of the number of public cancer centers from 2004 to 2020

Screening programs should also be expanded to other cancers such as colorectal cancer. Moreover, palliative care also needs to be improved and expanded to more Moroccan cancer patients. Finally, survival data is lacking for most cancers, which does not allow us to adequately evaluate the ongoing cancer programs.

The Moroccan government has recently validated the National Plan for Cancer Prevention and Control 2020–2029 with a specific focus on prevention and screening programs, improvement in national cancer management, investment in information technology, and advanced research programs. The Moroccan Government has committed in 2020 to make cancer care a national priority. A strong decision was made to create a national agency dedicated to the management of cancer care in Morocco under the presidency of the Prime Minister.

11.11 The Future of Cancer Care in Morocco

11.11.1 Quality Improvement

Standardization of cancer care is another challenge to improve patients' outcomes. Few guidelines for cancer management are produced by scientific societies, however, they are not endorsed by the authorities. There is a need for standardization of care to improve patients' outcomes.

11.11.2 Information Systems

The improvement at the national level of cancer care cannot be done without an efficient collection, analysis, and reporting system. The adoption of oncology information systems was late in Morocco. The National Institute of Oncology in Rabat was the first to set up a Hospital Information System (HIS), quickly followed by the regional oncology centers in Casablanca, Tangier, Benimellal, and soon in Agadir and Laayoune. This has made possible the streamline of the patient pathway, the improvement of traceability and information sharing, and the improvement of prescribing safety, particularly for cytotoxic drugs. The generalization of Hospital Information System (HIS) adoption is a fundamental step to improve patient care. It must include not only tertiary centers but also primary and secondary centers to coordinate the patient pathway from prevention, screening, treatment, and follow-up. This generalization is under evaluation in the country.

11.12   Conclusion

In the last 20 years, Morocco has improved cancer care with strong investments in infrastructure, human resources training, awareness, and screening programs. The adoption of the National Plan for Cancer Prevention and Control 2010–2019 was a major step forward by the Moroccan government to reach these achievements. Many challenges remain, such as early cancer diagnosis, follow-up pathways, investment in information technology, and better national management of cancer care. The strong commitment of the Moroccan Government and substantial collaboration with oncologists and international organizations, are major assets for Morocco to reach the goals of the next National Plan for Cancer Prevention and Control 2020–2029.

Conflict of Interest   Authors have no conflict of interest to declare.

References

1. High Commission for Planning (HCP). Final results of the national survey on demographic repeated passage in 2014. 2014
2. https://gco.iarc.fr/today/data/factsheets/populations/504-morocco-fact-sheets.pdf
3. https://www.worldbank.org/en/country/morocco/overview
4. Bouchbika Z, Haddad H, Benchakroun N, Eddakaoui H, Kotbi S, Megrini A, Bourezgui H, Sahraoui S, Corbex M, Harif M, Benider A. Cancer incidence in Morocco: report from Casablanca registry 2005-2007. Pan Afr Med J. 2013;29:16–31.
5. Tazi MA, Er-Raki A, Benjaafar N. Cancer incidence in Rabat, Morocco: 2006-2008. Ecancermedicalscience. 2013;7:338.
6. Lachgar A, Tazi MA, Afif M, Er-Raki A, Kebdani T, Benjaafar N. Lung cancer: incidence and survival in Rabat, Morocco. Rev Epidemiol Sante Publique. 2016;64(6):391–5.
7. Errihani H, Inrhaoun H, Boukir A, Kettani F, Gamra L, Mestari A, Jabri L, Bensouda Y, Mrabti H, Elghissassi I. Frequency and type of epidermal growth factor receptor mutations in Moroccan patients with lung adenocarcinoma. J Thorac Oncol. 2013;8(9):1212–4.
8. Khalil AI, Bendahhou K, Mestaghanmi H, Saile R, Benider A. Breast cancer in Morocco: phenotypic profile of tumors. Pan Afr Med J. 2016;6(25):74.
9. Mechita NB, Tazi MA, Er-Raki A, Mrabet M, Saadi A, Benjaafar N, Razine R. Survie au cancer du sein à Rabat (Maroc) 2005-2008 [Survival rate for breast cancer in Rabat (Morocco) 2005-2008]. Pan Afr Med J. 2016;25:144.
10. http://www.contrelecancer.ma/en/le_pnpcc
11. Fakhfakh R. Tobacco control in three north African countries: Tunisia, Algeria and Morocco. Tob Induc Dis. 2019;17(1):44.

12. El Rhazi K, Nejjari C, Zidouh A, Bakkali R, Berraho M, Gateau PB. Prevalence of obesity and associated sociodemographic and lifestyle factors in Morocco. Public Health Nutr. 2011;14(1):160–7.
13. Selmouni F, Zidouh A, Belakhel L, Sauvaget C, Bennani M, Khazraji YC, Benider A, Wild CP, Bekkali R, Fadhil I, Sankaranarayanan R. Tackling cancer burden in low-income and middle-income countries: Morocco as an exemplar. Lancet Oncol. 2018;19(2):93–101.
14. Basu P, Selmouni F, Belakhel L, Sauvaget C, Abousselham L, Lucas E, Muwonge R, Sankaranarayanan R, Khazraji YC. Breast cancer screening program in Morocco: status of implementation, organization and performance. Int J Cancer. 2018;143(12):3273–80.
15. Boutayeb S, Taleb A, Belbaraka R, Ismaili N, Berrada N, Allam W, et al. The practice of medical oncology in Morocco: the National Study of the Moroccan Group of Trialist in medical oncology (EVA-Onco). ISRN Oncol. 2013;2013:1–4.
16. Hrora A, Majbar AM, Elalaoui M, Raiss M, Sabbah F, Ahallat M. Risk factors for conversion and morbidity during initial experience in laparoscopic proctectomies: a retrospective study. Indian J Surg. 2017 Apr;79(2):90–5.
17. Majbar AM, Abid M, Alaoui M, Sabbah F, Raiss M, Ahallat M, Hrora A. Impact of conversion to open surgery on early postoperative morbidity after laparoscopic resection for rectal adenocarcinoma: a retrospective study. J Laparoendosc Adv Surg Tech A. 2016;26(9):697–701.
18. Serji B, Souadka A, Benkabbou A, Hachim H, Jaiteh L, Mohsine R, et al. Feasibility and safety of laparoscopic adrenalectomy for large tumours. Arab J Urol. 2016;14(2):143–6.
19. Benkabbou A, Souadka A, Serji B, Hachim H, El Malki HO, Mohsine R, Ifrine L, Belkouchi A. Laparoscopic liver resection: initial experience in a north-African single center. Tunis Med. 2015;93(8–9):523–6.
20. Rabiou S, Lakranbi M, Ghizlane T, Elfatemi H, Serraj M, Ouadnouni Y, Smahi M. Quelle chirurgie pour quelle tumeur du médiastin: expérience du service de chirurgie thoracique de CHU Hassan II de Fès [Which surgery for mediastinum tumor: experience of the Department of thoracic surgery of CHU Hassan II of Fès]. Rev Pneumol Clin. 2017;73(5):246–52.
21. Benkabbou A, Awab AM, Koraichi A, Souadka A, Alilou M, Sbihi L, Moatassim N, Rhou H, Afifi R, Essaid A, Belkouchi A. First case of successful liver transplantation performed by a Moroccan team. Arab J Gastroenterol. 2016;17(1):1–2.
22. Howard SC, Zaidi A, Cao X, Weil O, Bey P, Patte C, Samudio A, Haddad L, Lam CG, Moreira C, Pereira A, Harif M, Hessissen L, Choudhury S, Fu L, Caniza MA, Lecciones J, Traore F, Ribeiro RC, Gagnepain-Lacheteau A. The my child matters programme: effect of public-private partnerships on paediatric cancer care in low-income and middle-income countries. Lancet Oncol. 2018;19(5):252–66.
23. Hessissen L, Madani A. Pediatric oncology in Morocco: achievements and challenges. J Pediatr Hematol Oncol. 2012 Mar;34(Suppl 1):S21–2.
24. Mouh FZ, Slaoui M, Razine R, El Mzibri M, Amrani M. Clinicopathological, treatment and event-free survival characteristics in a moroccan population of triple-negative breast cancer. Breast Cancer (Auckl). 2020;14:1178223420906428. https://doi.org/10.1177/1178223420906428. eCollection 2020
25. Slaoui M, Mouh FZ, Ghanname I, Razine R, El Mzibri M, Amrani M. Outcome of breast cancer in Moroccan young women correlated to clinic-pathological features, risk factors and treatment: a comparative study of 716 cases in a single institution. PLoS One. 2016;11(10):e0164841.
26. Souadka A, Majbar MA, El Harroudi T, Benkabbou A, Souadka A. Perineal pseudocontinent colostomy is safe and efficient technique for perineal reconstruction after abdominoperineal resection for rectal adenocarcinoma. BMC Surg. 2015 Dec;15(1):40.
27. Essangri H, Majbar MA, Benkabbou A, Amrani L, Belkhadir Z, Ghennam A, Al Ahmadi B, Bougtab A, Mohsine R, Souadka A. Predictive factors of oncological and survival outcome of surgery on mid and low rectal adenocarcinoma in Morocco: single center study. J Med Surg Res. 2019;1(1):627–35.
28. Ettahri H, Berrada N, Tahir A, Elkabous M, Mrabti H, Errihani H. Palliative care, a reel challenge in income and middle countries. Example of Morocco. J Palliat Care Med. 2017;7(5):316.
29. Fourtassi M, Abda N, Bentata Y, Hajjioui A. Medical education in Morocco: current situation and future challenges. Med Teach. 2020;42(9):973–9.
30. https://www.irc.ma/en

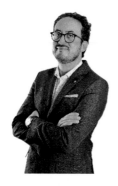

Saber Boutayeb is a Moroccan medical oncologist. He obtained his certification in medical oncology in 2008 after mixed training in Rabat and Paris and holds a Ph.D. in Clinical Epidemiology from the University Mohammed V (Rabat, Morocco). He currently serves as Manager of the Chemotherapy Day Hospital and co-referent of information systems at the Moroccan Institut National d'Oncologie. There, he specializes in treating gastrointestinal and breast cancers. In addition, he also holds a university position as Professor in Medical Oncology at University Mohammed V (Rabat, Morocco).

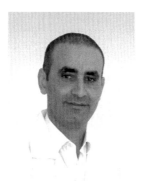

Mohammed Anass Majbar is a Moroccan surgeon. He obtained his certification in general surgery in 2011 after mixed training in Rabat and Paris and holds a level 2 master's in mini-invasive surgery and new technologies from Italy. He currently works as a surgeon in the Digestive Surgical Oncology department at the Moroccan Institut National d'Oncologie, with a focus on colorectal cancer and mini-invasive surgery. He is also a co-referent of information systems at the same institution. In addition, he holds a university position as Professor in general surgery at University Mohammed V (Rabat, Morocco).

Chapter 12
General Oncology Care in Oman

Itrat Mehdi ⓘ, Abdul Aziz Al Farsi, Bassim Al Bahrani,
and Shadha S. Al-Raisi

12.1 Oman Demographics

The Sultanate of Oman is an Arab country, bordering Saudi Arabia, UAE, and Yemen. The total area of Oman is about 309,500 km². Oman is more densely populated in its cities, where 80% of the population lives. The current population of Oman is 5,462,006 as of December 2020, males 3,222,910 (59%) and females 2,239,097 (41%), and rank 120 in the Global list [1–3]. The population density in Oman is 16 per km². The median age in Oman is 30.6 years (Fig. 12.1). Life Expectancy is 77.4 years, while the Population growth rate is 3.4% annually. The country has a fertility rate of 2.92 births per woman, as one of the fastest-growing populations [1, 2, 4]. Current projections believe that the growth rate will peak in 2020. After 2025 the growth rate will continue to slow, getting down to 0.62% by 2050 [4, 5].

Oman is an ethnically diverse country. There are 38.7% foreigners, mostly expatriate workers from Bangladesh, India, Pakistan, Philippines, and Egypt. Oman has a mortality rate of 3.3 deaths per 1000 populations. It is a relatively young population with 65% less than 30 years of age (Fig. 12.1). The literacy rate in Oman is 93%. The economy is based on agriculture, fishing, and overseas trading. Petroleum revenues account for 40% of GDP. The per capita income is 41,680 dollars [4, 6, 7].

I. Mehdi (✉) · A. A. Al Farsi · B. Al Bahrani
National Oncology Centre, The Royal Hospital, Muscat, Oman
e-mail: bassim.albahrani@moh.om

S. S. Al-Raisi
Department of Non-Communicable Diseases, Ministry of Health, Muscat, Oman

© The Author(s) 2022
H. O. Al-Shamsi et al. (eds.), *Cancer in the Arab World*,
https://doi.org/10.1007/978-981-16-7945-2_12

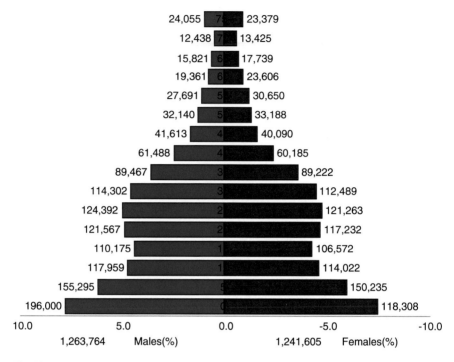

24,055 7 23,379
12,438 7 13,425
15,821 6 17,739
19,361 6 23,606
27,691 5 30,650
32,140 5 33,188
41,613 4 40,090
61,488 4 60,185
89,467 3 89,222
114,302 3 112,489
124,392 2 121,263
121,567 2 117,232
110,175 1 106,572
117,959 1 114,022
155,295 5 150,235
196,000 0 118,308

| 10.0 | 5.0 | 0.0 | -5.0 | -10.0 |
| | 1,263,764   Males(%) | | 1,241,605   Females(%) | |

Fig. 12.1 Population pyramid Oman 2017 (Used With Permission from MoH Oman) [3]

12.2 Cancer Statistics in Oman

Cancer is the leading cause of death with 6% of disease-related mortality [8]. The age-adjusted annual incidence of cancer ranges from 70 to 110 per 100,000 population, which is lower than other regional countries [9, 10]. The leading male cancers in order of prevalence are prostate, colorectal, liver, hematologic, gastric, and lung (Fig. 12.2). The leading female cancers in order of prevalence are breast, thyroid, colo-rectum, hematologic, and uterine (Table 12.3 and Fig. 12.3) [3, 5, 6, 11]. The already known and established risk factors for any cancer are diet, smoked and charcoal prepared food (Gastric Cancer and Colon Cancer), higher life expectancy, obesity, smoking, and diabetes [12].

An increasing number of patients are diagnosed with cancer every successive year (Fig. 12.2, Tables 12.1 and 12.2) [6]. The number of cancer cases registered in 2017 was 2101. Of these, 1892 (90.05%) were among Omanis (1005 females, 887 males), and 188 (8.95%) were among Non-Omanis (123 females, 65 males). One hundred and twenty-seven cases (6.7%) were reported in people aged below 14 years. The median age at cancer diagnosis was 53 years. The crude incidence rates for cancer in Oman were 70.2 per 100,000 for males and 80.9 per 100,000 for females. The Age Standardized Rate (ASR) was 113.3 per 100,000 for males and 114.2 per 100,000 for females. A total reported 193 males and 173 females died of

Yeras	2005	2006	2007	2008	2009	2010	2011	2012	2013	2014	2015	2016	2017
Frequency	958	903	939	964	1,020	1,059	1,346	1,309	1,426	1,537	1,726	1,880	1,892

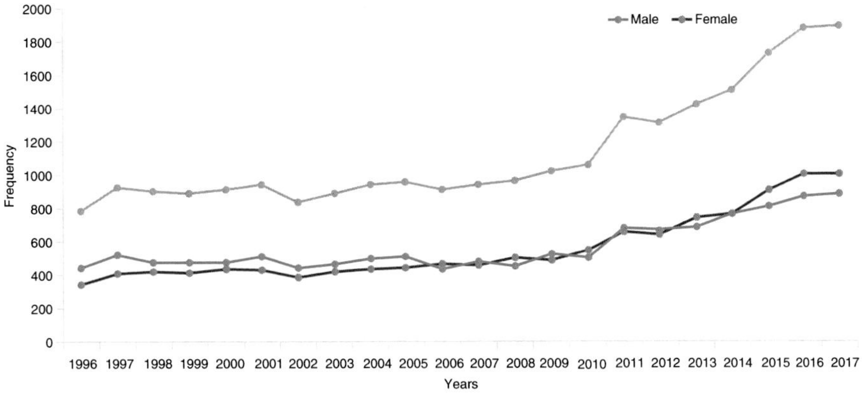

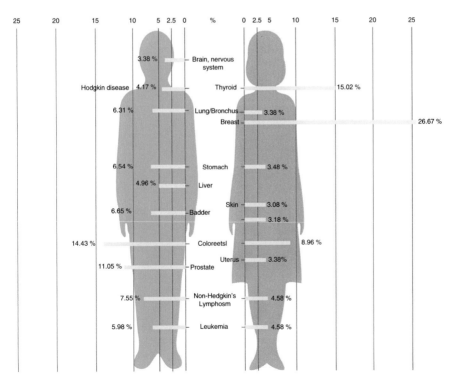

Fig. 12.2 Cancer trends 1996–2017 (used with permission from MoH Oman) [3]

Fig. 12.3 Ten most common cancers in Oman 2017 [6]

Table 12.1 Male cancers Oman 1996–2017 [3, 6]

Site	2005	2006	2007	2008	2009	2010	2011	2012	2013	2014	2015	2016	2017
Stomach	54	43	36	33	50	33	58	65	55	56	47	57	58
Lung and bronchi	30	30	40	29	30	25	44	33	42	50	45	57	56
Colon and rectum	37	37	32	29	42	43	63	71	71	71	88	81	128
Liver	34	18	20	30	18	19	29	34	31	57	51	67	44
Prostate	40	29	55	41	48	49	68	84	83	83	93	98	98
U. Bladder	28	27	33	25	26	36	35	35	48	53	43	50	59
NHL	43	41	43	45	41	41	57	54	55	62	68	64	67
CNS	17	10	14	14	23	18	20	29	18	29	24	31	30
Kidney	12	6	5	7	18	22	14	15	16	26	21	15	17
Leukemia	41	38	37	45	46	42	66	35	40	53	57	54	53
Esophagus	12	11	9	5	8	15	10	10	10	15	10	7	11
Pancreas	7	6	5	8	10	14	17	16	23	13	18	22	26
Skin	18	17	24	25	29	22	25	27	36	24	24	33	26
HL	14	20	11	18	17	17	23	27	20	25	30	36	37
Thyroid	10	6	7	12	13	3	12	17	19	32	31	46	29

Table 12.2 Frequency of female cancers 1996–2017 [3, 6]

Site	2005	2006	2007	2008	2009	2010	2011	2012	2013	2014	2015	2016	2017
Breast	99	101	108	125	124	139	164	159	182	174	220	272	268
Stomach	33	28	18	15	24	23	25	29	31	34	23	26	35
Lung and bronchi	9	13	6	11	15	18	14	20	17	16	19	16	34
Colon and rectum	21	25	32	30	36	36	39	59	52	72	70	78	90
Liver	9	11	4	5	16	15	10	14	17	32	29	35	20
Uterus	7	9	10	13	13	14	24	15	17	19	24	30	26
Cervix	26	30	25	30	13	36	31	26	26	32	34	34	32
U. Bladder	9	15	10	10	10	9	8	11	9	15	12	16	15
NHL	26	23	27	30	31	41	42	29	35	33	57	46	46
CNS	10	13	11	14	12	20	14	8	13	18	20	30	35
Kidney	11	4	6	17	8	9	21	10	16	15	17	10	17
Leukemia	23	23	30	38	26	33	32	34	37	46	42	36	46
Esophagus	5	6	1	6	8	5	4	9	3	3	5	3	3
Pancreas	8	4	11	7	4	5	8	9	15	11	11	12	14
Skin	17	15	11	18	21	26	24	21	25	20	36	29	31
HL	8	5	9	15	11	14	23	10	21	15	17	17	14
Thyroid	36	40	38	40	52	40	75	75	111	96	144	164	151

Table 12.3 Frequency of cancers 2017 [6]

Male			Female		
Topography	Frequency	Percentage	Topography	Frequency	Percentage
Colo-rectal	128	14.43	Breast	268	26.67
Prostate	98	11.05	Thyroid	151	15.02
Non-Hodgkin lymphoma	67	7.55	Colo-rectal	90	8.96
Urinary bladder	59	6.65	Non-Hodgkin lymphoma	46	4.58
Stomach	58	6.54	Leukemia	46	4.58
Bronchi and lung	56	6.31	Stomach	35	3.48
Leukemia	53	5.98	Uterus	34	3.38
Liver	44	4.96	Bronchi and lung	34	3.38
Hodgkin's lymphoma	37	4.17	Uterine cervix	32	3.18
Brain and nervous system	30	3.38	Skin	31	3.08

cancer in 2017 [3]. According to GLOBOCAN, the projected new cancer cases expected in 2030 and 2040 are 5761 and 8549 in Oman [5]. Over time, changing trends of incidence have been observed, as colorectal cancer has surpassed stomach cancer, lung cancer is being diagnosed 2–3 times more frequently, thyroid cancer in females has increased five times [6] (Table 12.3).

12.3 Healthcare System in Oman

Oman spent around 2.6% of its GDP (11% of the budget) on health care, rising by 12.9% annually. It is not possible to specifically tell about the amount spent in oncology. Firstly, the MoH and Ministry of Education are involved in cancer care services. Secondly, the diagnostic, screening, and treatment facilities are done by different sections of MoH. Oman has 69 hospitals (as in 2016), with a total of over 6400 beds, which are expected to grow at an annual rate of 3.1%. Only two hospitals have a cancer care services unit. The government operates 80% of hospitals [13–16]. The Omani government is inclined to increase the role of the private health sector, to cope with the increasing demand. New hospitals like Sultan Qaboos Medical City in Muscat, along with International Medical City in Salalah will contribute to meeting the increasing demand. The population growth is putting additional pressure on the health care system. An estimated 95% of the population now live within five miles of a medical center. Cancer care services visited in Oman are high, as the public healthcare system is free. This is saturating the system and increases healthcare costs. Omani nationals have free access to healthcare, though expatriates seek medical care in private hospitals. The insurance-financed healthcare and private hospitals are still far from comprehensive and do not cover all cancer treatment like expensive targeted therapy, and immunotherapy. There are NGOs and private charities which do help a number of patients [17].

In 2014, the government commenced a long-term plan for the healthcare sector entitled Health Vision 2050; including extension of existing cancer care services, establishment of two comprehensive care hospitals, and satellite oncology units [13, 14, 17]. The plan, which according to the World Health Organisation (WHO) serves "as a model for strategic planning in health," envisions large-scale investment in the healthcare sector to create a well-organized, equitable, efficient, and responsive health system. The Health Vision 2050 has pointed out the need to move part of cancer care out of the hospitals and closer to communities and homes, for better service and reduced burden. Oman requires an additional 7000 doctors by 2050. The country now has an accredited medical university and many Omani doctors have obtained their postgraduate medical training overseas in Australia, Canada, the United Kingdom, and the United States.

12.4 Oncology Care in Oman

12.4.1 Access to Cancer Care services

There is an integrated system of primary, secondary, and tertiary medical facilities with a reasonably well-organized referral system by e-referral portal of MoH. All hospitals are interlinked, and the patient's electronic medical records can be accessed by the treating team from anywhere. The MoH through treatment abroad committee sends patients abroad or to GCC for a treatment modality if it is not locally available. A small number of patients travel abroad on their own expenses, often treated at more than one center and in more than one country.

12.4.2 Multi-sectoral Efforts to Prevent and Control Cancer

The Ministry of Education, social welfare, environmental health, PDO all support a coordinated effort for prevention and control of cancer. Cancer prevention strategies include health education, vaccinations (HPV, Hepatitis), and regular primary health care follow-ups. There is an integrated referral pathway from primary to tertiary care. The treatment facility including oncology surgery, radiation oncology, stereotactic radiotherapy, systemic therapy, bone marrow transplant, and liver transplant is available. There are specialized sub-specialty hospitals for ENT, neurosurgery, dermatology, and orthopedics. There are oncology outreach clinics in Salalah. The prime pathology is Royal hospital for the main focal and referral point. The patients who are cured of cancer follow in an outpatient clinic as per protocol and long-term survivors are followed in survivorship clinics or shifted to tertiary/primary care. A dedicated palliative care team is there for pain management, palliative symptom care, and end-of-life care once the patient is transited to palliative symptomatic care [18, 19].

12.4.3   National Oncology Center: The Royal Hospital

The National Oncology Center (NOC) is the oldest center established in December 2004 by MoH, as an extension of the Royal Hospital in Muscat. The NOC comprises medical oncology, radiation oncology, hemato-oncology and BMT, pediatric hematology, and oncology. The center treats around 70% of all cancer cases in Oman. There are sub-specialty clinics for breast and gastrointestinal tumors. Combined clinics for breast, ear-nose-and-throat, gynae-oncology, pain clinics, and outreach clinics are routinely held. There is a multidisciplinary tumor board. Psycho-social support is available by social workers, counseling nurses, occupational therapists, speech therapists, and dieticians. The patients are given free accommodation during their treatment. The treatment facility for treatment, which is free of charge, is available to Omani nationals only. The NOC is a designated and approved center for Integrated Palliative care by ESMO (European Society for Medical Oncology) and is an approved center with UICC (Union Internationale Cancer Control).

12.4.4   Other Cancer Centers

As infectious diseases have been effectively abridged, Oman is now contending with the rise in Non-communicable diseases like diabetes, obesity, hypertension, and cancer. The hospitals in Oman provide high-quality healthcare. There are two cancer care hospitals in Muscat, The Royal Hospital, and the Sultan Qaboos University Hospital. The healthcare system is primarily in the public sector; the Ministry of Health (MoH), is the main health care provider especially the oncology services [14, 17, 20]. The MoH provides healthcare in a 3-tiered system: primary health care centers, secondary hospitals, and tertiary referral hospitals. Private hospitals and clinics, licensed by the MoH, are playing an increasingly important role in cancer care like Burjeel hospital, NMC, Al Hayat, and Muscat private hospital [7, 13]. The two cancer centers are supported by ancillary diagnostic facilities like radiology, pathology, gastroenterology, urology, respiratory medicine, genetics center, nuclear and molecular imaging centers [21].

12.4.5   National Cancer Registry

The Oman National Cancer Registry, established in 1985 as a hospital registry, helps guide policymakers in setting priorities for cancer control activities. The registry began functioning as a population-based registry in 1996 and publishes an annual report on cancer incidence. Cancer diagnosis notification was made mandatory in 2001. The registry also collects data from treatment abroad committees and

Omani patients diagnosed in Qatar [3, 6]. In 2002 and 2007, the International Agency for Research on Cancer (IARC) published Oman's data in its publication "Cancer incidence in five continents volume VIII and IX," Oman being the second Arab nation to contribute. In October 2019, on the 20-year anniversary cancer registry released a comprehensive 20 years compilation of cancer data on the trends of cancers and the lists of the most common cancers, and the regional distribution of cancer cases [3, 6, 10, 16].

12.4.6 Community Obligations

NOC along with Oman Cancer Association (OCA) helps to provide professional guidance by advocating community wellness. NOC liaises between different hospitals, polyclinics, community nursing, and social welfare in the care of oncology patients by providing only logistic and financial support. It works in association with MoH and cancer center for conferences and is not doing any research work. There is a patient awareness group at NOC and is actively involved in community awareness programs for different cancers, through print and electronic media. There is a need to develop patient support groups with the participation of educated and willing patients to help patients in coping with a cancer diagnosis, treatment, and treatment-related side effects. Patients with cancers are liable to develop psychological issues especially depression, with a need to incorporate psychologist's advice and support in managing cancer patients [19].

12.4.7 The Cancer Care Plan

A cancer care plan is based on need assessment of population for convenient and high-quality care focusing patients. It emphasizes the need for prevention, easy access to services, and a road map for future improvements in services. There is a need to streamline existing cancer care services, focusing on patient needs to ensure a continuum of care. The major focus of efforts should be on providing state-of-the-art services and searching for new partners in the public and private sectors to facilitate prompt diagnosis and treatment. It also aims to increase the public understanding of a healthy lifestyle and risk factors, screening, early diagnosis, and prompt treatment. This should translate into improved survival and outcome, decreasing the burden on the health care system. There is a need to bridge the gap in research and clinical practice. There are many taboos and false beliefs in society due to cultural influences, which need to be addressed. The Individual Cancer Care Plan, made for patients by treating physicians at NOC, should facilitate communication between caregivers and families/patients, at every step of management to enhance confidence in the health system and help them cope with the disease. We monitor it by setting targets of performance indicators every year, with a vision to improve it. Efforts should be directed to facilitate the establishment of hospice and home care services. The patients need to be educated about hospice care, and enrolment in trials [6].

12.5 Cancer Risk Factors

In Oman, chronic Non-Communicable Diseases related to lifestyle like coronary artery diseases, hypertension, diabetes mellitus, and cancer; are now emerging as significant potential health challenges [21]. The aging population along with factors like obesity (53%), lack of physical activity, smoking (15%), Westernized lifestyle, change in diet, and other environmental factors contribute to an increased cancer incidence [6, 11]. The International Agency for Research on Cancer (IARC) predicted the doubling of cancer cases in the period 2008–2020 from 1400 to 2500 [22].

12.6 Cancer Screening Programs

A pre-emptive screening for common cancers is integral to improve diagnosis at an early stage, decrease disease burden, improve outcome, and is cost-effective. The MoH and OCA (Oman Cancer Association) run breast cancer screening by mobile mammography services, and a vast number of female patients benefit from it. An analysis of the impact of screening on early-stage detection was submitted for publication, which showed that T1 increased from 28.70% to 71.30%, while T4 decreased from 61.48% to 38.52%. The N0 increased from 32.75% to 67.25%. A comprehensive guideline for breast screening is developed available at www.mog. gov.om. A cancer colon and Hepatocellular screening in susceptible population groups is evolving. A comprehensive Genetic center is recently established under MoH where tests and genetic counseling services are available for hereditary and familial cancers [18].

12.7 Cancer Prevention Programs

In 2018, Oman launched its national policy and action plan for the prevention and control of Non-Communicable Diseases including Cancer. This multisector plan was developed to reduce mortality of NCDs by 25% in 2025 through reinforcing the cooperation between stakeholders from industry, education, information, Sports affairs, Regional municipalities, Council for planning, civil society, and international organizations [13, 17, 21, 23]. These include Oman anti-smoking society, Oman Medical Association, Oman Cancer Association, World Health Organization

(WHO), and UNICEF [7, 13]. In addition, several departments in the MoH help in planning, implementation, and monitoring of cancer control and prevention activities like the National Oncology Centre, the directorate general of primary healthcare, and the directorate general of specialized services. This helps to ensure a coordinated and integrated approach between primary, secondary, and tertiary services. HPV vaccination is available but not mandatory at present for everyone.

12.8   Cancer Diagnosis

The cancer care services are supported by sophisticated pathology services including molecular, Fluorescent in situ hybridization (FISH), Immunohistochemistry (IHC), and cytogenetic testing facility. Some genetic tests are sent abroad as well like RAS, BRAF, Oncotype DX, PIK3C, etc. Nuclear imaging centers provide PET scan, bone scan, densitometry, MIBG, PSMA PET, and other scans. A genetic center is established for specialized genetic tests and genetic counseling [24]. The challenges in diagnosis are access, coping up with demand, and limited availability.

12.9   Treatment

The oncology services in Oman started in 1990, the Medical Oncology department was established in 1996 at the Royal hospital, and subsequently, National Oncology center was established in 2004 at the Royal Hospital under MoH. It has expanded to meet the ever-growing needs of the community. Omani nationals have free access to cancer care services. This includes sophisticated diagnostic services up to PET Scans and most recently incorporated therapeutic modalities like targeted therapy, bone marrow transplant, and immunotherapy. Enrolment in Clinical trials is a legitimate treatment option for many diseases and patients. Unfortunately, in Oman, we do not have access to clinical trials as would be desired.

12.9.1   Medical Oncology

Two centers in Oman have a medical oncology and chemotherapy facility, the Royal hospital National Oncology Centre under MoH and Sultan Qaboos University hospital (Ministry of Higher Education). In addition, there are satellite units in Salalah and Sohar. These provide outpatient clinics, diagnostic services, daycare treatment, and inpatient facilities. The chemotherapies are prepared within the NOC Pharmacy. Most state-of-art treatment options are available locally in Oman. Several patients are sent abroad for specialized management at high-volume specialized institutes if the required services are not available locally [6, 9, 11].

12.9.2   Radiation Therapy

National Oncology Centre—The Royal Hospital is the only center with a radiation oncology facility at present, while Sultan Qaboos University Hospital (SQUH) is likely to start radiation therapy in the near future. The two facilities are concentrated in Muscat and patients travel from all over Oman for treatment. The NOC has facilities for IMRT (Intensity Modulated Radiotherapy), Brachytherapy, and SBRT (Stereotactic Body Radiation Therapy). There are two Linear accelerators in NOC and two more are planned to be installed in SQUH [6].

12.9.3   Surgery

Oncologic surgery is still an evolving specialty in Oman, with countable oncology surgeons. They are in breast, colo-rectal, osteo-oncology, hepatobiliary, faciomaxillary, gynecologic-oncology, and uro-oncology. There are multi-modality and multi-specialty combined clinics like breast, ENT, and neuro-oncology. There is a multidisciplinary forum like the tumor board for discussion and consensus decision-making as per current guidelines [11].

12.9.4   Pediatric Oncology

There are two pediatric oncology units, one in NOC Royal Hospital and the other in SQUH dealing with hematologic and solid tumors. They also have inpatient services, outpatient specialty clinics, and daycare facilities. Adolescent oncology is evolving as a further subspecialty with a dedicated trained consultant and team [11].

12.9.5   Survivorship Track

The outcome and survival in malignant diseases have improved, thus increasing the number of long-term cancer survivors. These patients need to follow up due to the risk of relapse, chances of subsequent tumors, long-term sequel of cancer treatment, and their affiliation to a primary cancer care team. A survivorship clinic is run by NOC on a regular basis to cater services to these patients [6].

12.9.6 Palliative Care Track

Cancer patients often present with advanced-stage disease in the developing world, shifting the aim of management from curative to a palliative intent. Oman lacks the required palliative and hospice care, resulting in an increased burden on existing cancer care facilities and compromising the desirable care of potentially treatable cancers. The idea of hospice care is still not morally, socially, or religiously very acceptable in society, probably due to closed integrated families [6, 9]. There is a policy of DNR approved by MoH, ethical experts, and religious factions.

12.10 Research and Education

MoH has set guidelines and priorities for research [25, 26]. NOC is actively involved in undergraduate and postgraduate teaching. NOC has organized one to two international oncology conferences every year since 2009. NOC made several presentations in international conferences and meetings and has published over 150 articles in international journals [27–55]. The research areas of interest at present are Microsatellite Instability, Mismatch Repairs, Colorectal Tumour Bank, Stomach cancer, Breast cancer molecular subtypes, Bevacizumab in Ovarian Cancer, anti-EGFR (epidermal growth factor receptor) in mCRC, utilization of palliative chemotherapy near the end of life, Changing Trends, Management outcomes and survival of Common Cancers, Castration-Resistant Prostate Cancer, the Effect of Diet and Obesity On Colonic Cancer, Impact of Body Mass Index, diet and diabetes on incidence, RAS mutation and clinical outcome of colorectal cancer, Synchronous and metachronous tumors, Chemotherapy induced Neutropenic necrotic Enterocolitis, Rapid Rituximab infusion, Young age Breast Cancer in Oman, Prognostic determinants of gastric cancer, Renal cell carcinoma metastasizing to larynx, Does Traditional WASAM (Cautery Burn) Therapy Facilitate an Early and Extensive Loco regional Metastasis of Breast Cancer?, Primary Gastric Choriocarcinoma, Lean philosophy within cancer-care service in Oman, Breast cancer in Kindlers syndrome, Non-traumatic avascular necrosis of femoral head, Lobbying for regulatory reforms of narcotic analgesics in Middle East, Epidemiology of Lung Cancer in Oman, Cancer Incidence in Oman (1996–2015), and 20-year trends of cancer incidence in Omanis. A lot of presentations, both oral and abstract, were done in local, regional, and international meetings in the Gulf region, Europe, and the USA. The important ones were Outpatient Cisplatin Administration, stress and fatigue in Breast cancer, Brain metastasis in Her-2 (human epidermal growth factor receptor 2) positive Breast cancer, and RAS mutations and ethnicity [27–55].

12.11   Cost-Effective Cancer Care

Effective and prompt management of cancer is increasingly challenged with the escalating cost of diagnosis and treatment with the incorporation of new modalities of diagnosis and integration of more effective drugs. The management has to be balanced with resource allocation and cost-effectiveness due to increasing economic pressures. The paradigm is shifting to cancer prevention, screening, and genetic screening to reduce the economic burden. A comprehensive genetic center was established recently for genetic testing and counseling. The early-stage diagnosis cut down the management cost and was observed with breast screening programs. We are seeing a higher proportion of early-stage curable, treatable breast cancer with less frequency of a relapse. Oman is therefore allocating resources to health education, genetic testing, prevention, and screening with the objective of early detection and cost-effectiveness. These potential programs include familial and genetically determined tumors like colon, sero-positive hepatocellular carcinoma, gastric cancer, endometrial cancer, ovarian cancer, pancreatic cancer, and prostate cancer [54].

Oman is also introducing health economics principles in cancer care for expensive tests and medications in collaboration with the pharmaceutical industry. The country is expanding the use of approved generics and biosimilar. The authorities have developed and approved local institutional guidelines for management and follow-up with the objective of judicious and cost-effective use of laboratory, radiology, and healthcare services.

12.12   Challenges and Advantages

Oman has certain advantages and specific challenges in cancer care plans and services. Oman has a young population, with almost everyone being vaccinated for hepatitis. Local population has free access to comprehensive primary and specialized healthcare services. There is a facility to send patients abroad by MoH, if any needed treatment is not locally available.

The challenges are multi-dimensional and include a high population growth rate, traditional tribal system, social taboos, beliefs, herbal and traditional medications, and a tendency of health tourism. The literacy rate is half in the population over 65 years of age, who influence public opinion. There is a need to invest in health education, prevention and screening programs, diagnostic services, and therapeutic interventions. There is a need for capacity building by training the workforce and investing in cancer care. Increasing economic pressure globally is a challenge with resource allocation, better planning, setting priorities, and implementing cost-effectiveness. There is a need for continuing political will and support and commitment to achieve the set objectives [19, 25, 26].

12.13 The Future of Cancer Care in Oman

Cancer-related mortality is often predestined, but with the execution of the comprehensive Cancer Care Plan, there will be expectantly less mortality in the future. To accomplish these objectives all the partners (public and private, physicians, nurses, patients, and families) must operate concurrently to meet the challenges and realize the targets. There is a need to focus on strengthening the Cancer Control Program, improve Cancer Registry, focus on early detection and prevention, improve integrated cancer management, accessibility, establish integrated palliative care services, engage civil society, capacity building, human resource development, and improve public awareness.

Infrastructure development, lobby for funding, emphasis on research, need to develop clinical pathways and guidelines. There is a continued need for quality assurance, implementing Key Performance Indicators, performance monitoring, and improving patient experience. We need to make a prompt and swift access to cancer services individually or by an integrated referral pathway, decrease referral abroad, make new drugs available for treatment, empower more patients in decision-making, implement patient safety protocols, maintain, and get new certifications, and ensure effective capacity building [56, 57].

12.14 Conclusion

Cancer management is a very dynamic discipline due to a rapid pace of research and development. It is a challenge to offer state-of-the-art cancer care due to increasing cost and access to treatment. Each country has to balance its objectives and resources to have an optimal strategy. There is a necessity for capacity building, reinforcement of cancer control, concentrating on early detection and prevention, developing integrated management, developing local management guidelines, and authenticating palliative care services. Civil society and Non-Governmental Organizations should be involved to the optimum. There is a need for infrastructure improvement, lobby for funding, stress on research, need to develop clinical pathways, demand for quality assurance, implement performance indicators and monitoring, and improve patient experience. It is mandatory to make prompt and swift access to cancer services by everyone through an integrated referral pathway. All the new effective drugs should be made available for treatment, empower patients in decision-making, execute patient safety protocols, maintain and acquire new accreditations, and ensure capacity building.

Conflict of Interest Authors have no conflict of interest to declare.

References

1. Ševčíková H, Raftery AE. Probabilistic population projections. J Stat Softw. 2016;75(6):3849.
2. UN World Population Prospects. United Nations Department of Economic and Social Affairs. 2019.
3. Cancer incidence in Oman 2017, Directorate of Non-Communicable diseases, Ministry of health Sultanate of Oman; www.moh.gov.om.
4. Oman Popul Rev. 2020. Available at https://worldpopulationreview.com/countries/oman-population/.
5. GLOBOCAN database (September 2018)—https://gco.iarc.fr/today/home a--: GLOBOCAN database (September 2018)—https://gco.iarc.fr/today/home, Accessed July 21st 2020.
6. Al-Lawati JA, Al-Zakwani I, Fadhil I, Al-Bahrani BJ. Cancer incidence in Oman (1996–2015). Oman Med J. 2019;34(4):271–3.
7. Al Hasni ZS. The tourism sector, its importance in achieving economic growth in the sultanate of Oman. Int J Adv Res. 2019; https://doi.org/10.21474/IJAR01/9666. 5 Sept 2019
8. Chang Mo O, Lee D, Kong HJ, Lee S, Won YJ, Jung KW, Hyunsoon. Causes of death among cancer patients in the era of cancer survivorship in Korea: attention to the suicide and cardiovascular mortality. Cancer Med. 2020;9(5):1741–52. https://doi.org/10.1002/cam4.2813.
9. Al-Madouj AN, Eldali A, Al-Zahrani AS. 10-Year cancer incidence among nationals of the GCC states 1998-2007. Gulf Centre for Cancer Control and Prevention; 2009.
10. Khoja T, Zahrani A. Epidemiology on cancer in gulf region. 2010. http://www.Amaac.org.
11. Al-Lawati NA, Shenoy SM, Al-Bahrani BJ, Al-Lawati JA. Increasing thyroid cancer incidence in Oman: a join point trend analysis. Oman Med J. 2019;35(1):e98. https://doi.org/10.5001/omj.2020.16.
12. Song W, Powers S, Zhu W, Hannun YA. Substantial contribution of extrinsic risk factors to cancer development. Nature. 2016;529:43–7.
13. Al-Riyami A. Health vision 2050 Oman: a committed step towards reforms. Oman Med J. 2012;27(3):190–1.
14. World Health Organization. Health system profile: Oman 2015. 2015.
15. Ghannem H, Becerra-Posada F, IJsselmuiden C, Helwa I, de Haan S. National research for health system mapping in 5 countries in the eastern Mediterranean region and perspectives on strengthening the systems. East Mediterr Health J. 2011;17(3):260–1.
16. Oman Health Vision 2050. Under secretariat for Planning Affairs, Ministry of Health Sultanate of Oman. 2014. Available from: https://www.moh.gov.om/documents/16506/119833/Health+Vision+2050/7b6f40f3-8f93-4397-9fde34e04026b829.
17. Al Mawali AHN, Al Qasmi AM, Al Sabahi SMS, Idikula J, Elaty MAA, Morsi M, Al Hinai AT. Oman Vision 2050 for Health Research: a strategic plan for the future based on the past and present experience. Oman Med J. 2017;32(2):86–96.
18. Al-Azri M, Al-Rubaie K, Al-Ghafri S, Al-Hinai M, Panchatcharam SM. Barriers and attitudes toward breast cancer screening among Omani women. Asian Pac J Cancer Prev. 2020;21(5):1339–47. https://doi.org/10.31557/APJCP.2020.21.5.1339.
19. Al-Azri M, Al-Awisi H, Al-Rasbi S, El-Shafie K, Al-Hinai M, Al-Habsi H, Al-Moundhri M. Psychosocial impact of breast cancer diagnosis among Omani women. Oman Med J. 2014;29(6):437–44.
20. Al-Maawali A, Al Busadi A, Al-Adawi S. Biomedical publications profile and trends in gulf cooperation council countries. Sultan Qaboos Univ Med J. 2012;12(1):41–7.
21. World Health Organization. Non-communicable Diseases Country Profiles 2011 WHO Global Report 2011. 2011.
22. Latest Global Cancer Data. Cancer burden rises to 19.3 million new cases and 10.0 million cancer deaths in 2020. International Agency for Research on Cancer—World Health Organization. 2020. Press release No. 292, Lyon France. 15 Dec 2020.

23. Sabah Al-Bahlani and Ruth Mabry. Preventing non-communicable disease in Oman, a legislative review. Health Promot Int. 2014;29(suppl 1):i83–91. https://doi.org/10.1093/heapro/dau041.
24. Anna Rajab I, Rashdi A, Al Salmi Q. Genetic services and testing in the Sultanate of Oman. Sultanate of Oman steps into modern genetics. J Community Genet. 2013;4(3):391–7. https://doi.org/10.1007/s12687-013-0153-1.
25. Guidelines for Responsible Conduct of Clinical Studies & Trials. Centre of Studies and research. Directorate General of Planning and Studies. Ministry of Health, Oman. 2016. Available from: http://mohcsr.gov.om/clinical-trials-and-studies-guideline/.
26. Health Research Priorities. Centre of studies and research. Directorate General of Planning and Studies, Ministry of Health, Oman. 2014. Available from: http://mohcsr.gov.om/health-research-priorities/.
27. Mehdi I, Shah AH, Moona MS, Verma K, Abussa A, Elramih R, El-Hashmi H. Synchronous and metachronous tumors—expect the un-expected. J Pak Med Assoc. 2010;60:905–9.
28. Moona MS, Al R, Alarabi R, Hussain A, Ahmed M, Mehdi I. Study of ER (estrogen receptor), PR (progesterone receptor), and Her-2/Neu status in patients with breast cancer. JMJ. 2010;10(2):141–3.
29. Moona MS, Mehdi I. Nasopharyngeal carcinoma presented as cavernous sinus tumor. J Pak Med Assoc. 2011;61:1235–6.
30. Aromatase inhibitors, a viable option for recurrent granulose cell tumor ovary: overview and case report. J Pak Med Assoc. 2012;62(5):505–7.
31. Anaplastic large cell lymphoma of scrotal skin. J Pak Med Assoc. 2011;61:1140–3.
32. Renal cell carcinoma metastasizing to larynx. Gulf J Oncolog. 2012;11:70–4.
33. Chemotherapy induced neutropenic necrotic enterocolitis—review article. J Pak Med Assoc. 2012;62:718–23.
34. Mehdi I, Kashmiri AH. Chronic myeloid leukemia in Libya. South Asian J Cancer. 2012;1(1):25–6. www.Journal.sajc.org Thursday June 28, 2012: IP: 37.40.61.242
35. Monem EA, Al-Bahrani B, Mehdi I, Nada A. Rapid rituximab infusion: local center experience. Gulf J Oncolog. 2013;14:52–6.
36. Mehdi I. Be a true listener, rather than a good conversationalist. South Asian J Cancer. 2013;2(4):218–9.
37. Kamal V, Itrat M, Nazhia I, Hussein H. Unusual presentation of cancer colon. J Obstet Gynecol. 2013; https://doi.org/10.1007/S13224-013-0436-9. On line ISSN 0975-6434. Print ISSN 0971-9202
38. Mehdi I, Monem EA, Al Bahrani BJ, Al Kharusi S, Nada AM, Al Lawati J, Al Lawati N. Young age breast cancer in Oman: issues and implications. South Asian J Cancer. 2014;3(2):101–6. https://doi.org/10.4103/2278-330X.130442.
39. Mehdi I, Monem AA, Al Bahrani B, Ramadhan F. Molecular subtypes of breast cancer in Oman. Correlation of age, stage, and outcome—an analysis of 542 cases. Gulf J Oncolog. 2014;15:38–48.
40. Monem EA, Mehdi I, Al Bahrani BJ, Nada AM, Al Kharusi S. Utilization of chemotherapy at the end of life (EOL): a local experience. J Pak Med Assoc. 2014;64:863–8.
41. Baraka BA, Al Bahrani BJ, Al Kharusi SS, Mehdi I, Nada AM, Rahabi NH. The external Auditory Canal as an unusual site for metastasis of breast cancer: a case report. Gulf J Oncolog. 2015;17:85–7.
42. Al-Lawati T, Mehdi I, Al Bahrani B, Al-Harsi K, Al Rahbi S, Varvaras D. Does alternative and traditional WASAM (local cautery) therapy facilitate an early and more extensive loco-regional metastasis of breast cancer? Gulf J Oncolog. 2016;22:37–42.
43. Essam AM, Venniyoor A, Nagdev S, Mehdi I, Al Bahrani B. Long term survival in a case of metastatic papillary renal cell carcinoma. South Asian J Cancer. 2017;6(1):19–24. https://doi.org/10.4103/2278-330X.202562.
44. Venniyoor A, Essam AM, Ramadhan F, Keswani H, Mehdi I, Al Bahrani B. High occurrence of non-clear cell renal cell carcinoma in Oman. Asian Pac J Cancer Prev. 2016;17(6):2801–4.

45. Venniyoor A, Mehdi I, Balakrishnan R, Al Bahrani B. Early chemotherapy in metastatic prostate cancer improves survival: a quick note to surgical colleagues. Indian J Surg. 2020;82(6):1206. https://doi.org/10.1007/s12262-020-02213-y.
46. Venniyoor A, Mehdi I, Balakrishnan R, Al Bahrani B. Long term survival in a case of metastatic papillary renal cell carcinoma. 2017;6(1):19–24. https://doi.org/10.4103/2278-330X.202562.
47. Mehdi I, Al Bahrani BJ. Are we prepared to implement a lean philosophy within cancer-care service in Oman? Saudi Med J. 2017;38(7):691–8. https://doi.org/10.15537/smj.2017.7.17712.
48. Mehdi I, Al Bahrani BJ, Al Lawati TM, Mandhari ZA, Al Lawati FR. Breast cancer in a patient with kindlers syndrome. J Pak Med Assoc. 2017;67(8):1283–6.
49. Mehdi I, Al Bahrani BJ, Kamona A, Al Lawati FR, Vennyor AJ. Non-traumatic avascular necrosis of femoral head in malignant disease: is it disease induced or treatment related? J Pakistan Med Assoc. 2018;68(2):310–7.
50. Mehdi I, Al Bahrani B. Lobbying for regulatory reforms of narcotic analgesics in the current social environment of the Middle East. Gulf J Oncolog. 2018;27:52–9.
51. Mehdi I, Al Bahrani B. Expanding role of bio markers in Colo-rectal cancer (CRC). Int J Cell Sci Mol Biol. 2017;3(1):1–5. https://doi.org/10.19080/IJCSMB.2017.03.555605.
52. Mehdi I, Al Bahrani B. Fast food chains and obesity in Oman. J Cancer Epidemiol Prev. 2020;5(4):1–6. https://doi.org/10.36648/cancer.5.4.6.
53. Mehdi I, Al Bahrani B. Medical tourism in Oman. Cancer Rep Rev. 2020;4:1–5. https://doi.org/10.15761/CRR.1000212.
54. Al Bahrani BJ, Mehdi I. A potential 2nd wave of COVID-19: an approaching reality. J Pak Med Assoc. 2020;70(12):2299–301.
55. Al Bahrani BJ, Mehdi I, Monem EA, Al Farsi AAM, Al Lawati N, Nada AM. Laterality of colorectal cancer (CRC) in Oman. Cancer Sci Res. 2021;4(1):1–7.
56. Burney IA. The trend to seek a second opinion abroad amongst cancer patients in Oman, challenges and opportunities. Sultan Qaboos Univ Med J. 2009;9(3):260–3.
57. Al Balushi M, Al Mandhari Z. Radiation oncology in Oman: current status and future challenges. Int J Radiat Oncol Biol Phys. 2020;108(4):851–5. https://doi.org/10.1016/j.ijrobp.2020.05.059. Epub 2020 Jul 11

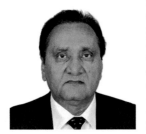

Itrat Mehdi has postgraduate training in the UK, having vast experience in clinical Oncology, research, and postgraduate teaching. He is a member of international organizations like ASCO, ESMO, ESACC, SGM, etc. He is on the editorial board and is a reviewer of many international indexed journals like BMJ, JPMA, JPMR, World Journal series, SQUMJ, OMJ, J Nephrology Urology and Transplant, and GJO. He has been part of many collaborative studies and clinical trials, supervised many postgraduate students, and been an examiner in Oncology. He has presented numerous papers at local and international meetings. He has over 70 publications in local and international journals.

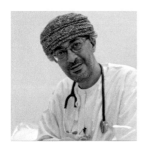

Abdul Aziz Al Farsi, MD, MRCP(UK), FRCPC, graduated from the college of medicine SQUH in 2001. He joined the Internal Medicine Program OMSB in 2003. He became a member of the Royal College of Physicians UK in 2006 and joined the department of medical oncology at the Royal Hospital that year. Dr. Aziz completed his studies at McMaster University, Hamilton, Canada where he finished internal medicine and medical oncology residency from 2010 till 2015. He completed research and clinical fellowship in thoracic malignancies at the same university in June 2017. Currently, he works as Senior Consultant and Head of Adult Oncology, National Oncology Center, Muscat, Oman.

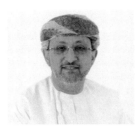

Bassim Al Bahrani, a Senior Medical Oncologist at the Royal Hospital in Oman. A visiting Professor at the postgraduate program on Health Economics, Management and Policy at the University of Peloponnese in Corinth, Greece. He has done his advanced training in Medical Oncology in Australia and earned a fellowship from the Royal Australasian College of Physicians year 2000. He is an honorary Fellow of the Royal College of physicians and surgeons of Glasgow, ESMO Certified, and a Ph.D. from the University of Rome Tor Vergata. He is a member of many international Oncology associations and the author of over 56 research articles published in peer-reviewed international journals.

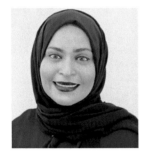

Shadha S. Al-Raisi, is the Director of Non-Communicable Diseases (NCD) in the Ministry of Health, Oman. She is involved in the management of NCDs and mental illness in PHC, the provision of services for people living with disabilities, and the development of a surveillance system for NCDs in the country. Among a number of committees, she is the rapporteur of the National NCD committee and a member of the GCC NCD committee. Dr. Al-Raisi has degrees in Medicine and Biomedical science from the University College of Cork, Ireland, and a master's degree in Public Health from the London School of Hygiene & Tropical Medicine.

Chapter 13
General Oncology Care in Palestine

Khalid Halahleh, Niveen M. E. Abu-Rmeileh, and Mohammad M. Abusrour

13.1 Demographics of the State of Palestine

At present, the state of Palestine is referred to the areas of historic Palestine that are controlled by the Palestinian authority, namely the West Bank, including East Jerusalem, and the Gaza Strip. The state of Palestine is located at the eastern coast of the Mediterranean Sea to the West of the Jordan River. The state includes 16 governorates—11 in the West Bank and 5 in the Gaza Strip. According to the Palestinian Central Bureau of Statistics, the total population in 2020 is estimated to be about 5.1 million; 3.05 million live in the West Bank and 2.05 live in the Gaza Strip, with an average age of 21 years. This indicates that 66% of the population is under 30. Males make up 51% of the population and females 49%, whereas the sex ratio stands at 103.4; meaning that there are 103 males for every 100 females. The Gross Domestic Product (GDP) per capita is estimated to be $3378 in 2019 [1].

K. Halahleh
Medical Oncology Hematology Section, Hematopoietic Cell Transplantation and Cell Therapy Unit-King Hussein Cancer Center, Amman, Jordan

N. M. E. Abu-Rmeileh
Institute of Community and Public Health, Berzeit University, Birzeit, Palestine

M. M. Abusrour (✉)
Augusta-Victoria Hospital, Jerusalem, Palestine
e-mail: mabusrour@doh.gov.ae

© The Author(s) 2022
H. O. Al-Shamsi et al. (eds.), *Cancer in the Arab World*,
https://doi.org/10.1007/978-981-16-7945-2_13

13.2   Cancer Statistics in Palestine

13.2.1   Cancer Epidemiology

It was challenging to receive accurate data on cancer incidence and mortality in the occupied Palestinian territory until 1998. The Ministry of Health has published the first cancer report, including statistics for both the West Bank and the Gaza Strip [2]. This report was the first product of the Palestinian Cancer Registry (PCR). The registry was based at two hospitals: one in the West Bank and one in the Gaza Strip. From the establishment of the registry until 2008, the data of both locations were combined in one report. Afterward, data was reported separately for the West Bank and the Gaza Strip.

Although the Palestinian Cancer Registry is almost 25 years old, the reported statistics are still elementary and limited to incidence rate and percentage of site-specific cancer stratified by age and sex. Survival statistics, case fatality statistics, and age at diagnosis and recovery in addition to effective management plans are not reported.

13.2.2   Cancer Statistics

The cancer incidence rate was 117.8 per 100,000 population in 2019. The rate has a steady slow increase compared with 2013 (79.5 per 100,000 population) and 2016 (86.4 per 100,000). It is not clear whether this is an actual increase in cancer cases or is it due to an improvement in the reporting system.

In the West Bank, breast cancer was the most common cancer, 16.9% of all cancer cases in 2019 (incidence rate was 19.9 per 100,000 population). The second most common cancer was colorectal cancer, 12.6% of all cancer cases (Incidence rate was 14.8 per 100,000 population). The third highest incidence rate was lung cancer 8.4 per 100,000 population (7.2% of all cancer cases). (Table 13.1) [3, 4]. Similarly, in the Gaza Strip, breast cancer (18.0%) and colon cancer (10.7% of all cancer cases) were at the top [5].

The most common cancer among females was breast cancer [3, 4] (40.0% in the West Bank and 32.3% in the Gaza Strip), colorectum cancer (15.6% in the West Bank and 9.2% in the Gaza strip), and thyroid cancer (9.2% in the West Bank and 7.7% in the Gaza Strip) [3, 4]. These three types were common cancers reported among females in the last 10 years.

Among males, the most common cancers in the West Bank were lung cancer [3, 4] (14.1%), colorectum cancer (14.1%), prostate cancer (9.9%), and bladder cancer (9.8%). While in the Gaza Strip, the most common cancers were colorectum cancer (13.1%), lung cancer (11.5%), leukemia (9.2%), Non-Hodgkin's Lymphoma (7.8%), and prostate cancer (7.6%).

Table 13.1 Percentage of reported cancer cases by sex and diagnosis, West Bank, Palestine 2019 [3, 4]

Site	IDCO3	Male	%	Female	%	Total	%	Incidence rate per 100,000
Lip, oral cavity & pharynx	C00-C08	21	0.7	13	0.4	34	1.1	1.3
Oropharynx & nasopharynx	C10-C11	11	0.4	1	0.0	12	0.4	0.4
Esophagus	C15	11	0.4	4	0.1	15	0.5	0.6
Stomach	C16	43	1.4	35	1.1	78	2.5	2.9
Small intestine	C17	5	0.1	8	0.3	13	0.4	0.5
Colorectal	C18-C20	194	6.1	206	6.5	400	12.6	14.8
Anus	C21	3	0.1	1	0.0	4	0.1	0.1
Liver	C22	36	1.1	15	0.5	51	1.6	1.9
Gallbladder & biliary	C23-C24	12	0.4	16	0.5	28	0.9	1.0
Pancreas	C25	57	1.8	33	1.0	90	2.8	3.3
Ill-defined digestive organs	C26	6	0.2	2	0.1	8	0.3	0.3
Nose & nasal sinuses	C30-C31	5	0.2	3	0.1	8	0.3	0.3
Larynx	C32	35	1.1	4	0.1	39	1.2	1.4
Trachea, bronchus & lung	C33-C34	194	6.2	33	1.0	227	7.2	8.4
Thymus, adrenal gland & other endocrine glands	C37, C74-C75	6	0.2	11	0.3	17	0.5	0.6
Heart, mediastinum & pleura	C38	4	0.1	2	0.1	6	0.2	0.2
Bones	C40-C41	24	0.7	15	0.5	39	1.2	1.4
Melanoma	C43	3	0.1	5	0.2	8	0.3	0.3
Skin	C44	87	2.8	74	2.3	161	5.1	6.0
Mesotheliom	C45	3	0.1	0	0.0	3	0.1	0.1
Kaposi sarcoma	C46	1	0.1	1	0.0	2	0.1	0.1
Retroperitonium	C48	1	0.1	1	0.0	2	0.1	0.1
Connective & soft tissue	C49	18	0.6	16	0.5	34	1.1	1.3
Breast	C50	7	0.2	529	16.7	536	16.9	19.9
Vulva	C51	0	0.0	3	0.1	3	0.1	0.1
Vagina	C52	0	0.0	1	0.0	1	0.0	0.0
Cervix uteri	C53	0	0.0	16	0.5	16	0.5	0.6
Uterus	C54-C55	0	0.0	112	3.5	112	3.5	4.2
Overy	C56	0	0.0	53	1.7	53	1.7	2.0
Fallopian tube	C57	0	0.0	2	0.1	2	0.1	0.1
Prostate	C61	136	4.3	0	0.0	136	4.3	5.0
Testis	C62	40	1.3	0	0.0	40	1.3	1.5
Kidney, renal pelvis & ureter	C63-C64	37	1.2	29	0.9	66	2.1	2.4
Bladder	C67	134	4.3	14	0.4	148	4.7	5.5
Eye & adnexa	C69	3	0.1	1	0.0	4	0.1	0.1

(continued)

Table 13.1 (continued)

Site	IDCO3	Male	%	Female	%	Total	%	Incidence rate per 100,000
Brain & nerves system	C70-C72	67	2.1	−56	1.4	11	3.5	4.1
Thyroid	C73	44	1.4	122	3.8	166	5.2	6.2
Malignant neoplasm without specification of site	C80	12	0.4	10	0.3	22	0.7	0.8
Hodgkin's disease	C81	46	1.5	45	1.4	91	2.9	3.4
Non-Hodgkin's lymphoma	C82-C85, C96	68	2.2	64	2.0	132	4.2	4.9
Multiple myeloma	C90	30	0.9	16	0.5	46	1.4	1.7
Leukemia	C91-C95	83	2.6	74	2.3	157	4.9	5.8
Other hematologic disorders	C42	23	0.8	30	0.9	53	1.7	2.0
Total		1510	47.6	1664	52.4	3174	100.0	117.8

The percentage of cancer among children is relatively low compared to those of older ages in 2019. The most common cancer among children was leukemia (42% of all cancers in the West Bank and 26% of all cancers in the Gaza Strip). The second most common pediatric cancer in the West Bank was brain and nervous system cancers (33% of all cancers), followed by Non-Hodgkin's Lymphoma (17%) [4]. While in the Gaza Strip, brain and nervous system cancers accounted for 16.5% of all cancers and Non-Hodgkin's Lymphoma 17.1% [3].

Regional variations between governorates within the West Bank and the Gaza Strip were reported on:

- http://site.moh.ps/Content/Books
- http://www.moh.gov.ps/portal/wp-content/uploads/2020/06/MOH-Annual-Report-2019.pdf

However, these variations were not consistent over time and the interpretation of high or low percentages in certain areas was difficult to interpret.

13.2.3 Cancer Mortality

Mortality in Palestine is mainly due to Non-Communicable Diseases (NCDs). In 2019, cardiovascular diseases were the leading cause of death in the West Bank (29.9%) and the Gaza Strip (49.6%). Cancer was the second leading cause of death which accounted for 16% of the total deaths in the West Bank (Cancer mortality rate was 42.9 per 100,000) and 10.3% of total deaths in the Gaza Strip [3]. Lung cancer (17%), colon cancer (14.9%), and breast cancer (11.2%) were the leading causes of death among other cancers in the West Bank (Table 13.2) [4].

Table 13.2 Percentage of top reported cancer deaths by sex and site, West Bank, Palestine 2019 [3, 4]

Site	IDCO3	Male	Female	Total	%
Lip, oral cavity, & pharynx	C00-C14	6	1	7	0.6
Esophagus	C15	7	3	10	0.9
Stomach	C16	21	26	47	4.1
Colon	C18	87	85	172	14.9
Rectum	C20	6	10	16	1.4
Liver	C22	35	29	64	5.5
Gallbladder	C23	9	8	17	1.5
Pancreas	C25	31	23	54	4.7
Nasal cavity & middle ear	C30	0	1	1	0.1
Larynx	C32	7	1	8	0.7
Lung	C33-C34.9	160	36	196	17.0
Thymus	C37	1	2	3	0.3
Bones	C40-C41.9	14	7	21	1.8
Skin	C43-C44	9	4	13	1.1
Retroperitoneum & peritoneum	C48	0	1	1	0.1
Connective & soft tissue	C49	5	4	9	0.8
Breast	C50	0	130	130	11.2
Vulva	C51	0	1	1	0.1
Uterus	C53- C55.9	0	25	25	2.2
Overy	C56	0	23	23	2.0
Prostate	C61	48	0	48	4.2
Testis	C62	1	0	1	0.1
Kidney	C64	14	6	20	1.7
Urinary bladder	C67	36	5	41	3.5
Eye	C69	0	1	1	0.1
Brain & other nerves system	C70-C72.9	44	38	82	7.1
Thyroid gland	C73	1	4	5	0.4
Adrenal gland	C74	1	3	4	0.3
Lymph nods	C77	2	0	2	0.2
Without specification of site	C80	2	5	7	0.6
Hodgkin's disease	C81	3	5	8	0.7
Non-Hodgkin's lymphoma	C82-C85.9	7	6	13	1.1
Leukemia	C90-C95.9	53	38	91	7.9
Lymphoid, hematopoietic & related tissue	C96	5	10	15	1.3
Total in West Bank		615	541	1156	100.0
Total in Gaza		2842 (9.9%)	2477 (10.8%)	5319	33.7 per 100,000

13.3   Cancer Risk Factors

Few studies reported cancer risk factors in Palestine. Most of them were focused on breast cancer risk factors. A cross-sectional study was conducted in the Gaza Strip, in 2014, reported selected risk factors. Positive family history of breast cancer, high Body Mass Index (BMI), hypertension and diabetes are common risk factors for breast cancer among Palestinian women [6].

Classical cancer risk factors such as tobacco control, obesity, and unhealthy nutrition habits were studied separately or with other Non-Communicable Diseases. The rate of tobacco smoking among adults ($\geq$18) was 36.7%. Cigarette smoking was 28.2%, while waterpipe tobacco smoking was 12.9% [7]. The prevalence of current waterpipe tobacco smoking among university students aged 18–25 years old was 24.4%, which was higher than the prevalence of current cigarette smoking (18.0%). The prevalence of waterpipe tobacco smoking (36.4%) and cigarette smoking (32.8%) was higher among men compared to women (18.0%, 3.6%, respectively) [8]. The prevalence of tobacco smoking was reported high among students 12–15 years old in 2016, where 17.5% of the students (28.6% of boys and 7.1% of girls) were current cigarette smokers [9].

The WHO STEPS survey was conducted in Palestine in 2010–2011. The prevalence of overweight (BMI $\geq$25 kg/m^2) and obesity (BMI $\geq$30 kg/m^2) was 57.8% and 26.8% among adults, those between 15 and 64 years old. The prevalence of obesity was higher among women than men (30.8% vs. 23.3%) [10].

13.4   Cancer Screening Programs

In Palestine, cancers that are amenable to early detection are being diagnosed at a later stage than in high-income countries. The establishment of early detection programs may be the most feasible strategy in the country. The only active screening program in Palestine is for breast cancer. The Palestinian Breast Cancer Program (PBCP) is a national program, established in 2008, for early breast cancer detection.

The program introduced a mobile mammography unit with centralized image reading taking place at the Palestinian Ministry of Health. The Ministry of Health began providing free mammograms for women younger than 40 years old and for young women who were considered at high risk in 2008–2009 in the West Bank and in 2010 in Gaza. In 2014, Augusta-Victoria Hospital (AVH) and national PBCP introduced a mobile mammography unit with centralized reading at AVH to increase patient access to breast cancer screening. There are 19 mammographic machines in the West Bank and 20 mammographic machines in Gaza (19 in the government sector, with the remainder in the private and non-governmental sector) [5].

Although the Palestinian Breast Cancer Program has been relatively successful in detecting cancers at an early stage; it still needs considerable improvement to be truly effective. Indeed, there are financial constraints. However, a major challenge is in public education to overcome cultural barriers against screening.

13.5   Cancer Prevention Programs

In Palestine, cancer care is focused on treatment with little emphasis on other elements of the cancer care continuum that includes screening and prevention. For instance, there is no cancer control plan for preventable cancers such as lung, head and neck, tobacco-related cancers, alcohol-related cancers, or cervical cancer.

Particular attention is needed to combat rising cancer rates in the future [6]. Over one-third of cancers can be prevented through controlling known risk factors [7]. Unfortunately, many cost-effective prevention measures have yet to be implemented in Palestine. Lung, breast, and colon cancer are three of the most top 10 common cancers in Palestine that could be prevented. Unfortunately, there are no effective national programs addressing preventable cancer risks in Palestine.

Although smoking rates remain high in the region, there has been some progress in combating smoking in Palestine. In 2015, taxes on tobacco products have also increased. Unfortunately, there are currently no smoking cessation clinics available for counseling.

No organized programs for cervical cancer screening or for Human Papillomavirus (HPV) vaccination in young people currently exist in Palestine. More pressingly, given the unique situation in Gaza as a conflict zone, there is an important public health requirement that needs to be addressed to adequately educate the population that might have been exposed to increased levels of potentially carcinogenic and toxic materials.

13.6   Cancer Diagnosis

13.6.1   Imaging Diagnosis

Cancer diagnosis is an extremely complex task, requiring advanced radiological, nuclear diagnostics, and cyto-molecular markers. Almost every specialized hospital has a conventional diagnostic section, including general X-rays machines, Computed Tomography (CT) scans, Magnetic Resonance Imaging (MRIs). However, fragmented biopsies can be performed safely by experienced radiologists. Recently, the use of advanced imaging modalities such as Positron Emission Tomography (PET/CT) scan was introduced in Palestine, in 2018. However, the country lacks expert personnel. Nuclear medicine specialists are not available in Palestine. Consequently, all images are to be reviewed and reported by doctors abroad. Currently, three PET-CT scans are available in the country. All three are located outside the Ministry of Health. Fortunately, one is in the most comprehensive cancer center at AVH in East Jerusalem. AVH has a strong collaborative agreement with the King Hussein Cancer Center (KHCC) in Amman. All images are being reviewed and reported by experts on nuclear medicine at KHCC. The second is in a general hospital in the south of Palestine and a third is in a private diagnostic center in the north. Regulations pertaining to the use of advanced imaging modalities such as PET/CT scans have been implemented, approved, and regulated by the referral department, Ministry of Health medical committee [11].

13.6.2 Cytogenetics and Molecular Genetics

Treating cancer or hematological conditions requires an established cytogenetic-molecular laboratory for the Next-Generation Sequencing (NGS). In Palestine, most cancer departments lack such facilities. The only established advanced diagnostic laboratory is at August-Victoria Hospital- East Jerusalem, which was established in 2016. The laboratory has conventional cytogenetic, Fluorescence in situ Hybridization (FISH) analysis and molecular tests for most of the hematological disorders and some solid tumors like lung and colon cancer. Despite the progress we have achieved, we are still lacking more sophisticated diagnosis methods such as liquid biopsy or evaluating circulating tumor DNA (ct-DNA) components. It is difficult to access specialized laboratories equipped for either ct-DNA detection or molecular testing on cancer specimens, leading to most of the specimens being referred outside.

13.7 Treatment

13.7.1 Medical Oncology

Nowadays, there are two main branches of cancer care in Palestine: governmental and non-governmental branches. For those who have not been referred elsewhere, there are four government hospitals in the West Bank and three in the Gaza Strip that are able to treat most of the patients. These hospitals have small oncology and hematology units (10–15 beds), without specialized pathology laboratories or advanced diagnostic facilities. However, surgery and chemotherapy facilities are generally available in these hospitals, but no radiotherapy services are present on-site.

Recently, two non-governmental hospitals have opened their oncology and hematology services, National University Hospital in Nablus, and Al-Istishari Hospital in Ramallah city. Each has a limited vacancy with 20 beds for inpatients and 10–15 beds for outpatient's chemotherapy infusion. Both hospitals are equipped with pathology and advanced conventional laboratory sections with two pathologists on-site in each hospital.

Currently, Augusta-Victoria Hospital Cancer Care Center, located in East Jerusalem, is the only comprehensive cancer center in Palestine. It was established in 2006, after the introduction of radiotherapy services, supported by the Norwegian government and operated by the Lutherian Federation. This center includes more advanced pathology, cytogenetic-molecular facilities, apheresis unit (1 machine), and (1) PET-CT scan. The AVH has two departments for oncology and hematology with 10–15 beds, more expanded outpatient care, a radiotherapy unit with three linear accelerators, and isolated Bone Marrow Transplantation (BMT) units of 4 beds for high-dose chemotherapy consolidation.

13.7.1.1 Hematology

Before 2008, most hematology patients were referred to neighboring countries like Jordan, Egypt, and occupied 1948 land hospitals. Despite the progress we have made in medical oncology, advanced hematology and Bone Marrow Transplantation services are still lacking. There are fragmented hematology services in most government hospitals. Two non-government hospitals operate and serve hematology services. However, not in a systematic and complete manner. An additional sophisticated hematology department was established in AVH, in 2016, helped by a European Union's (EU) grant for complete hematology and Bone Marrow Transplantation services. The hematology section contains 10–15 beds for inpatients, larger outpatient care and Hematopoietic Cell Transplantation units of four isolated beds for stem cell infusions [12].

Bone marrow Hematopoietic Cell Transplants (HCTs) are available in Palestine, by using high-dose chemotherapy infusions (autologous transplants). Adult and pediatric patients requiring Hematopoietic Cell Transplant must be referred to neighboring countries' hospitals in occupied Palestine 1947 land or travel abroad to Jordan or Egypt. This entails significant distress and cost to the patient, their families, and the Health Care Providers (HCPs). Several models have been initiated, leading the Palestinian government to establish a Hematopoietic Cell Transplant to cover this demand in collaboration with Al-Najah National University Hospital (NNUH) and Augusta-Victoria Hospitals (AVH). Each unit has only four beds isolated for high-dose chemotherapy. This situation will change soon as several leading hospitals announced plans to include Bone Marrow Transplant services shortly. They will include different types of allogeneic transplants: matched, mismatched, unrelated, and haploidentical transplants.

13.7.1.2 Immunotherapy/Targeted Therapy/Biological Agents

Conventional oncology drugs are available in each hospital with occasional shortages in Gaza Strip hospitals due to logistical and political reasons. In Palestine, it is extremely difficult to have access to approved and highly expensive medications, including the newer immunotherapy drugs and targeted agents. Not all United States Food and Drug Administration (FDA) approved medications are easily accessible to patients. Patients are mainly offered medications (not listed in the formulary list of the Ministry of Health) after gaining special approval from the referral department's medical committee in the Ministry of Health on specific medication or intervention, "Referral path in MoH." All these immunotherapy drugs and targeted agents given to a selected limited number of patients have no universal use in governmental and non-governmental hospitals due to the high cost. Cost-effective analysis is yet to be made. Hospitals offering those drugs usually request them directly from the pharmaceutical companies and, if indicated, the drug cost would be covered.

13.7.2 Radiation Oncology

In Palestine, radiation therapy services are extremely limited. Radiation oncology is currently offered in one facility with only three linear accelerators available in East Jerusalem to serve all Palestinian oncologic needs (1/1,000,000 inhabitants). 3D, Intensity-modulated radiation therapy (IMRT) planning is implemented. There is no brachytherapy available, and all patients must be referred abroad. The problem is not just the lack of new radiation therapy machines. Introducing isotopic machines in the West Bank is not just a money shortage issue. The military occupation and the daily obstacles prevent patients from freely moving, also affect cancer care outcomes. Although financial investment in technology is undeniably necessary, many deaths from untreated cancer also occur for political reasons in the form of the deliberate denial of access to care [13].

13.7.3 Surgery

In Palestine, there are no structured oncology surgery services, and we are lacking in specialized centers for oncology surgery. The surgery is getting a step forward to improving in the form of acquiring new physicians, specialized in oncology surgery, and subspecialized in breast surgery for instance. There was an established collaborative training program for oncology surgery with King Hussein Cancer Center in Jordan. Two physicians have just graduated and started their mission in Palestine. However, there are no robotic surgeries for cancer or Hyperthermic Intraperitoneal Chemotherapy (HIPEC) procedures available. Oncology patients can have their surgeries in governmental and non-governmental hospitals, where they are being treated for their cancers.

13.7.4 Pediatric Oncology

The incidence of pediatric hematology and oncology cases is within the expected range, with a total of 170 children in the West Bank, reportedly (aged 0–17), diagnosed with cancer in Palestine in 2019 [14, 15]. There is underreporting of children cancer cases in the Gaza Strip. By contrast to high-income countries, 10% of new cancer patients were children less than 17 years of age. The three most common cancers in children are leukemia (30%), brain and other central nervous system tumors (20%), and lymphomas (14%) [16].

There are three pediatric oncology departments in the West Bank and one in the Gaza Strip, located in both public and private hospitals. In 2012, Huda Al Masri Pediatric Cancer Department was the first and only public cancer department for children in Huda's name at Beit-Jala Hospital. Two other facilities were established in East Jerusalem and in the north of Palestine-Nablus. These facilities are well staffed with pediatric oncologists, nursing staff, therapists, and only in East Jerusalem is equipped with radiation oncology. However, the most significant limitation in pediatric oncology in Palestine remains the lack of coordination and lack of Hematopoietic Cell Transplant centers.

13.7.5   Palliative Care Track

Palliative care is an emerging specialty in Palestine with no organized national program in place to date [17]. Several small non-profit organizations exist, but their efforts are limited by several factors that include financial constraints and general societal aversion to the notion of palliation [18]. There is an urgent need for a comprehensive palliative care platform for hospital and home-based care, as well as a need for psychosocial programs and integrated research for end-of-life care [17–20].

There are two palliative care facilities in the West Bank and East Jerusalem. Al-Sadeel Society, registered as Non-Governmental Organization (NGO), provides palliative care services in Bethlehem city, focusing on educating physicians, nurses, patients, and their families about the fundamental practices [18]. The second is within AVH in East Jerusalem with a dedicated, though small inpatient service, but with no at-home care available. The Lutheran World Federation has secured the permits necessary and begun construction of the Elder Care and Palliative Medicine Institute (ECPMI) in 2019. This 144-bed facility on the Mount of Olives will nearly double the capacity of AVH [21, 22].

Recently, a training program was opened in collaboration within the three facilities Al-Sadeel, Palestinian, MoH, Augusta Victoria Hospital at Ibn-Sina College for Health Sciences to train undergraduate nursing students on palliative care [20]. Hospice and end-of-life care services are not available for terminally ill Palestinian patients.

13.8   Research and Education

Despite the improved cancer care in Palestine, it was not integrated with the health research. There is a mismatch between the distribution of disease burden and diseases investigated in published articles from Palestine between 2000 and 2015 [20]. The number of published Palestinian medical and health research articles increased over time, almost doubling every 5 years (13% between 2000 and 2004, 32% between 2005 and 2010, and 55% between 2011 and 2015). However, cancer research is one of the most understudied fields relative to cancer burden, representing only 3% of the total health research compared to infectious (20%), nutritional (11%), and mental and substance use (11%). The highest priority should be given to research investigating conditions that most substantially contribute to disease burden. Cancer is one of the leading causes of death in Palestine approaching 14% [23]. This gap can be explained by several factors that include researchers' interest and expertise. Limited research infrastructure and funding resources drive researchers to accept the funder agenda that is not commonly aligned with local community needs. This should be implicated in establishing a national medical and health research priority-setting in Palestine. This fosters a dialog between researchers, policymakers, funders, and end-users/patients [24].

Despite the relatively limited research capacity, recent publications led by investigators in Palestine are appearing in premiere medical journals [20, 23–25]. Research specifically targeting the Palestinian population should be undertaken to establish a proper future cancer care plan, which will likely be different from other societies. Therefore, treatment protocols based on a western population must be modified to fit the unique patient population in Palestine with different genetic makeup.

There are two Palestinian medical schools in the West Bank and one in Gaza. In 2005, the Palestinian Oncology Society was established with a total of 59 members, including medical oncologists, hematologists, general surgeons, and pathologists. The mission is educational and has no major effects on policymakers. In Palestine, there is only one medical oncology training program for 3 years with 1 year abroad, registered under the Palestinian Medical Council (PMC). One or two graduates annually. We do not currently have an established training program in both hematology and Bone Marrow Transplantation.

Further, epidemiology cancer research in Palestine is in its early stages, utilizing descriptive types of studies. The available research is limited to knowledge, perception, and attitude about cancer types and their symptoms. Most of the research was focused on breast cancer [26–29].

13.8.1 Publications

A list of publications is provided in Appendix.

13.9 Cost-Effective Cancer Care

Healthcare in Palestine has been a major concern of the Palestinian government since 1994, when the Palestinian authorities took over the administration of healthcare after the signing of the Oslo Accords. Investment in healthcare has been supported by the World Health Organization (WHO) and foreign donors, especially the United States Agency for International Development. Despite major challenges, primary healthcare in Palestine is among the best in its neighboring Arab countries in terms of life expectancy and maternal, infant, and child mortality rates. Cancer treatment is covered by the government health insurance in Palestine and in neighboring countries. About 13.5% of the healthcare budget goes to patients with malignant tumors.

13.10 Challenges and Advantages

13.10.1 Specialized Oncology Services

Before 2000, cancer care in Palestine was fragmented with no cooperation between oncologists, pathologists, surgeons, and radiologists. Cancer care focuses on treatment with little emphasis on other elements of the cancer care continuum, such as prevention, early detection, screening, and diagnosis. Comprehensive cancer care centers were not present. Cancer care was given in isolated sections in government hospitals only. Few support services were in place, such as palliative care, nutritional and psychosocial support, or rehabilitation services. Because of the lack of specialized services, most of our patients were referred to neighboring countries.

In 2008, the Ministry of Foreign Affairs (MFA) of Norway funded a 6-year program. This project has been implemented through Norwegian Church Aid. The aim was to establish a comprehensive cancer center for adults and pediatrics in East Jerusalem at Augusta-Victoria Hospital (AVH). AVH is a non-profit, Non-Governmental Organization, operated by the Lutheran World Federation. The hospital will cooperate with the Palestinian Ministry of Health. Aside from cancer care, the center planned to provide training and conduct research also [30].

13.10.2 Oncology Physicians

The shortage of cancer specialists in the region is acute, with only 5 radiation oncologists, 6 pediatric hematologists, 20 medical oncologists, 6 hematologists, 7 surgical oncologists, and 15 surgical pathologists, with little hemopathology training, registered in the Department of Health in Palestine and Palestinian Medical council [31]. Consequently, only one radiation oncologist and two medical oncologists are available per 100,000 population, which is half the number seen in the USA and the EU. However, it is like neighboring countries like Lebanon [32, 33]. Most oncologists and hematologists receive their training in different parts of the world, such as Europe, Jordan, specifically at the King Hussein Cancer Center, and other neighboring countries.

13.10.3 Cancer Care Capacity Building

Besides government hospitals located in the West Bank (N-3), Gaza Strip (N-3), and East Jerusalem (N-1), there are centers serving cancer patients in the private sector (N-3). In the West Bank, there are three oncology departments including Ramallah Medical Complex, Al-watani, and Jenin Hospitals in North Palestine. Three Gaza Strip centers, including Ranteesy Hospital, European Gaza Hospital, and the recently opened Children cancer department in the children's hospital. There are two medical oncology departments in the West Bank, Al-Najah National University Hospital, and a recently opened department in Al-Istishari hospital in the heart of Ramallah city. There is a comprehensive cancer center in East Jerusalem, Augusta-Victoria Hospital cancer care center (AVH CCC). There is a strong collaboration between governmental and non-governmental sectors through the referral department in the Ministry of Health.

In 2006, the first radiation service in Palestine was opened and accredited by the Joint Commission International, with the help of WHO and the International Atomic Energy Agency at AVH CCC. However, despite substantial progress, Augusta-Victoria Hospital Cancer Center is the most qualified cancer center with established advanced diagnostic services and imaging studies like PET-CT scans. In 2017, Al-Najah National University Hospital opened an oncology-hematology service with preliminary autologous Hematopoietic Cell Transplantation (HCT). In 2020, a third department was opened in Al-Istishari Hospital.

13.11 The Future of Cancer Care in Palestine

Cancer care in Palestine is improving and there is a strong collaboration between public and private facilities. This led to the creation of an organized referral system between the Ministry of Health hospitals, non-government, and private sectors. Collaborative efforts have been made to reduce the population's demands for cancer care.

Several new cancer care facilities have been announced to open in both public and private hospitals. One of the major advances is the plan to develop a national comprehensive cancer center in Ramallah City in the heart of the West Bank-Khalid Al-Hasan Cancer Center-currently on-hold. The design is already completed, and the center will initially operate with 250 beds, with plans to expand to 500 in the future. Specialized units for radiotherapy, medical and surgical oncology, hematology, palliative care, and Hematopoietic Cell Transplantation are planned with a projected opening within 10 years. Besides providing much-needed oncology care, the center will train medical graduates for careers in medical oncology, hematology, radiation oncology, and others. This will foster progress toward more integrated clinical care. A research network will be formed to partner with national and international leading cancer centers [34].

13.12   Conclusion

The Palestinian healthcare system is improving, despite the political and financial constraints. Primary healthcare is amongst the best five healthcare systems in the Arab region. Cancer care is available in several public and private healthcare facilities. However, lacking a more specialized cancer subspecialty, for example, Hematopoietic Cell Transplantation. Comprehensive oncology care is present in one large cancer center in East Jerusalem and plans to open new facilities soon, Khalid Al-Hassan cancer Center. Highly trained Health Care Providers (HCPs), along with government financial and logistic support, have improved cancer care in Palestine. Strong national and international collaborations will enhance comprehensive cancer care and research initiatives with Arab and other countries.

Conflict of Interest   Authors have no conflict of interest to declare.

Appendix: List of Publications

1. Cancer care in the Palestinian Territories. Lancet Oncol. 2018;19(7):e359–64. https://doi.org/10.1016/S1470-2045(18)30323-1.
2. Cancer care in the Palestinian territories—the ASCO post. 25 Oct 2018 https://ascopost.com. Accessed 28 May 2021.
3. The Palestinian National Institute of Public Health. Performance of mammography screening in the Palestinian National Institute of Public Health. http://pniph.org/site/article/15. Accessed 7 June 2018.
4. Azaiza F, Cohen M, Awad M, Dauod F, et al. Factors associated with low screening for breast cancer in the Palestinian. Cancer 2010;116:4646–55.
5. Al Waheidi S, McPherson K, Chalmers I, Sullivan R, Davies EA. Mammographic screening in the occupied Palestinian Territory: a critical analysis of its promotion, claimed benefits, and safety in Palestinian Health Research. JCO Global Oncol. 2020;6:1772–90.
6. Black WC, Haggstrom DA, Welch HG. All-cause mortality in randomized trials of cancer screening. J Natl Cancer Inst. 2002;94:167–73.
7. Gøtzsche PC, Jørgensen KJ. Screening for breast cancer with mammography. Cochrane Database Syst Rev. 2013;13(6):CD001877.
8. Marmot MG, Altman DG, Cameron DA, et al. The benefits and harms of breast cancer screening: an independent review. Br J Cancer 2013;108:2205–40.
9. Mittra I. Breast cancer screening in developing countries. Prev Med. 2011;53:121–2.
10. Mukhtar TK, Yeates DRG, Goldacre MJ. Breast cancer mortality trends in England and the assessment of the effectiveness of mammography screening: population-based study. J R Soc Med. 2013;106:234–42.
11. Portaluri M, Abu-Rmeileh N, Gianicolo E. Radiation therapy in palestine: not only money, but also real accessibility. Int J Radiat Oncol Biol Phys. 2017;98(3):504–5. https://doi.org/10.1016/j.ijrobp.2017.03.038.

12. Abu-Rmeileh NM, Gianicolo EA, Bruni A, et al. Cancer mortality in the West Bank, occupied Palestinian territory. BMC Public Health 2016;16:76.
13. Seir RA, Kharroubi A. Implementation of palliative care in Palestine: cultural and religious perspectives. Open J. 2017. https://doi.org/10.17140/PMHCOJ-SE-1-102.
14. Ambroggi M, Biasini C, Toscani I, Orlandi E, Berte R, Mazzari M, Cavanna L. Can early palliative care with anticancer treatment improve overall survival and patient-related outcomes in advanced lung cancer patients? A review of the literature. Support Care Cancer 2018;26(9):2945–53.
15. Khleif M, Dweib A, et al. Palliative Care and Nursing in Palestine. J Palliat Care Med. 2015;S4:003. https://doi.org/10.4172/2165-7386.1000S4003.
16. Khleif M, Imam A, et al. Quality of life for Palestinian patients with cancer in the absence of a palliative-care service: a triangulated study. Lancet. 2013;382:S23.
17. Khleif A, Shawawreh M, et al. Palliative care situation in Palestinian Authority. J Pediatr Hematol Oncol. 2011;33:S64–7.
18. Albarqouni L, Elessi K, Abu-Rmeileh NME. A comparison between health research output and burden of disease in Arab countries: evidence from Palestine. Health Res Pol Syst. 2018;16:25.
19. Abdalla B, Mansour M, Ghanim M, Aia B, Yassin M. The growing burden of cancer in the Gaza Strip, vol 20, www.thelancet.com/oncology. August 2019.
20. Giacaman R, Khatib R, Shabaneh L, Ramlawi A, Sabri B, Sabatinelli G. Health status and health services in the occupied Palestinian territory. Lancet. 2009;373:837–49.
21. Atrash F, Gil Z, Nammour W, Billa S. Building independence in health care and a partnership between Nations, vol 19. www.thelancet.com/oncology. July 2018.
22. Ashour A, Safi J, et al. Environmental risk factors associated with breast cancer in Gaza strip. Arch Food Nutr Sci. 14 Jan 2019.
23. Panato C, Abusamaan K, Bidoli E, Hamdi-Cherif M, Pierannunzio D, Ferretti S, Daher M, Elissawi F, Serraino. Survival after the diagnosis of breast or colorectal cancer in the GAZA Strip from 2005 to 2014. BMC Cancer. 2018;18(1):632. https://doi.org/10.1186/s12885-018-4552-x.
24. Economics of pediatric cancer in four eastern Mediterranean countries: a comparative assessment. JCO Glob Oncol. 2020;6:1155–70. https://doi.org/10.1200/GO.20.00041.
25. AlWaheidi S. Breast cancer in Gaza-a public health priority in search of reliable data. Ecancermedicalscience. 2019.
26. Qumseya BJ, Tayem YI, Dasa OY, Nahhal KW, Abu–Limon IM, Hmidat AM, Al–Shareif AF, Hamadneh MK, Riegert–Johnson DL, Michael B. Wallace barriers to colorectal cancer screening in Palestine: a national study in a medically underserved population. Clin Gastroenterol Hepatol 2014;12:463–9.
27. Genomic analysis of inherited breast cancer among Palestinian women: genetic heterogeneity and a founder mutation in TP53. Int J Cancer. 2017;141(4):750–6. https://doi.org/10.1002/ijc.30771.

28. Baloushah S, Salisu WJ, Elsous A, Muhammad Ibrahim M, Jouda F, Elmodallal H, Behboodi Moghadam Z. Practice and barriers toward breast self-examination among Palestinian women in Gaza City, Palestine. Sci World J. 2020:7484631. https://doi.org/10.1155/2020/7484631

References

1. The Palestinian Central Bureau of Statistics (PCBS). http://www.pcbs.gov.ps
2. Health inforum: the first report on oncology in Palestine. 1(15). 15 Nov 2002. Available at www.who.int/disasters/repo/8485.doc. Accessed 8 Oct 2018.
3. Ministry of Health, Health Annual Report, Palestine 2019, June 2020.
4. Ministry of Health, health annual report, Gaza, Palestine 2019, April 2020.
5. UNFPA and Palestinian Ministry of Health. Pathway to survival: the story of breast cancer in Palestine. https://healthclusteropt.org/admin/file_manager/uploads/files/1/2-BC in Palestine, Final for print 2019.pdf.
6. Katzke VA, Kaaks R, Kühn T. Lifestyle and cancer risk. Cancer J. 2015;21(2):104–10. https://doi.org/10.1097/PPO.0000000000000101.
7. Cancer Control. Knowledge into action. WHO guide for effective Programmes. Module 2: prevention. World Health Organization; 2007.
8. Tucktuck M, Ghandour R, Abu-Rmeileh NME. Waterpipe and cigarette tobacco smoking among Palestinian university students: a cross-sectional study. BMC Public Health. 2017;18(1):1.
9. Global Youth Tobacco Survey. West Bank 2016. Fact sheet.
10. Palestine STEPS Surveu 2010-0211. Fact Sheet.
11. The Use of Positron Emission Tomography (PET) for Cancer Care Across Canada, Time for a National Strategy, Susan D. Martinuk, 2011. https://www.triumf.ca/sites/default/files/TRIUMF-AAPS-Martinuk-PET-Across-Canada-REPORT.pdf. Accessed 1 July 2020.
12. Closeout Audit of Fund Accountability Statement of Augusta Victoria Hospital, New Bone Marrow Transplantation Program in West Bank and Gaza, Cooperative Agreement AID-294-A-13-00001, May 1, 2015, to August 31, 2016 https://www.oversight.gov/report/usaid/closeout-audit-fund-accountability-statement-augustavictoria-hospital-new-bone-marrow
13. Abu-Rmeileh NM, Gianicolo EA, Bruni A, et al. Cancer mortality in the West Bank, occupied Palestinian territory. BMC Public Health. 2016;16:76.
14. The Palestine Information Centre. Ministry of health reveals statistics about cancer in the Palestinian Territories. https://English.palinfo.com/news/2017/2/5/ministry-of-health-reveals-statistics-about-cancer-in-palestine.
15. http://site.moh.ps/index/Books/BookType/2/Language/ar. Accessed 19 Apr 2021.
16. https://www.pcrf.net/huda-al-masri-pediatric-cancer-department.
17. Khleif M, Dweib A, et al. Palliative care and nursing in Palestine. J Palliat Care Med. 2015;S4:003. https://doi.org/10.4172/2165-7386.1000S4003.
18. Khleif M, Imam A, et al. Quality of life for Palestinian patients with cancer in the absence of a palliative-care service: a triangulated study. Lancet. 2013;382:S23.
19. Seir RA, Kharroubi A. Implementation of palliative Care in Palestine: cultural and religious perspectives. Open J. 2017; https://doi.org/10.17140/PMHCOJ-SE-1-102.
20. Khleif A, Shawawreh M, et al. Palliative care situation in Palestinian Authority. J Pediatr Hematol Oncol. 2011;33:S64–7.
21. Elder Care and Palliative Medicine Institute (ECPMI). https://jerusalem.lutheranworld.org. Accessed 28 May 2021.
22. Albarqouni L, Elessi K, Abu-Rmeileh NME. A comparison between health research output and burden of disease in Arab countries: evidence from Palestine. Health Res Pol Syst. 2018;16:25. https://doi.org/10.1186/s12961-018-0302.

23. Al Waheidi S, McPherson K, Chalmers I, Sullivan R, Davies EA. Mammographic screening in the occupied Palestinian Territory: a critical analysis of its promotion, claimed benefits, and safety in Palestinian Health Research. JCO Glob Oncol. 2000;6:1772–90.
24. Abdalla B, Mansour M, Ghanim M, Aia B, Yassin M. The growing burden of cancer in the Gaza Strip, vol 20. www.thelancet.com/oncology. Aug 2019.
25. Khalid Halahleh MD, Robert Peter Gale MD. Cancer care in Palestinian Territories. Lancet Oncol. 2018;19:e359–64.
26. Pathway to survival: the story of breast cancer in Palestine. 2018.
27. Azaiza F, Cohen M, Awad M, et al. Factors associated with low screening for breast cancer in the Palestinian authority: Wiley Subscription Services, Inc., A Wiley Company, p. 4646–55.
28. Nissan A, Spira RM, Hamburger T, et al. Clinical profile of breast cancer in Arab and Jewish women in the Jerusalem area. Am J Surg. 2004;188(1):62–7.
29. Bendel M. Breast cancer in the Gaza strip: a death foretold. Physicians for Human Rights–Israel; 2005, p. 1–27.
30. Evaluation of the Strategic Cancer Care Initiative (SCC, Phase I&II evaluation-of-the-strategic-cancer-care-initiative-SCCI-phase-III). 22 Dec 2016.
31. American Society of Clinical Oncology. The state of cancer care in America, 2017: a report by the American Society of Clinical Oncology. J Oncol Pract. 2017;13(4):e353–94.
32. Zeidan YH, Geara F. Lebanon: an evolving hub for radiation therapy in the Arab world. Int J Radiat Oncol Biol Phys. 2015;91:888–91.
33. Corn BW, Symon Z. Radiation therapy in the Middle East: local and regional targets. Int J Radiat Oncol Biol Phys. 2014;90(5):975–8. https://doi.org/10.1016/j.ijrobp.2014.06.029.
34. Qatar Red Crescent Society Call No. (RES/QRC/2020/11). Call for Scientific Papers on Cancer in Palestine. https://www.jobs.ps/tenders/call-for-scientific-papers-on-cancerin-palestine-2579.html

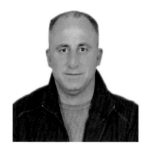

Khaled Halahleh is a senior consultant Medical Oncologist Hematologist. He served as the Head of the Hematology section at August-Victoria Hospital Cancer Care Center, Jerusalem (2007–2013). Dr. Halahleh holds specialty certificates from the Jordanian Board of Medical Oncology and the Palestinian Board of Medical Oncology and Hematology. Currently, he serves as a senior consultant in Medical Oncology Hematology and Bone Marrow Transplantation Program at King Hussein Cancer Center, Jordan. He is an active member of several KHCC's institutional committees, including the Institutional Review Board, Drugs and Therapeutics Committee and Venous Access Device Committee. He is the author of 11 peer-reviewed articles and publications. His research interest is allotransplants in myeloid and lymphoid malignancies.

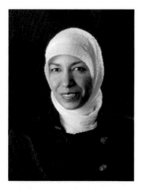

Niveen M.E. Abu-Rmeileh is a Professor of Epidemiology and Public Health at Birzeit University. She obtained her doctoral degree from the University of Glasgow. She has led national, regional, and international research. She is a board member of the Global Implementation Society (GIS). She is a member of the Eastern Mediterranean-Advisory Committee for Health Research (EM-ACHR) and the WHO-Eastern Mediterranean Research Ethics Review Committee (ERC). Dr. Abu-Rmeileh was ranked among the 100,000 most cited scientists, top 2 percent in their sub-fields. Her research interest is focused on three broad categories: Non-Communicable Diseases (with special focus on diabetes, cancer, and tobacco smoking), Reproductive Health, and Information Systems for Health.

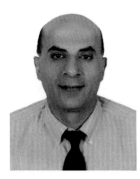

Mohammad M. Abusrour was born and raised in Palestine. He is a graduate of Columbia University, USA, with a master's degree in Medical Physics. Mr. Abusrour has extensive experience in Nuclear Medicine Technology, Diagnostic Imaging Physics and Radiation Therapy Physics. Mr. Abusrour worked in hospitals in the USA and Palestine. He worked for Augusta-Victoria Hospital in Jerusalem (2006–2008). Mr. Abusrour has participated in IAEA projects to establish reference dose levels for patients in diagnostic radiology. Currently, he works as a senior specialist in healthcare quality related to diagnostic imaging and radiation oncology. Moreover, he serves as a member of the National Radiation Protection Committee in the UAE and other working groups.

Chapter 14
General Oncology Care in the Kingdom of Saudi Arabia

Atlal Abusanad, Majed Alghamdi, Mohammed Bakkar, and Abdul Rahman Jazieh

14.1 The Kingdom of Saudi Arabia Demographics

The Kingdom of Saudi Arabia (KSA) is in the southwest of Asia. It extends over four-fifths of the Arabian Peninsula, stretching over a land area of 2,149,700 square kilometers and it is divided into 13 administrative regions. Riyadh city is the capital of the KSA. The country has the two holy mosques of Islam in Makkah and Al-Madinah. The estimated population for Saudi Arabia in 2016 was 31,787,580. Saudi nationals were estimated to be 20,081,582 of these 10,231,364 (51%) were males and 9,850,218 (49%) were females. The Non-Saudi population was 11,705,998 of these 8,028,355 (69%) were males and 3,677,643 (31%) were females [1].

A. Abusanad (✉)
Faculty of Medicine, King Abdulaziz University and Hospital, Jeddah, Saudi Arabia
e-mail: Aabusanad@kau.edu.sa

M. Alghamdi
Department of Internal Medicine, Medical College, Al Baha University,
Al Baha, Saudi Arabia

Ministry of National Guard, Radiation Oncology, Princess Norah Oncology Center, King Abdulaziz Medical City, Jeddah, Saudi Arabia

M. Bakkar
Prince Mohammed Bin Nasser Hospital, Jazan, Saudi Arabia
e-mail: mmbakkar@moh.gov.sa

A. R. Jazieh
Ministry of National Guard Health Affairs, Department of Oncology, King Abdullah International Medical Research Center, King Abdulaziz Medical City, King Saud bin Abdulaziz University for Health Sciences, Riyadh, Saudi Arabia

© The Author(s) 2022
H. O. Al-Shamsi et al. (eds.), *Cancer in the Arab World*,
https://doi.org/10.1007/978-981-16-7945-2_14

215

14.2 Cancer Statistics in Saudi Arabia

14.2.1 Cancer Incidence

In 1992, The Saudi Cancer Registry (SCR), a population-based registry, was established under the authority of the Ministry of Health (MOH). In 2014, SCR was moved to the Saudi Health Council under the Department of National Registries in the National Center for Health Information. According to the most recent cancer incidence report by SCR in 2016, the total number of newly diagnosed cancer cases reported to the Saudi Cancer Registry (SCR) was 17,602. Overall, cancer cases were more among women than men; it affected 8044 (45.7%) males and 9558 (54.3%) females (Fig. 14.1). A total of 13,562 cases were reported among Saudi nationals, 3834 among non-Saudi, and 206 of unknown nationality. The crude incidence rates (CIR) of all cancers were 56.6/100,000 in males and 74.5/100,000 in females. The overall age-standardized incidence rate (ASR) was 74.7/100,000 in males and 91.3/100,000 in females. Eastern region reported the highest ASR among males and females, whereas Jazan region reported the lowest ASR among males and females (Fig. 14.2). The median age at diagnosis was 57 years with a range of (0–116) for males and 51 years with a range of (0–116) for females (Table 14.1).

The most common malignancies among the overall population are breast cancer, colorectal, and thyroid cancer (Table 14.2). The top three reported cancers among Saudi females are breast, thyroid, and colorectal cancers in descending order. Cancers among Saudi males are topped with colorectal cancer, lymphoma (Non-Hodgkin's), and prostate cancer. Non-Saudi males manifested colorectal followed by prostate and skin cancers, while non-Saudi females showed similar distribution to the Saudi females. A detailed report of SCR can be found online.

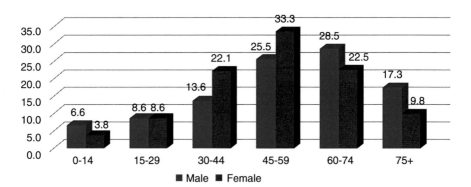

Fig. 14.1 Distribution of cancer cases among Saudi nationals by gender and age groups, 2016. *Source*: Cancer Incidence Report Saudi Arabia 2016 [1]

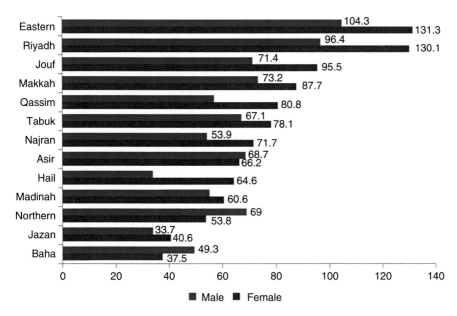

Fig. 14.2 Age Standardized Rate (ASR)* of all cancer sites among Saudi nationals, 2016. *Source*: Cancer Incidence Report Saudi Arabia 2016 [1]

14.2.2   Cancer Mortality

The percentage of deaths due to cancer increased steadily between 1990 and 2016. In 1990, the total percentage of deaths due to cancer was approximately 5% and increased to 12% in 2016 [2]. There were 36,951 deaths from Noncommunicable Diseases, and cancer accounted for 19.1% as per WHO cancer country profile 2020 [3, 4].

14.3   Oncology Care in Saudi Arabia

Oncology care across the Kingdom is provided through multiple public sectors, including the Ministry of Health, Ministry of Higher Education via university hospitals and specialized hospitals serving different governmental sectors (e.g., the Military, the National Guard Ministry, Arabian American Oil Company (ARAMCO), and the Ministry of Interior). Another providing partner is the Al-Faisal organization through the world-renowned King Faisal Specialist Hospitals and Research Centers (KFSH&RC) in Riyadh, Jeddah, and a recent branch in Al-Madinah cities. All cancer care facilities are freely accessible to citizens. Furthermore, private

Table 14.1 Number, percentage, CIR, ASR, and Cumulative Rates (per 100,000) among Saudi Nationals by primary cancer site and gender, 2016. Source: Cancer Incidence Report Saudi Arabia 2016 [1]

ICD-10	Site	Male						Female					
		No.	%	Crude Rate	ASR World	Cumulative Rate		No.	%	Crude Rate	ASR World	Cumulative Rate	
						0-64	0-74					0-64	0-74
All	All sites Total	5803	100.00%	56.6	74.7	39.95	81.8	7358	100.00%	74.5	91.3	62.75	99.35
Not C44	All sites but C44	5596	96.40%	54.6	72	39.05	79.3	7192	97.70%	72.9	89.2	61.7	97.2
C00	Lip	16	0.30%	0.2	0.2	0.125	0.205	6	0.10%	0.1	0.1	0.025	0.055
C01-C02	Tongue	60	1.00%	0.6	0.8	0.34	1.045	47	0.60%	0.5	0.7	0.435	0.83
C03-C06	Mouth	59	1.00%	0.6	0.8	0.39	0.95	60	0.80%	0.6	0.8	0.46	0.925
C07-C08	Salivary glands	23	0.40%	0.2	0.3	0.135	0.28	30	0.40%	0.3	0.4	0.255	0.33
C09	Tonsil	3	0.10%	0	0	0.03	0.03	2	0.00%	0	0	0.005	0.05
C10	Other Oropharynx	4	0.10%	0	0.1	0.015	0.06	2	0.00%	0	0	0.015	0.015
C11	Nasopharynx	154	2.70%	1.5	1.8	1.425	1.895	59	0.80%	0.6	0.7	0.535	0.745
C12-C13	Hypopharynx	7	0.10%	0.1	0.1	0.035	0.125	14	0.20%	0.1	0.2	0.08	0.2
C14	Pharynx unspec.	2	0.00%	0	0	0.02	0.02	1	0.00%	0	0	0.01	0.01
C15	Oesophagus	78	1.30%	0.8	1.1	0.53	1.055	50	0.70%	0.5	0.7	0.275	0.69
C16	Stomach	207	3.60%	2	2.9	1.26	3.32	111	1.50%	1.1	1.5	0.765	1.615
C17	Small intestine	37	0.60%	0.4	0.5	0.27	0.645	32	0.40%	0.3	0.4	0.27	0.44
C18	Colon	581	10.00%	5.7	7.8	4.595	8.96	447	6.10%	4.5	6.1	4.09	7.13
C19-C20	Rectum	374	6.40%	3.6	5.1	2.945	6.1	257	3.50%	2.6	3.4	2.34	3.685
C21	Anus	24	0.40%	0.2	0.3	0.165	0.37	11	0.10%	0.1	0.2	0.15	0.18
C22	Liver	290	5.00%	2.8	4.2	1.805	4.885	127	1.70%	1.3	1.9	1.005	2.585
C23-C24	Gallbladder etc.	80	1.40%	0.8	1.2	0.555	1.675	113	1.50%	1.1	1.7	0.73	2.305
C25	Pancreas	170	2.90%	1.7	2.5	1.285	3.26	104	1.40%	1.1	1.5	0.71	1.985
C30-C31	Nose, sinuses etc.	18	0.30%	0.2	0.2	0.115	0.345	5	0.10%	0.1	0.1	0.055	0.1
C32	Larynx	69	1.20%	0.7	0.9	0.58	1.175	7	0.10%	0.1	0.1	0.025	0.1
C33-C34	Trachea,Bronchus,Lung	298	5.10%	2.9	4.4	2.13	5.42	148	2.00%	1.5	2	1.185	2.355
C37-C38	Other Thoracic organs	16	0.30%	0.2	0.2	0.135	0.18	10	0.10%	0.1	0.1	0.095	0.17
C40-C41	Bone	93	1.60%	0.9	0.9	0.535	0.71	53	0.70%	0.5	0.5	0.305	0.35
C43	Melanoma of Skin	14	0.20%	0.1	0.2	0.04	0.12	25	0.30%	0.3	0.3	0.125	0.28
C44	Other Skin	207	3.60%	2	2.7	0.955	2.555	166	2.30%	1.7	2.1	1	2.135
C45	Mesothelioma	11	0.20%	0.1	0.2	0.015	0.24	7	0.10%	0.1	0.1	0.085	0.085
C46	Kaposi sarcoma	27	0.50%	0.3	0.4	0.175	0.505	4	0.10%	0	0.1	0.01	0.055
C47;C49	Connective,Soft tissue	89	1.50%	0.9	1	0.57	0.925	70	1.00%	0.7	0.8	0.415	0.645
C50	Breast	42	0.70%	0.4	0.6	0.41	0.59	2240	30.40%	22.7	27.2	21.46	29.67
C51	Vulva	-	-	-	-	-	-	9	0.10%	0.1	0.1	0.1	0.145
C52	Vagina	-	-	-	-	-	-	8	0.10%	0.1	0.1	0.06	0.06
C53	Cervix Uteri	-	-	-	-	-	-	111	1.50%	1.1	1.4	0.83	1.475
C54	Corpus Uteri	-	-	-	-	-	-	454	6.20%	4.6	6.6	4.76	8.475
C55	Uterus unspec.	-	-	-	-	-	-	40	0.50%	0.4	0.5	0.349	0.605
C56	Ovary	-	-	-	-	-	-	219	3.00%	2.2	2.7	1.755	3.075
C57	Other Female Genital	-	-	-	-	-	-	18	0.20%	0.2	0.2	0.17	0.245
C58	Placenta	-	-	-	-	-	-	4	0.10%	0	0	0.02	0.02
C60	Penis	4	0.10%	0	0	0.045	0.045	-	-	-	-	-	-
C61	Prostate	405	7.00%	4	6.3	1.87	7.76	-	-	-	-	-	-
C62	Testis	123	2.10%	1.2	1.1	0.695	0.795	-	-	-	-	-	-
C63	Other male genital	3	0.10%	0	0	0.03	0.065	-	-	-	-	-	-
C64	Kidney	196	3.40%	1.9	2.6	1.635	3.065	138.0	0.0	1.4	1.8	1.16	1.89
C65	Renal Pelvis	7	0.10%	0.1	0.1	0.08	0.08	2.0	0.0	0.0	0.0	0.02	0.065
C66	Ureter	8	0.10%	0.1	0.1	0.03	0.155	0.0	0.0	0.0	0.0	0	0
C67	Bladder	229	3.90%	2.2	3.2	1.725	3.465	59.0	0.0	0.6	0.8	0.39	0.89
C68	Other Urinary organs	7	0.10%	0.1	0.1	0.065	0.1	2	0.00%	0	0	0.035	0.035
C69	Eye	30	0.50%	0.3	0.3	0.17	0.17	16	0.20%	0.2	0.2	0.095	0.14
C70-C72	Brain, Nervous system	212	3.70%	2.1	2.3	1.625	1.965	155	2.10%	1.6	1.8	1.18	1.755
C73	Thyroid	222	3.80%	2.2	2.5	1.7	2.47	854	11.60%	8.7	8.9	7.005	7.985
C74	Adrenal gland	22	0.40%	0.2	0.2	0.14	0.14	19	0.30%	0.2	0.2	0.095	0.095
C75	Other Endocrine	5	0.10%	0	0.1	0.04	0.04	6	0.10%	0.1	0.1	0.035	0.035
C81	Hodgkin disease	265	4.60%	2.6	2.6	1.675	2.135	230	3.10%	2.3	2.3	1.535	1.825
C82-C85;C96	Non-Hodgkin lymphoma	469	8.10%	4.6	5.6	3.195	5.795	372	5.10%	3.8	4.9	3.01	5.435
C88	Immunoproliferative dis.	0	0.00%	0	0	0	0	0	0.00%	0	0	0	0
C90	Multiple Myeloma	72	1.20%	0.7	1	0.505	1.165	48	0.70%	0.5	0.6	0.455	0.775
C91	Lymphoid Leukaemia	165	2.80%	1.6	1.8	0.915	1.36	105	1.40%	1.1	1.2	0.635	0.97
C92-C94	Myeloid Leukaemia	142	2.40%	1.4	1.5	1.02	1.42	158	2.10%	1.6	1.7	1.275	1.62
C95	Leukaemia unspec.	27	0.50%	0.3	0.3	0.18	0.305	13	0.20%	0.1	0.1	0.05	0.095
Other	Other & unspecified	137	2.40%	1.3	1.7	1.12	1.76	110	1.50%	1.1	1.5	0.605	1.895

CIR crude incidence rate, *ASR* age-standardized incidence rate

cancer care is available and covered by insurance. The national cancer institute of Saudi Arabia (SANCI) was founded following a royal decree in 2016 under the authority of the Saudi Health Council. It serves as a consultive entity to develop national strategies to control and combat cancer in coordination with other health authorities and related agencies in the Kingdom.

Table 14.2 Most common cancers among Saudi, 2016 (Source: Cancer Incidence Report Saudi Arabia 2016) [1]

Site	Male	Female	All	%
Breast	42	2240	2282	17.3
Colorectal	955	704	1659	12.6
Thyroid	222	854	1076	8.2
NHL	469	372	841	6.4
Leukaemia	334	276	610	4.6
Hodgkin's lymphoma	265	230	495	3.8
Corpus Uteri	0	454	454	3.4
Lung	298	148	446	3.4
Liver	290	127	417	3.2
Prostate	405	0	405	3.1

The Saudi MOH designates the oncology facilities based on the range of the provided oncology services. There are three models of the oncology facilities; comprehensive oncology centers, specialized oncology departments, and oncology service units; the latter two are built within a hospital and are utilizing shared resources with the other hospital subspecialties. Also, there are other public non-MOH comprehensive oncology centers. Specialized oncology departments are found in MOH hospitals and other non-public MOH hospitals. The third model is oncology service units, which applies the hub-and-spoke design. This model arranges service delivery assets into a network consisting of an anchor establishment (hub) which offers a full array of services, complemented by secondary establishments (spokes) which offer more limited services.

14.4   Cancer Risk Factors

14.4.1   Obesity

The Saudi Health Interview Survey (SHIS) from 2013 showed high rates of obesity in the Kingdom. The prevalence of obesity, defined as a BMI of 30 kg/m^2 was 28.7%. It was higher among females than males, 33.5% vs. 28.7%. It increased with increasing age, being the highest among those aged between 55 and 64 years, reaching up to 48%. Obesity is reported to be the leading risk factor for disability-adjust life years (DALYs), accounting for 11.8% and 11.1% DALYs among males and females, respectively. In 2017, the Population-Attributable Fraction (PAF) of obesity was reported at 6.8% for cancer cases [3–5].

14.4.2 Smoking/Tobacco Use

Overall, 12.1% of the population reported tobacco use. The prevalence was 23.7% and 1.5% among men and women, respectively. Individuals aged 55–64 years old reported the highest tobacco use, with 24.7% in men and 4.2% in women. Different tobacco use was reported, including cigarette 11.4% with an average of 15 cigarettes/day, Shisha smoking in 11.2%, and smokeless tobacco in 0.3%. The average age of starting smoking is 18.7 years. Secondhand smoke exposure is reported among 17.2% at home and 14.8% at work. In 2017, the Population-Attributable Fraction (PAF) of tobacco use was reported at 10% for cancer deaths [3, 4, 6].

14.4.3 Low Physical Activity

The Saudi Health Interview Survey (SHIS) from 2013 reported a high percentage of individuals reporting low physical activity; overall, 60% reported a sedentary lifestyle. The estimated PAF in Saudi Arabia was 19.9% for breast cancer, 20.4% for colon cancer, and 18.4% for all-cause mortality due to physical inactivity [7, 8].

14.4.4 Infections

The infection PAF is 12% for cancer cases in Saudi Arabia. Seventy-five percent of Hepatocellular Carcinoma (HCC) cases in Saudi Arabia are attributed to viral hepatitis (hepatitis B and C) with a more recent dominance of HCV over HBV. HCC is rated sixth in Saudi males and ninth in Saudi females among all cancers, with an age-standardized incidence rate of 4.8/100,000 for males and 2.4/100,000 for females [9]. HBV vaccination has become a mandatory requirement for all Saudi children at school entry in addition to a free mass vaccination program among adults in 1989–1990. HPV prevalence among women with normal cervical cytology in Saudi Arabia is 28.6%, among women with invasive cervical cancer in Saudi Arabia is 76%. However, cervix uteri cancer is not common among Saudi females accounting for 1.6% of cancer incidence [10, 11].

14.5 Cancer Screening Programs

14.5.1 Breast Cancer

Several pilot screening projects in different regions—Riyadh, Dammam, Jeddah, and Al-Qassim-were initiated as early as 1997 [12]. All commonly reported low uptake rates and low cancer detection compared to Western countries; however, follow-up periods were short ranging from 2 to 5 years [13]. In 2012, the MOH initiated a nationwide Breast Cancer Early Detection (BCED) project to promote primary prevention through advertising awareness of modifiable risk factors associated with breast cancer, and secondary prevention through mammography for average-risk women [14]. Designated facilities, including mobile units across the Kingdom equipped with mammograms, were made available and accessible free of charge for citizens. The month of October is recognized nationally as the breast cancer awareness month, mirroring the international cancer calendar. Nonetheless, screening facilities are accessible throughout the year. Other nonprofit governmental and private initiatives for early detection of breast cancer are available, too [15, 16].

14.5.2   Colorectal Cancer

The Colorectal Cancer Early Detection Project was initiated by the MOH recently (2017) and aimed at average-risk individuals and the ones at increased risk of developing colorectal cancer [17]. Several healthcare centers provide the screening through fecal occult blood test and proctoscopy according to the individualized risk.

14.5.3   Cervical Cancer

Although there is no nationwide campaign advertising screening, pap smear with and without HPV testing is available in both the public and private sectors.

14.5.4   Other Screenable Cancers

A National program to screen for lung and prostate cancers is not activated. However, individualized screening as per a physician's recommendation or a patient's desire is available by the corresponding screening tools.

14.6   Cancer Prevention Programs

The Ministry of Health has been advocating a healthy lifestyle with a healthy diet, physical activity, maintaining ideal body weight, and smoking cessation to decrease noncommunicable diseases, including cancer. Anti-smoking clinics were made widely accessible to assist individuals who desire to quit smoking with behavioral and pharmacologic therapy. Saudi Food and Drug Authority (SFDA) mandates that nutritional facts and calories are listed on the product to inform the consumer choices of a healthy diet. Successful control of obesity and tobacco use may reduce cancer incidence and mortality as the tobacco use PAF is 10% for cancer deaths and the obesity PAF is 6.8% for cancer cases.

HBV and HPV are recognized infections that lead to cancer development in Saudi Arabia [9, 10]. Interventions to limit the risk of contracting these infections were implemented. HBV vaccination has become a mandatory requirement for all Saudi children at school entry in addition to a free mass vaccination program among adults that was launched in 1989–1990. HPV vaccination was included in the national immunization schedule for females at 11–12 years old. Different healthcare sectors, including the private sector, offer HPV vaccination at charge for desiring individuals but it is not covered by health insurance.

14.7 Cancer Diagnosis

14.7.1 Imaging (Access to Imaging for Diagnosis and Later for Staging)

Imaging facilities are available throughout the country. There are 81.7 mammographs, 251.6 CT scanners, and 158.5 MRI scanners per 10,000 cancer patients. There are 17 functioning PET CT machines in the Kingdom 13 in Riyadh, 3 in Dammam, and one in Jeddah with access time 2–3 weeks. Expanding in PET CT scans is limited due to the unavailability of radiopharmaceutical substances and cyclotrons. Nevertheless, there is a national plan to increase the number of PET CT scans in the next 5 Years.

14.7.2 Laboratory

Most immunohistochemical staining and anatomical pathology studies are performed in all tertiary cancer facilities in the Kingdom. Historically, molecular and genetics studies were done in a reference laboratory in Europe and the USA and supported by industry. However, over the last 3 years, in-house molecular studies, especially Next-Generation Sequencing (NGS) are being performed in some tertiary facilities. Many of the tests performed locally or internationally are supported by industry grants.

14.8 Treatment

14.8.1 Medical Oncology

14.8.1.1 MOH-Cancer Care Facilities

Anti-neoplastic therapies are available and administrated in all models of the cancer care facilities that have been described in Sect. 14.3. Comprehensive care centers are independently regulating and purchasing their formulary. In comparison, oncology departments and units serve a prespecified MOH essential list of anti-neoplastic agents. An essential list of anti-neoplastic agents with selected chemo-therapies and targeted therapies is updated periodically to inform the must-have agents in stocks. In case there is a need for unlisted medication, an application is submitted to the central MOH oncology pharmacy for approval and supply. Anti-neoplastic agents for new or expanded indications, including chemotherapies, bio-logics, and immunotherapies are promptly reviewed by the SFDA for approval as they become supported by scientific evidence.

14.8.1.2   Non-MOH Cancer Care Facilities

These cancer care providers operate according to the corresponding founding gov-ernmental authority and regulate their formulary according to internal advisory committees.

14.8.1.3   Medical Oncology Workforce

Although there are local fellowship programs and several opportunities for abroad scholarships and careers in medical oncology, the number of native medical oncolo-gists is still below what is needed to meet the increasing number of cancer patients. Therefore, nearly 85–90% of the medical oncology workforce in Saudi Arabia are non-Saudi. Unfortunately, incorrect perception of medical oncology as a depressing subspeciality might have contributed to this [18]. Better advertisement and incen-tives to recruit trainees to the specialty are essential.

14.8.1.4   Stem Cell Transplant and High Dose Chemotherapy

Saudi Arabia was the first Arab state to perform Hematopoietic Stem Cell Transplantation (HSCT) in 1984. 6184 HSCTs were performed in Saudi Arabia between 1984 and 2016; 3586 were performed in adults and 2598 were performed in the pediatric population. In adults, 2179 were allo-HSCTs and 1407 were auto-HSCTs. In pediatric patients, the majority (2326) were allo-HSCTs, while the auto-HSCT represented a small proportion (272). In pediatric patients, a high proportion of HSCT is performed for nonneoplastic hematologic indications, including hemo-globinopathies, primary immunodeficiency disorders, thalassemia, and bone mar-row failure syndromes [19]. Five centers are providing stem cell transplant services in Riyadh, two in Jeddah, and one in Dammam. These centers provide both autolo-gous and allogeneic stem cell transplantation distributed between MOH and other public non-MOH sectors. New services limited to autologous stem cell transplant in Makkah and Al-Madinah cities are being introduced [20]. A national marrow donor registry is being established to facilitate matched unrelated donor transplant. Also, umbilical cord blood banks are available in KFSH&RC, Riyadh.

14.8.2 Radiation Therapy

Currently, 32 linear accelerators are operational with a few more being in commissioning or planning phases. These machines are distributed in four provinces, Riyadh, Makkah, Eastern region, and Tabuk. Specialized and dedicated available radiotherapy machines included 4 Cyberknife, 6 intraoperative radiotherapy units, 4 brachytherapy units, and 1 Gamma Knife. Most existing linear accelerators can perform 3-D, IMRT, VMAT, and SBRT treatments. Around 60 radiation or clinical oncologists are currently licensed in Saudi Arabia in treating patients with radiation therapy. The Saudi Proton Therapy Center at King Fahad Medical City, Riyadh, has the first proton therapy facility in the Arab world and the Kingdom [21]. This project is going to be operational very soon.

14.8.3 Surgery

Surgical oncology is available throughout the comprehensive cancer centers and the specialized oncology departments at both MOH and public non-MOH facilities as well as the private sector. Complex oncologic procedures are referred to tertiary centers; for instance, the first two cytoreductive surgery and Hyperthermic Intraperitoneal Chemotherapy (HIPEC) were done in 2008 at KFSH&RC and King Fahad Medical City, followed by King Abdullah medical city, Makkah, King Abdulaziz University Hospital, Jeddah and King Saud University Hospital, Riyadh. More recently, King Khalid hospital, Najran, is providing PIPAC. Some of the centers receive patients from neighboring countries. Up to date, over 1,200 cases were performed [22].

14.8.4 Pediatric Oncology

A total of 803 cancer cases were diagnosed among children aged between 0 and 14 years, accounting for 4.6% of the total number of cancers reported to Saudi Cancer Registry in 2016. The reported incidents show that cancer was more common among boys than girls, 463 (57.6%) cases were reported among boys and 340 (42.4%) were reported among girls. A total of 664 cancer cases were reported among Saudi children, 129 were among non-Saudis, and 10 cases were with unknown nationality. The leading cancer among Saudi children was leukemia (30.4%), followed by brain tumors (14.6%), then Hodgkin's lymphoma (11.6%), and NHL (9.1%) [1].

Centers that provide comprehensive pediatric cancer care are in Riyadh, Jeddah, Dammam, and Al-Qassim. There are six centers in Riyadh, three centers in Jeddah, one in Dammam, and one in Al-Qassim under the authority of MOH and other governmental non-MOH sectors.

14.8.5   Survivorship Track

Several survivorship clinics caring for long-term survivorship issues are operational within some of the specialized cancer centers. Generally, global guidelines are widely adopted to guide these issues. However, national dedicated guidelines and strategies on long-term survivorship planning and related issues in patients of different age groups who survived a cancer diagnosis have yet to be generated. Some cancer care professionals and nonprofit organizations' efforts to advocate survivorship awareness are on the horizon [23]. The need to develop a national survivorship strategy tailored to cancer, cultural and population characteristics is necessary to optimize holistic cancer care delivery [24].

14.8.6   Palliative Care Track

An effective palliative care system is essential for cancer patients diagnosed in advanced stages, suffering pain, and having end-of-life issues, especially a higher proportion of our patients are presenting in advanced stages than in western societies. The palliative care service in Saudi Arabia was started over two decades ago at the KFSH&RC in Riyadh with the progressive expansion of the specialty all over the Kingdom. Currently, there are 10 palliative care units are built-in in hospitals. They operate through consultation service within the hosting hospital, outpatient clinics, home healthcare program, and an outreach program in some. Although there are more advanced stage cancers, the per capita consumption of morphine in the country is below the mean global consumption of 6.11 mg [25]. Several factors contribute to the observed underuse of opioids, including poor awareness, the misconception on addiction, life-threatening adverse events, and strict prescribing policy. Initiatives directed toward improving education, awareness, and modifying prescribing policies to suit local cancer trends are underway [26]. The Saudi health council has issued a Do-Not-Resuscitate (DNR) policy to limit inconsistency and have a standardized approach across the healthcare facilities. Likewise, the Saudi Commission for Health Specialties (SCHS) published educational material on DNR to assist decision-making [27, 28].

14.9   Research and Education

Local training programs are available for all oncology subspecialties, including medical oncology, hematology, bone marrow transplant, pediatric hematology-oncology, radiation oncology, palliative care, and surgical oncology. These programs are mostly consistent with programs in North America. They are accredited and supervised by SCHS [29]. All training programs are considered fellowship/subspecialty training after successful completion of general specialty training except radiation oncology [30]. For example, a medical oncology fellowship is a 2-year program following an internal medicine residency [31]. Likewise, the hematology-oncology program requires a 2-year training after internal medicine residency with another optional year of further training in bone marrow transplant [32]. Surgical oncology often requires 3–5-year training after general surgery board certification. The pediatric hematology-oncology program is a 3-year program after completion of training in pediatrics [33]. Palliative care training (1 year fellowship) requires a background in family medicine, internal medicine, pediatric, general surgery, emergency, or anesthesia specialties. However, radiation oncology is a residency program of 5 years, starting after completing the internship year [30]. Local training programs are reviewed and accredited by the SCHS [29]. Governmental scholarships to international oncology training programs are also attainable.

Alghamdi et al. [34], recently reviewed all oncology publications from Saudi Arabia over 10 years. There was an increase in the volume of oncology publications comparing two time periods; 2008–2012 and 2013–2017. However, research quality remained the same. These findings call for a national strategy to improve cancer research. With more observed international collaboration, cancer research in Saudi Arabia is expected to continue growing in terms of quality and quantity, especially with improving research funds [35]. Funding is often secured through individual universities or dedicated research centers. Many clinical trials with and without international collaborations are open in multiple cancer centers in Saudi Arabia. Not surprisingly, the increasing research productivity in oncology reflects the increase in overall healthcare research activities, including basic sciences in Saudi Arabia [36].

14.10   Cost-Effective Cancer Care

Jazieh et al. [37] analyzed the future projection of cancer incidence and economic burden concluded that a projected additional increase of 63% cancer incidence is associated with increasing costs of 56% in 2030 compared to 2015. Managing costs of healthcare is one of the main focuses of the Kingdom's Vision 2030 and the national transformation program. Many strategies have been postulated, including increasing private sector share of spending in healthcare generally and in oncology care specifically, encouraging the privatization of the medical cities through a Public–Private Participation (PPP) scheme, mandating health insurance for all citizens, and broader utilization of digital health solutions to improve accessibility with reducing costs. Besides, continuing, and growing efforts to promote a healthy lifestyle, primary prevention, and early detection of noncommunicable diseases, including malignancies.

There is no Health Technology Assessment (HTA) for the cost-effectiveness of oncology medication in the Kingdom of Saudi Arabia; however, the SFDA is in the process of registration and negotiating the pricing issues. There is a national agency to purchase medications, the National Unified Procurement Company for Medical Supplies (NUPCO). It will be the universal agent to purchase oncology medications and other medications in the Kingdom of Saudi Arabia, which will give strong bargaining power and obtain the best deals for the medication in the country.

14.11 Challenges and Advantages

The geographic nature of Saudi Arabia, with central cities being urbanized disproportionally to the peripheral ones, produced difficulties with equal care accessibility, timely referral to the higher specialized cancer center, and inadequate therapeutic supply on occasions. A digital referral program (Ehalati) linking peripheral to higher centers was implemented to overcome the issue. The program is directed toward all health specialties, including cancer cases requiring immediate care. Additionally, the outreach (spoke-hub) model is being applied. Other inherited challenges are the young population (70% of the Saudi population is younger than 40 years), with a life expectancy that is expected to increase to 78.4 (males) and 81.3 (females) by 2050 and increasing population capacity coupled with the projected increase in cancer incidence by 60% in 2030 compared to 2015 [37]. Saudi Arabia has many out-of-the country workers, the non-Saudi population estimated at one-third of the total (nearly 12 Million). Medical expenses have to be managed reasonably to avoid loading the healthcare system. Hence, expanding the private healthcare investment in cancer has been encouraged recently when the Council of Cooperative Health insurance mandated private healthcare insurance providers to cover cancer care expenses for insured patients up to 500,000 SAR.

People's awareness and misconceptions surrounding cancer diagnosis and treatment contribute to the late-stage presentation, DALYs, and loss of productivity. Altogether, reflecting poorly on survival and costs. A significant deficiency in the native oncology workforce and expertise resulting in out-of-the-country recruitment is a considerable challenge. The desire of some cancer patients to be treated abroad (medical tourism) is an issue that has been regulated strictly over the past years in light of treatment availability at home. Although only 1800 cases in 2016 were granted such governmental sponsorship, the cost to cases ratio is still huge. Saudi cancer registry shows progressive improvement in cancer incidence reporting; however, data collection and accuracy on patient demographics, primary tumor site, tumor morphology, stage at diagnosis, the first course of treatment, and follow-up with patients for vital status are yet to be optimized.

There are multiple healthcare sectors in KSA, and coordination is essential to avoid duplicate efforts. This is being achieved via the Saudi Health Council and its sub, the Saudi NCI. Many newly approved medications are readily available in KSA, matching their availability in other developed world countries after being reviewed by the SFDA.

14.11.1   Quality of Cancer Care

The practice of oncology in Saudi Arabia is provided at a high standard and assurance of adherence to the latest advances of care. Well-trained oncologists provide cancer care with all different specialties that most of them are trained in North America (Canada or the USA). The tertiary hospitals usually have multidisciplinary teams to discuss complex cases and generally, oncologists adhere to National Comprehensive Center Network (NCCN) guidelines. In that regard, the first and only center for coordination of NCCN collaboration outside the USA was established in Saudi Arabia to adopt the NCCN guidelines to the Middle East and North Africa in 2010. There are multiple national guidelines developed over the last couple of decades by different entities, such as the Saudi Lung Cancer Association, Saudi Oncology Society [38, 39]. Lately, the Saudi NCI launched an initiative for national guidelines in 2018 [40].

The MOH adopted several Key Performance Indicators (KPIs) for their cancer care providers to assess care quality. Additionally, both MOH and non-MOH, including private cancer care providers must meet the accreditation requirement by the Saudi Central Board for Accreditation of Healthcare Institutions (CBAHI) [41].

Several comprehensive cancer care facilities in KSA are accredited and certified by international oncology societies. There are three ESMO designated oncology centers in KSA [42]. Besides, King Abdulaziz Medical City, Ministry of National Guard, Riyadh being the first in the Middle East and North Africa to receive ASCO's standards for quality cancer care delivery (QOPI) certification. Likewise, The KFSH&RC, Riyadh, was the first center outside Europe to obtain the Joint Accreditation Committee of the ISCT and the EBMT (JACIE) in 2010.

14.12   The Future of Cancer Care in Saudi Arabia

The Saudi Ministry of Health has led many initiatives to transform oncology care in the Kingdom starting from 2016. Several workshops, stakeholder meetings, global experts, and patients' interviews have been conducted. Several themes have been identified to shape the cancer care transformation strategy, including promoting general health awareness and primary prevention, improving early detection and screening, ensuring care accessibility, equality and quality, mobilizing and utilizing resources effectively, avoiding fragmented services, expanding services and bed capacity, measuring patients satisfaction, optimizing outcomes; specifically survival and quality of life, establishing guidelines/pathways, incorporating tele-health, and encouraging different sectors collaboration [43].

14.13 Conclusion

The Kingdom of Saudi Arabia is a pioneer in regional cancer care. Continuous advances are spanning a half-century (Fig. 14.3), with significant strides recently stirred by the national cancer care transformation strategy which is exploring challenges and solutions to improve cancer care further.

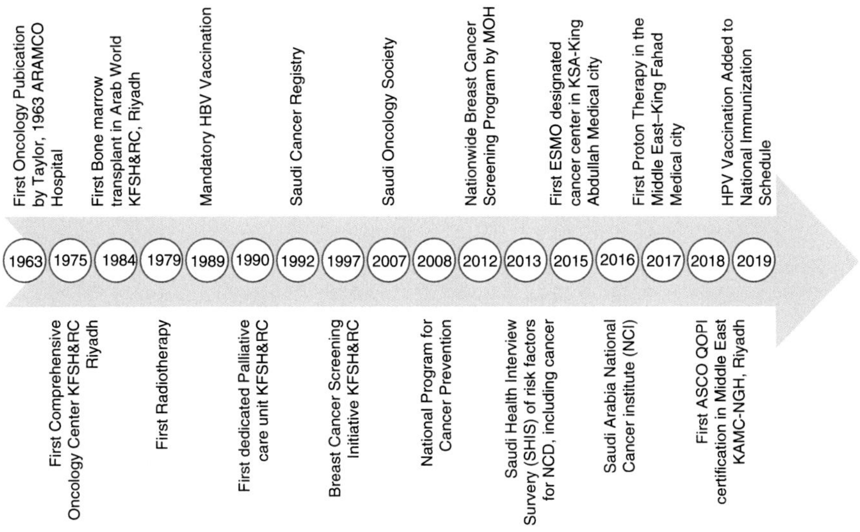

Fig. 14.3 Timeline of cancer care milestones in the Kingdom of Saudi Arabia

Conflict of Interest Authors have no conflict of interest to declare.

References

1. Saudi Arabia Cancer Incidence Report 2016, Saudi Cancer Registry (SCR). http://nhic.gov.sa/en/eServices/Documents/2016.pdf
2. Althubiti MA, Nour Eldein MM. Trends in the incidence and mortality of cancer in Saudi Arabia. Saudi Med J. 2018;39(12):1259–62. https://doi.org/10.15537/smj.2018.12.23348.
3. WHO Cancer Country Profile 2020, Saudi Arabia. https://www.who.int/cancer/country-profiles/SAU_2020.pdf
4. WHO international agency of research on cancer, Saudi Arabia. https://gco.iarc.fr/today/data/factsheets/populations/682-saudi-arabia-fact-sheets.pdf
5. Obesity at glance: findings from the Saudi health information survey for non-communicable diseases 2013. https://www.moh.gov.sa/Ministry/Statistics/Documents/obesity.pdf
6. Smoking in the Kingdom of Saudi Arabia: findings from the Saudi health information survey for non-communicable diseases 2013. https://www.moh.gov.sa/Ministry/Statistics/Documents/smoking.pdf
7. Alahmed Z, Lobelo F. Physical activity promotion in Saudi Arabia: a critical role for clinicians and the health care system. J Epidemiol Glob Health. 2018;7(Supplement 1):S7–S15., ISSN 2210-6006. https://doi.org/10.1016/j.jegh.2017.10.005.
8. The Saudi health information survey for non-communicable diseases 2013 https://www.moh.gov.sa/Ministry/Statistics/Documents/Final%20book.pdf
9. Aljumah AA, Kuriry H, Faisal N, Alghamdi H. Clinicopathologic characteristics and outcomes of hepatocellular carcinoma associated with chronic hepatitis B versus hepatitis C infection. Ann Saudi Med. 2018;38(5) September-October 2018 https://doi.org/10.5144/0256-4947.2018.358.
10. Alsbeih G. HPV infection in cervical and other cancers in Saudi Arabia: implication for prevention and vaccination. Front Oncol. 2014;31(4):65. https://doi.org/10.3389/fonc.2014.00065.
11. Bruni L, Albero G, Serrano B, Mena M, Gómez D, Muñoz J, Bosch FX, de Sanjosé S. ICO/IARC Information Centre on HPV and Cancer (HPV Information Centre). Human Papillomavirus and Related Diseases in Saudi Arabia. Summary Report 17 June 2019. https://hpvcentre.net/statistics/reports/SAU.pdf
12. Knoll SM. Breast cancer screening and a comprehensive breast cancer program in Saudi Arabia. Ann Saudi Med. 1997;17(1):1–3. https://www.annsaudimed.net/doi/full/10.5144/0256-4947.1997.1
13. Abulkhair OA, Al Tahan FM, Young SE, Musaad SMA, Jazieh A-RM. The first national public breast cancer screening program in Saudi Arabia. Ann Saudi Med. 2010;30(5):350–7. https://doi.org/10.4103/0256-4947.67078.
14. Ministry of Health, Saudi Arabia. MOH initiatives & projects, breast cancer early detection https://www.moh.gov.sa/en/Ministry/Projects/breast-cancer/Pages/default.aspx
15. Sheikh Mohammed Hussien AL-Amoudi Center of Excellence in Breast Cancer. https://ala-moudi-breastcenter.kau.edu.sa/Default-905-AR
16. Abdullateef Cancer Screening Center. https://www.saudicancer.org/index.php/2014-11-17-06-36-18/2014-11-30-13-30-00
17. The Saudi Ministry of Health. MOH initiatives & projects, colorectal cancer early detection https://www.moh.gov.sa/en/Ministry/Projects/Colorectal-Cancer-Awareness/Pages/default.aspx
18. Abusanad A. Only if you view it through a different lens. Curr Oncol. 2018;25(5):299. Epub 2018 Oct 31. https://doi.org/10.3747/co.25.4073.
19. Shaheen M, Almohareb F, Aljohani N, et al. Hematopoietic stem cell transplantation in Saudi Arabia between 1984 and 2016: experience from four leading tertiary care hematopoietic stem

cell transplantation centers. Hematol Oncol Stem Cell Ther. 2021;14(3):169–78. https://doi.org/10.1016/j.hemonc.2020.07.008.

20. Al-Hashmi H, Alsagheir A, Estanislao A, et al. Establishing hematopoietic stem cell transplant programs; overcoming cost through collaboration. Bone Marrow Transplant. 2020;55(4):695–7. https://doi.org/10.1038/s41409-020-0793-9.

21. Saudi Proton Therapy Center. https://sptc.med.sa/en/home-en/

22. Alyami M, Mercier F, Traiki TB, Trabulsi N, Al-Alem I, Alzahrani A, Alqannas M, Almohaimeed K. The current status of peritoneal surface oncology in Saudi Arabia. Indian J Surg Oncol. 2019;10(Suppl 1):33–6. https://doi.org/10.1007/s13193-019-00876-y. Epub 2019 Jan 15

23. Abusanad A. "Najia" story: a WhatsApp support group for patients with breast cancer. Innovations in Digital Health, Diagnostics, and Biomarkers. 1(1):16–8. https://doi.org/10.36401/IDDB-20-01.

24. G20 discusses support for cancer survivors post treatment. https://www.arabnews.com/node/1745586/saudi-arabia

25. World Health Organization population data 2013, Pain and Policy Studies Group: 2011 EMRO Consumption of Morphine. International Narcotics Control Board. http://www.painpolicy.wisc.edu/sites/www.painpolicy.wisc.edu/files/EMRO_morphine_2011%20[Compatibility%20Mode].pdf

26. Alshammary SA, Abdullah A, Duraisamy BP, Anbar M. Palliative care in Saudi Arabia: two decades of progress and going strong. J Health Specialties. 2014;2(2):59.

27. The Saudi Commission for Health Specialties, Department of Medical Education & Postgraduate Studies, Code of Ethics for Healthcare Practitioners. http://docplayer.net/11868886-Code-of-ethics-for-healthcare-practitioners-the-saudi-commission-for-health-specialties-department-of-medical-education-postgraduate-studies.html

28. Arabi YM, Al-Sayyari AA, Al Moamary MS. Shifting paradigm: from "no code" and "do-not-resuscitate" to "goals of care" policies. Ann Thorac Med. 2018;13:67–71. https://doi.org/10.4103/atm.ATM_393_17.

29. The Saudi Commission for Health Specialties, programs accreditation. https://www.scfhs.org.sa/en/education/ProgramsAccreditation/Pages/default.aspx

30. The Saudi Board of Radiation Oncology. https://www.scfhs.org.sa/MESPS/TrainingProgs/TrainingProgsStatement/Documents/Radiation%20Oncology%20Residency.pdf

31. The Saudi Board of Medical Oncology. https://www.scfhs.org.sa/MESPS/TrainingProgs/TrainingProgsStatement/Documents/بطب%20الدمى%20وأورام%20الكبار.pdf

32. Adult Hematology Fellowship Program. https://www.scfhs.org.sa/MESPS/TrainingProgs/TrainingProgsStatement/Documents/أمراض%20الدمم%20الدمى%20الكبار.pdf

33. Pediatrics Hematology/Oncology Fellowship Program. https://www.scfhs.org.sa/en/MESPS/TrainingProgs/TrainingProgsStatement/ChildBloodDises/Documents/Program%20Booklit.pdf,

34. Alghamdi MA, Alzahrani RA, Alhashemi HH, et al. Oncology research in Saudi Arabia over a 10-year period. A synopsis. Saudi Med J. 2020;41(3):261–6.

35. Alabdula'aly AI. Experience of King Abdul-Aziz City for science and technology in funding medical research in Saudi Arabia. Saudi Med J. 2004;25(1 Suppl):S8–12.

36. Ul Haq I, Ur Rehman S, Al-Kadri HM, Farooq RK. Research productivity in the health sciences in Saudi Arabia: 2008-2017. Ann Saudi Med. 2020;40(2):147–54. https://doi.org/10.5144/0256-4947.2020.147.

37. Jazieh A, Da'ar OB, Alkaiyat M, Zaatreh Y, Saad AA, Bustami R, Alrujaib M, Alkattan K. Cancer incidence trends from 1999 to 2015 and contributions of various cancer types to the overall burden: projections to 2030 and extrapolation of economic burden in Saudi Arabia. Cancer Manag Res. 2019;11:9665–74. https://doi.org/10.2147/cmar.s222667.

38. Howington J. The first Saudi lung cancer guidelines. Ann Thorac Med. 2008;3(4):127. https://doi.org/10.4103/1817-1737.43155.

39. Bazarbashi SN. Saudi Oncology Society clinical management guidelines development. Saudi Med J. 2014;35(12):1524–6.

40. The Saudi Arabia National Cancer Institute. https://shc.gov.sa/en/NCC/Activities/Pages/ScientificTeams.aspx
41. The Saudi Central Board for Accreditation of Healthcare Institutions. https://portal.cbahi.gov.sa/english/home
42. ESMO Accredited Designated Centres. https://www.esmo.org/for-patients/esmo-designated-centres-of-integrated-oncology-palliative-care/esmo-accredited-designated-centres
43. Ministry of Health, Saudi Arabia. Health transformation strategy. https://www.moh.gov.sa/en/Ministry/vro/Documents/Healthcare-Transformation-Strategy.pdf

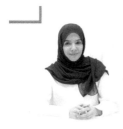

Atlal Abusanad , MBBS, MSc, ABIM, FRCPC, CIP, is working as a consultant in Internal Medicine and Medical Oncology, Oncology Division, Department of Medicine. She is also a Faculty of Medicine, King Abdulaziz University Hospital, Jeddah, Saudi Arabia. Dr. Abusanad specializes in breast and GI cancers and completed a Clinician-investigator fellowship (CIP) at McGill University, along with an MSc in experimental medicine and molecular oncology. Her scientific interests include clinical breast cancer, molecular oncology, translational research, cancer survivorship, communication, narrative medicine, and oncologists' burnout. She is the head of the breast cancer unit in KAUH and a member of the oncology pharmacy committee in the ministry of health.

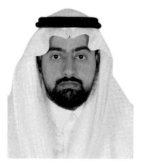

Majed Alghamdi is an assistant professor and consultant radiation oncologist with a sub-specialization in treating central nervous system tumors and stereotactic radiosurgery. He completed his residency training at the University of Calgary, Alberta, Canada, in 2016 and his fellowship training at the University of Toronto, Ontario, Canada in 2017. He holds the Canadian and American boards in radiation oncology. He is working as an assistant professor at Al-Baha University and consultant radiation oncologist at King Abdulaziz Medical City, Ministry of National Guard-Heath affairs, Jeddah, Saudi Arabia. He has published two textbook chapters and several peer-reviewed manuscripts that mainly focused on CNS oncology.

Mohammed Bakkar is a consultant in hematology at Prince Mohammed Bin Nasser Hospital, Jazan. He graduated from the college of medicine, King Saud University Riyadh, in 2004. He did residency training at KAMC for the national guard, Riyadh, Saudi Arabia. He passed the Saudi board of Internal medicine in 2009. Dr. Bakkar completed his hematology fellowship at the University of Ottawa, Ottawa, ON, Canada, in July 2014, followed by malignant hematology and BMT fellowship from the University of Ottawa, ON, Canada July 2015.

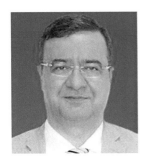

Abdul Rahman Jazieh is the Director of Innovations and Research and Director of International Program at Cincinnati Cancer Advisors, Cincinnati, OH, USA. He is the CEO of Innovative Healthcare Institute, Cincinnati, OH, USA. Additionally, he is the Editor-in-Chief, *Global Journal on Quality and Safety in Healthcare*. Dr. Rahman was a former Chairman of the Department of Oncology and a Professor at King Saud bin Abdulaziz University for Health Sciences, Riyadh, Saudi Arabia, between 2006 and 2020. He was also the former Professor and Chief of the Hematology Oncology Division at the University of Cincinnati. Dr. Jazieh founded the MENA-NCCN Collaborating Center (KSA) and the Association of VA Hematology Oncology (USA).

Chapter 15
General Oncology Care in Somalia

Hussein Abshir Hassan, Ikram Abdikarim, Nur Yassin, and Amin

15.1 Somalia Demographics

Africa's easternmost country, Somalia, has a land area of 637,540 km², slightly less than that of the state of Texas. Somalia occupies the tip of a region, commonly referred to as the Horn of Africa, because of its resemblance on the map to a rhinoceros's horn, which also includes Ethiopia and Djibouti [1]. Somalia's terrain consists mainly of plateaus, plains, and highlands. To the far north, the rugged east-west ranges of the Karkaar Mountains lie at varying distances from the Gulf of Aden coast. The weather is hot throughout the year, except at the higher elevations in the north. Rainfall is sparse, and most of Somalia has a semiarid to an arid environment suitable only for the nomadic pastoralism practiced by well over half the population. Only in limited areas of moderate rainfall in the northwest, and particularly in the southwest, where the country's two perennial rivers are found, is agriculture practiced to some extent [1]. The local geology suggests the presence of valuable mineral deposits. As of 1992, only a few significant sites had been located, and mineral extraction played a very minor role in the economy [1].

H. A. Hassan (✉) · Amin
University of Somalia, Mogadishu, Somalia

Uniso Hospital, Mogadishu, Somalia
e-mail: drhussein.abshir@uniso.edu.so

I. Abdikarim
Erdogan Hospital, Mogadishu, Somalia

N. Yassin
Faculty of Medicine, University of Somalia, Mogadishu, Somalia
e-mail: dryassin.nur@uniso.edu.so

© The Author(s) 2022
H. O. Al-Shamsi et al. (eds.), *Cancer in the Arab World*,
https://doi.org/10.1007/978-981-16-7945-2_15

Somalia's long coastline (3025 km) has been of importance, chiefly in permitting trade with the Middle East and the rest of East Africa. The exploitation of the shore and the continental shelf for fishing and other purposes had barely begun by the early 1990s. Sovereignty was claimed over territorial waters up to 200 nautical miles [1].

Somalia has an estimated population of around 15 million and has been described as Africa's most culturally homogeneous country [2–5]. Around 85% of its residents are ethnic Somalis who have historically inhabited in the country's north. Ethnic minorities are largely concentrated in the south [6, 7]. The official languages of Somalia are Somali and Arabic [6]. Most people in the country are Muslims. Many of them are Sunni [8].

The current population of Somalia is 16,149,487, as of February 1, 2021. Somalia's population in 2020 is estimated at 15,893,222 people in midyear according to UN data. The country's population is equivalent to 0.2% of the total world population. Somalia ranks 73rd in the list of countries (and dependencies) by population [2]. The population density in Somalia is 25 per Km^2 (66 people per mi^2). The total land area is 627,340 Km^2 (242,217 sq. miles). 46.8% of the population is urban (7,431,038 people in 2020). The median age in Somalia is 16.7 years. In 2019, Somalia's female population accounted for approximately 7.74 million, while the male population accounted for approximately 7.7 million inhabitants (Table 15.1) [9]. Table 15.2 shows the top 10 most populated cities in Somalia [10].

Table 15.1 Total population from 2017 to 2019, by gender (in millions) [9]. Prepared by Dr. Hussein Abshir. February 2021

Year	Female	Male
2017	7.31	7.28
2018	7.52	7.48
2019	7.74	7.7

Table 15.2 Top ten most populated cities in Somalia [10]. Dr. Hussein Abshir February 2021

S. No	City name	Population
1	Mogadishu	2,587,183
2	Hargeisa	477, 876
3	Berbera	242, 344
4	Kismayo	234,852
5	Marka	230, 100
6	Jamaame	185,270
7	Baydoa	129,839
8	Buro'	99,270
9	Bosaaso	74,287
10	Afgoi	65,461

15.1.1   Population Fertility Rate in Somalia

The current fertility rate for Somalia in 2021 is 5.845 births per woman, a 1.53% decline from 2020 whereas in 2020, it was 5.936 births per woman, a 1.53% decline from 2019. The fertility rate for Somalia in 2019 was 6.028 births per woman, a 1.5% decline from 2018 and in 2018 it was 6.120 births per woman, a 1.58% decline from 2017 [11].

15.1.2   Life Expectancy in Somalia

The life expectancy of both sexes is 58.3 years (life expectancy at birth, both sexes combined). The life expectancy of females is 60.1 years (life expectancy at birth, females). The life expectancy of males is 56.6 years. Infant mortality in Somalia is 62.8 (infant deaths per 1000 live births). The number of deaths under the age of 5 years is 104.6 (per 1000 live births) [12].

Until the collapse of the federal government in 1991, the organizational and administrative structure of Somalia's healthcare sector was overseen by the Ministry of Health. Regional medical officials enjoyed some authority, but healthcare was largely centralized. The socialist government of former President of Somalia Siad Barre had put an end to private medical practice in 1972 [13]. An exceptional amount of the national budget was devoted to military expenditure, leaving few resources for healthcare, among other services [14].

Somalia's public healthcare system was largely destroyed during the ensuing civil war. As with other previously nationalized sectors, informal providers have filled the vacuum and replaced the former government monopoly over healthcare, with access to facilities witnessing a significant increase. Many new healthcare centers, clinics, hospitals, and pharmacies have in the process been established through homegrown Somali initiatives [15]. The cost of medical consultations and treatment in these facilities is low at $5.72 per visit in health centers (with population coverage of 95%), and $1.89–3.97 per outpatient visit and $7.83–13.95 per bed day in primary through tertiary hospitals [16].

15.2   Cancer Statistics in Somalia

According to the estimate of the International Agency for Research on Cancer (IARC), in 2018, there were 17.0 million new cancer cases and 9.5 million cancer deaths worldwide. By 2040, the global burden is expected to grow to 27.5 million new cancer cases and 16.3 million cancer deaths, simply due to the growth and aging of the population [17].

15.2.1 Cancer Burden in Somalia

The total number of cancer cases in 2018 was 9942, while the total number of cancer deaths in that year was 8198. The future burden will probably be even larger due to the increased prevalence of factors that escalate risks, such as smoking, unhealthy diet, physical inactivity, and fewer childbirths, in economically transitioning countries [17].

Since there is no national cancer registry system in Somalia, the population-based cancer incidence is unknown. Dr. Bas of Erdogan Hospital and Dr. Hussein Abshir of UNISO Hospital have conducted the first study followed by other studies to evaluate the cancer incidence in Somalia, especially in the capital Mogadishu and its surroundings. The first study was conducted between January 01, 2016 and March 01, 2017. The results showed the 10 most common types of cancers were: esophageal ($n = 130$, 32.3%), Non-Hodgkin lymphoma ($n = 35$, 8.7%), liver ($n = 26$, 6.5%), breast ($n = 24$, 6.0%), skin ($n = 17$, 4.2%), thyroid ($n = 13$, 3.2%), brain ($n = 12$, 3.0%), bone ($n = 11$, 2.7%), colorectal ($n = 11$, 2.7%), and soft tissue ($n = 11$, 2.7%). The most common site of cancer in both males and females was the esophagus [18]. Table 15.3 shows the cancer incidence rate in Somalia, 2020 [23].

The second study was done by Erdogan Hospital in Mogadishu/Somalia, titled *Cancer Incidence and Distribution at a Tertiary Care Hospital in Somalia*, published on September 28, 2020, Volume 2020:12 PP. 8599–8611.

These studies aimed to determine both the cancer types and the distribution of cancers by age and gender in patients diagnosed at Somalia Turkey Recep Tayyip Erdogan Education and Research Hospital (STRTEH) and UNISO University Teaching Hospital. Both studies indicated the high incidence rate of esophageal cancer among the Somali population [19]. Due to limited number of patients, the results were not sufficient to reflect the real situation for the whole population. However, the studies can be considered as the first comprehensive retrospective studies on cancer incidence in the region. Furthermore, previous cancer incidence studies related to the population in Somalia were conducted with immigrants living in the United States of America (USA), and mostly focused only on women and on a single type of cancer, e.g., cervical or breast cancer [20].

Thus, a definitive conclusion has not yet been made regarding the incidence of all cancers in Somalia. Because Somali governments in the past and present did not

Table 15.3 Cancer incidence rate in Somalia 2020 [23]. Copyright—Dr. Hussein Abshir

Incidence	Country specific data source	Method	Total population	No. of new cases	No. of deaths	No. of prevalent cases (5- year)
Actual incidence is not known it is just an estimation	Not available	The rates are those of neighboring countries or registries in the same area	15,893,219	10,134	7439	13,212

pay much attention to support cancer programs (it could be due to lack of capacity or resources). Hence, there is no national data available on cancer statistics in Somalia. Somalia never had cancer centers, cancer registries, cancer research centers, cancer control programs, or national cancer policy. The country's government did not formulate a national cancer institution that could deal with the cancer problem. Also, international donors, governments, and Non-Governmental Organizations (NGOs) that assist Somalia, never considered cancer as a priority, which should be dealt immediately. Therefore, currently, there is no national cancer data in Somalia [21]. However, some Somali individual cancer specialists and private hospitals have started a few research studies related to oncology. A Somali doctor who specialized in medical oncology (Dr. Hussein Abshir) came back to Somalia from the diaspora and established the first cancer service center in Somalia in 2014, in collaboration with the University of Somalia, Mogadishu/Somalia. The center started offering chemotherapy services and improved diagnostic accuracy by working with the newly established radiology center, i.e., Kaamil Diagnostic Center. Additionally, the center has started working with some histopathologists who established their private practice. Currently, there are five histopathology labs in Mogadishu/Somalia. There is also one in Hargeisa/Northern Somalia. At present, these labs and the medical oncology center are working together closely by referring patients to each other and consulting with each other to improve the young cancer service that is emerging in Somalia [22].

15.2.2 Upcoming Projects

Some individuals and foreign companies are planning to establish modern private cancer centers and registries. These centers will focus on cancer diagnosis, treatment, and collection of data on cancer issues in Somalia.

15.3 Cancer Risk Factors

1. Infections—Such as viral hepatitis and Human Papillomavirus (HPV), cause 23.7% of the cancer cases in Somalia.
2. Tobacco—7.3% of the cancer cases.
3. UV—6.3%.
4. Obesity—1.2%.
5. Alcohol—0.8%.
6. Occupational risk—0.7% [24].

It is usually not possible to know exactly why one person develops cancer and another does not. However, research has shown that certain risk factors may increase a person's chance of developing cancer. In Somalia, suspected cancer risk factors include age, alcohol, cancer causing substances, chronic inflammation, diet, hormones, immunosuppression, infectious agents, obesity, radiation, sunlight, tobacco, and chewing a plant called khat. Alcohol consumption is on the rise in Somalia. Cheap alcoholic beverages come from neighboring countries, including Ethiopia and Kenya. Although it is illegal to import alcoholic beverages into Somalia, they are being smuggled in large numbers. The borders are porous, and the Somali coast is largely unguarded.

Smoking is not very common in Somalia, but tobacco is consumed in different ways; for example, a lot of Somalis chew tobacco which increases the risk of developing oral cancers. Unfortunately, using water-pipes (shisha) is becoming more and more popular. It is known that the risk of water-pipe is greater than simply smoking cigarettes. Somalis drink extremely hot beverages, especially hot tea, that has greatly increased the risk of developing esophageal carcinoma, which is the most common cancer in Somalia.

Moreover, Somali people eat a lot of red meat, since meat is cheap in Somalia and available everywhere. The Somali diet is typically deficient in vegetables and fruits, which may lead to an increased risk of developing cancer. Somali people are usually thin and not obese. However, this tendency is changing now. The new trend indicates Somali people are becoming more obese and sedentary, because of massive urbanization and the prevailing insecurity, which is scaring people away from sports and recreational activities [25].

15.4   Cancer Screening Programs

Cancer screening programs are just at the initial stage in Somalia. The past governments of Somalia never came up with a public health policy that would include screening programs. Currently, the most important screening program is for the Hepatitis B virus. According to the current statistics, 20% of the Somali people are carriers of Hepatitis B virus and are at risk of developing Hepatocellular Carcinoma (HCC) any time in the future. Pap smear screening for cervical cancer is now available and more women are becoming aware of the benefits of this screening. Some health facilities have started screening patients for cancers like HCC, breast, and cervical cancers. Women are being taught to do breast self-examination, from the age of 20 and above. A few private hospitals in Mogadishu and Hargeisa have started screening people for the Hepatitis B virus and vaccinating those who are negative for the virus. There are a lot of obstacles and challenges that are not permitting proper cancer screening programs to be established and operated in Somalia. Some of them are mentioned here:

- The Somali government and its institutions lack the financial and human resources needed to fight cancer in Somalia. Only some private nonprofit organizations and concerned individuals are leading the initiatives.
- A large part of the Somali population is ignorant of the disease and its dangers. There is a great need to educate the public about the disease and its impact on the life and the economy of the country. Even if there are programs in place, the public is not aware of the benefits and the importance of the screening programs.

- There is a lack of funding for screening programs. Donor organizations have other priorities for funding. They are not interested in funding such cancer screening programs. There is a need to solicit funders and local philanthropists to get engaged in the funding of these programs.

15.5   Cancer Prevention Programs

Currently, there is no national cancer control program in place. Only some volunteer organizations, for instance, the Somali Cancer Society, Hagarla Institute, and others are trying to provide beneficial services for the society. These voluntary organizations are conducting health education through local media, by organizing seminars, and by sending messages through social media. Some private hospitals have started vaccinations for Human Papillomavirus (HPV) and Hepatitis B virus. Women are being encouraged to do breast self-examination from the age of 20 and up and seek medical attention if they feel any suspicious lump or unusual swelling.

15.5.1   Obstacles and Challenges

- The Ministry of Health in Somalia lacks the capacity to participate in the prevention and control of the incidence of this deadly disease. The government budget cannot cover these programs.
- The majority of Somali people are not aware of the risk factors of this disease and ways and means of avoiding these factors and behaviors.
- There is a need to launch a massive health education to make people aware of the risk factors and avoid them. There is a need to fund programs that could identify risk factors and educate people about these risk factors.

15.6   Cancer Diagnosis

15.6.1   Laboratory

Until 2014, there was no proper diagnosis of cancer in Somalia. There was only one histopathologist in Somalia, but he was killed in an explosion together with other prominent intellectuals. Fortunately, there has been progress in this area. There are currently six pathology labs in Mogadishu that are conducting histopathological diagnoses. Most of these labs have qualified histopathologists (Table 15.4). There is no molecular testing, cytogenetic, and molecular genetic testing available in the country. Figure 15.1 shows the peripheral blood film of a child indicating Acute Lymphoblastic Leukemia (ALL).

Table 15.4 Number of histopathology labs in Mogadishu/Somalia (Source: According to my knowledge of the city). Copyrights—Dr. Hussein Abshir 2021

Name of the Doctor	Name of the facility	Location	Services offered	Price range	Waiting time
Dr. Sagal	Sagal pathology	Hodan district	FNA and histopathology	50–90 US $ per patient.	1–4 days
Dr. Mohamed.	Liibaan	Yakhshid district	FNA and histopathology	70–100 US $	1–7 days
Dr. Wehliye	Veritas	Hodan district	FNA and histopathology	50–90 US $	1–7 days
Dr. Abdullahi	Herd mark	Hodan	FNA and histopathology	50–90 US $	1–7 days
Erdogan Hospital staff	Erdogan Hospital	Hodan district	Cytology and histopathology	20–30 US $ per patient	1–10 days

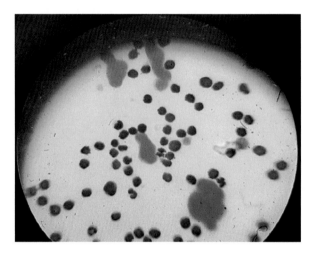

Fig. 15.1 Peripheral blood film of a child indicating Acute Lymphoblastic Leukemia (ALL) Copyright—Dr. Hussein Abshir, 2021

15.6.2 Imaging

Before 2010, there was no single Computed Tomography (CT) scan in Somalia. Today, there are CT scans along with four diagnostic centers that have Magnetic Resonance Imaging (MRI) scans (Table 15.5). The availability of modern imaging equipment and histopathology labs has greatly increased the diagnostic accuracy of cancer in Somalia. Some challenges that the country is facing are as mentioned:

- People are not aware of the importance of seeking diagnosis early enough, mainly because they cannot afford the cost of the tests.

Table 15.5 Number of imaging/radiology centers in Mogadishu/Somalia (Source: Myself; According to my knowledge of the city). Copyright—Dr. Hussein Abshir, 2021-02-09

Name	Location	Services	Price range	Waiting time
Kaamil	Hodan	CT, MRI & sonography	$100–200	1–2 days
Jasiira	Warta	CT	$120	1–2 days
Shaafi	Hodan	CT	$150	1–2 days.
Somali Sudanese	Hodan district	CT	$150	1–2 days
HawoAbdi	Hodan	MRI	$150	1–2 days

- Even if people can afford the cost of the diagnosis, the majority do not understand the importance of early diagnosis. These two factors have caused cancer to be diagnosed at an advanced stage, mostly at stage three or four.
- There is also stigma attached to this disease; a lot of people think this is a contagious disease. Others think this is totally incurable, so there is no need to diagnose them.

15.7   Treatment

15.7.1   Medical Oncology

There is only one medical oncologist in Somalia who is male and trained in China and Canada, Dr. Hussein Abshir Hassan. Currently, the only health facility that is providing cytotoxic chemotherapy treatment is in Mogadishu/Somalia. This is called UNISO Hospital and is a teaching hospital for the University of Somalia. It is attended by Somalia's only medical oncologist, Dr. Hussein Abshir Hassan. At present, there are no facilities that provide high-dose chemotherapy and Stem Cell Transplant (SCT). There is no advanced systemic therapy treatment or availability of immunotherapy/targeted therapy/biological agents.

Accessing these services is a challenge for the financially less fortunate patients, as there is no public coverage for these services. Most of the patients are poor and cannot afford the cost of chemotherapy. Currently, there is only one medical oncologist in Somalia, which is me, Hussein Abshir Hassan. I was trained in China as a medical oncologist (At Wuhan University, Wuhan city, China).

15.7.2   Radiation Therapy

Currently, there are no facilities that provide radiation therapy. However, there is a plan to establish a center soon in Mogadishu/Somalia. There is no availability of functional Linear Accelerators/gamma knife/cyberknife, neither has the country the facility of Brachytherapy. There are no registered radiation oncologists or clinical oncologists who provide radiation in Somalia.

15.7.3   Surgery

There are several centers for oncological surgery in Mogadishu and Hargeisa. However, there are no robotic surgeries for cancer available in Somalia. Hyperthermic Intraperitoneal Chemotherapy (HIPEC) procedure is not available.

15.7.4   Pediatric Oncology

Somalia does not have the facility of pediatric oncology in the country. There are no centers providing comprehensive pediatric cancer treatment. The statistics of pediatric oncology are not available in Somalia.

15.7.5   Survivorship Track

There is only one hospital performing posttreatment surveillance in Somalia, i.e., the University of Somalia Teaching Hospital.

15.7.6   Palliative Care Track

Palliative care service is offered at UNISO Hospital, the same hospital that is offering chemotherapy and posttreatment surveillance. There is no country-specific palliative care in Somalia.

15.8   Research and Education

The only cancer education that is available in Somalia is a clinical oncology course, given in one semester each year at Somali National University, located in Mogadishu/Somalia. The course is given by Somalia's only cancer specialist, Dr. Hussein Abshir Hassan. This course is given to undergraduate students who are in the final year of their MBBS program. There are two facilities in Mogadishu/Somalia that are involved in cancer research.

- Erdogan Hospital, run by the Turkish government
- University of Somalia teaching hospital

The research activities in these centers are focused on identifying the most common cancers in Somalia and their distribution in the country. At present, there are no clinical trials that are going on in Somalia.

15.8.1 Publications

- Baş, Y., Hassan, H. A., Adıgüzel, C., Bulur, O., Ibrahim, I. A., & Soydan, S. (2017, June). The distribution of cancer cases in Somalia. In Seminars in oncology (Vol. 44, No. 3, pp. 178–186). WB Saunders.
- Tahtabasi, M., Abdullahi, I. M., Kalayci, M., Ibrahim, I. G., & Er, S. (2020). Cancer Incidence and Distribution at a Tertiary Care Hospital in Somalia from 2017 to 2020: An Initial Report of 1306 Cases. Cancer Management and Research, 12, 8599.

15.9 Cost-Effective Cancer Care

Neither the Somali government nor international donors are spending any money to cover even partially the cost of effective cancer care in Somalia. Patients and their family members are shouldering the burden of cancer care-related problems in Somalia. Currently, the Somali government has no plans to tackle the increasing cancer care costs, increase in utilization of expensive medications (such as immunotherapy), radiation fractionation, etc.

15.10 Challenges and Advantages

Somalia is recovering from a devastating civil war that continued for 30 years. This war has destroyed all the health facilities in the country and since then, the country has not been able to reestablish the healthcare system. This healthcare system has affected cancer care in the country. There is only one facility in the entire country where cancer care is given, UNISO Hospital in Mogadishu/Somalia. This facility has only chemotherapy and surgical services. No radiation therapy service is available in this facility.

Somali people are extremely generous and giving. They are kind and caring when it comes to sick people. They are the ones paying for the cost of cancer care in Somalia. Most Somali cancer patients go to India for medical treatment. It is estimated that they spend over one billion US dollars in India alone, excluding other countries like Malaysia, Turkey, Thailand, Egypt, China, and Saudi Arabia.

There is an extreme lack of human resources in Somalia for cancer care. Only one medical oncologist and some nurses trained by him are available in the country. The expertise that is available in Somalia for cancer patients includes chemotherapy, surgery, biopsy, histopathology, and imaging services.

The cancer care coverage is private, i.e., payment is paid by patients and their families and, fortunately, there is some outside assistance.

15.10.1   Medical Tourism for Cancer (Either to or from the Country)

Most Somalis travel abroad for cancer treatment after local diagnostic centers diagnose the disease. Top destination countries for medical treatment include India, Turkey, Malaysia, China, Thailand, Egypt, and Saudi Arabia. Some Kenyan and Ethiopian patients come to Mogadishu for medical tourism (ethnically Somalis).

15.10.2   Conflicts and War Effects on Cancer Care

The civil war in Somalia has destroyed the entire healthcare system and still is a major challenge to the restoration of the system. Somalia needs assistance with everything that concerns cancer care.

15.11   The Future of Cancer Care in Somalia

The future of cancer care in Somalia is bright as more doctors are planning to specialize in cancer and more investors are planning to invest privately in the healthcare sector, especially cancer care. Also, as the Somali government is getting stronger, it is hoped the government will play a bigger role in cancer care in Somalia.

Some suggestions to improve cancer care over the next decade in Somalia are mentioned here:

- Somalia needs to train more professionals who can deal with cancer care issues.
- Somalia needs to invest more money in cancer care to provide basic cancer care and diagnostic services, e.g., screening and prevention programs.

- Availability of early detection systems and reliable diagnostic facilities.
- Establishment of cancer centers like radiotherapy centers, cancer care centers, and palliative care centers.
- Research and clinical trials to identify the most common cancers in the country, their risk factors, and to allocate budget according to the distribution of the cancers.

15.12 Conclusion

Cancer is a major health challenge in Somalia. The cancer incidence rate is on the rise in Somalia. Cancer in this country is a neglected national health problem and there is no national cancer control program. The most common cancer in Somalia is Esophageal Cancer (EC) in both male and female patients. EC peaks in the fifth decade, and the most common histological type is squamous cell carcinoma. Liver cancer is the second most common cancer overall and is more common in men. Cervical cancer is the second most common cancer among women. Breast cancer is the third most common overall and in women. Other common cancers are Non-Hodgkin Lymphoma, pancreatic cancer, skin, thyroid, brain, bone, colorectal, and soft tissue. Because of the 30 years of conflict, Somalia has lost its healthcare system, including cancer care services. Currently, Somalia has no effective cancer care system and is up to the challenge of dealing with the increasing cancer cases in Somalia.

At present, Somalia has only one cancer specialist doctor, who is trying to provide basic cancer care services, e.g., chemotherapy, palliative care, and public health education through the media. There is no radiotherapy service, no reliable diagnostic centers, no national reliable data, no cancer registries, or cancer centers. The Somalia government and the international Non-Governmental Organizations have other priorities and are not involved in the fight against cancer in Somalia. According to the cancer studies done in Somalia, there is a high incidence rate of esophageal cancer and strongly suggests that environmental risk factors and nutritional habits have a strong impact on the population. Serious and extensive research on the etiology of esophageal cancer is required.

Conflict of Interest Authors have no conflict of interest to declare.

References

1. Source: Us Library of Congress.
2. World Population Prospects—Population Division. Population.un.org. United Nations Department of Economic and Social Affairs Population Division. Retrieved 9 Nov 2019.
3. Jump up to "Overall total population"—World Population Prospects: The 2019 Revision (xslx). population.un.org (custom data acquired via website). United Nations Department of Economic and Social Affairs, Population Division. Retrieved 9 Nov 2019.

4. Ismail AA. Somali state failure: players, incentives and institutions. What is more puzzling is how this could happen in a country like Somalia, the most homogeneous country in Africa both ethnically, religiously, culturally, and linguistically. 2010.
5. Woldemichael B. Decentralisation amidst poverty and disunity: the Sudan, 1969–1983. Somalia, the only homogeneous country in Africa—all its people being ethnic Somalis speaking the same language and professing the same religion. 1993.
6. The World Factbook. Somalia: Central Intelligence Agency. www.cia.gov. Archived from the original on 10 July 2014. Retrieved 10 Nov 2020.
7. Abdullahi. 2001. p. 8–11.
8. Middle East Policy Council—Muslim Populations Worldwide. Mepc.org. 1 December 2005. Archived from the original on 14 December 2006. Retrieved 27 June 2010.^ Jump up to:[a][b] Abdullahi 2001, p. 1.
9. World Population Prospects: The 2019 Revision—United Nations Population Division, World Urbanization Prospects—Population Division—United Nations, GeoNames, United Nations Statistics Division, World Bank, Organization for Economic Co-operation, and Development (OECD).
10. According to UN Population Statistics.
11. United Nations Projections. Chart and table of the Somalia fertility rate from 1950 to 2021.
12. Life expectancy at birth. Data based on the latest United Nations Population Division estimates.
13. Barre MS. My country and my people: the collected speeches of Major-General Mohamed Siad Barre, President, the Supreme Revolutionary Council, Somali Democratic Republic, vol. 3. Ministry of Information and National Guidance; 1970. p. 141.
14. Better off stateless: Somalia before and after government collapse (PDF). Retrieved 27 June 2010.
15. Entrepreneurship and statelessness: a natural experiment in the making in Somalia. Scribd. com. 1 October 2008. Retrieved 30 Dec 2010.
16. Estimates of unit costs for patient services for Somalia. World Health Organization. 6 December 2010. Retrieved 12 June 2011.
17. The International Agency for Research on Cancer (IARC), in 2018.
18. Seminars in oncology, vol 44(3), p. 178–86; 2017.
19. Seminars in oncology, vol 44(3), p. 178–86; 2017 and Cancer Incidence and Distribution at a Tertiary Care Hospital in Somalia Published 28 September 2020, vol 12 p. 8599–8611.
20. Barriers to screening in the Somali Community in Minnesota. J Immigr Minor Health. Author manuscript; available in PMC 2016 Jun 1. Published in final edited form as: J Immigr Minor Health 2015;17(3): 722–8. https://doi.org/10.1007/s10903-014-0080-1.
21. There is no country-specific data source, source: WHO/Cancer Country Profile 2020-Somalia.
22. Source: The author himself. (According to his knowledge of the health situation in Somalia).
23. Globocan-2020. https://who.int-Som_2020.
24. WHO/Cancer Country Profile 2020-Somalia.
25. Baş Y, Hassan HA, Adıgüzel C, Bulur O, Ibrahim İA, Soydan S. The distribution of cancer cases in Somalia. In: Seminars in oncology, vol 44(3). WB Saunders; 2017. p. 178–86

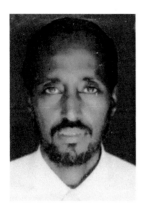

Hussein Abshir Hassan is an associate professor at the UNISO. He is an oncologist at the UNISO Hospital, Somalia. He took his primary education at an Egyptian school (Jamal Abdinasir) in Mogadishu/Somalia. He finished middle school in July 1977. He went to Benadir Secondary school in Mogadishu, Somalia from 1978 to 1981. Dr. Abshir studied the MBBS program at Fudan University, Shanghai, China. He started the profession of oncology at the Wuhan University, China in 2003 and finished in 2011. Currently, he is working at the University of Somalia, Mogadishu, Somalia as an associate professor., and Medical oncologist at Uniso Hospital of University of Somalia. Senior oncology lecturer at Somali National University, and Benadir University. His publications include Distribution of Cancer cases in Somalia, oncology care in the Arab league-Somalia's chapter. Few publications are pending.

Ikram Abdikarim was a surgeon in Mogadishu Somalia, Turkey Recep Erdogan Education and Research hospital in Mogadishu. She holds an MSc in General Surgery, from Jilin University (2016), MBBS in Medicine and Surgery, from Banadir University (2003). She is the author/co-author of articles published in international scientific journals. Developed teaching activities in the Curricular Units of the Bachelor of Medicine and Surgery in the Faculty of Medicine at Benadir University and co-supervised undergraduate students. Since 2016, she has been a surgeon at Mogadishu Somalia Turkey Recep Erdogan Education and Research Hospital in Mogadishu. She is in America now.

Nur Yassin was born in Belet Weyne, Somalia, in 1955. He is a graduate from Somali National University (MBBS), a Master in medical microbiology (virology), from Erasmus medical center, Erasmus university, worked for the WHO reference laboratory for measles and arboviruses and later on as a consultant virologist at King's College Hospital (Dulwich site) in UK. He has been Dean Faculty of Medicine and surgery, University of Somalia, since 2014.

Chapter 16
General Oncology Care in Sudan

Hussein AwadElkarim Hussein Maki

16.1 Sudan Demographics

Sudan, officially the Republic of the Sudan, was the largest country in Africa and the Arab world by area before the secession of South Sudan in 2011. The geographical location on the global map is a country in North-East Africa. It occupies 1,886,068 km² (728,215 square miles), making it Africa's third largest country and also the third largest in the Arab world [1].

The population of Sudan is estimated to be about 42 million, after the secession of South Sudan in July 2011. The last census was in 1993, no one carried out since that time due to the political Sudanese civil war. The rapidly increasing population in the capital of Sudan Khartoum (including Khartoum, Omdurman, and Khartoum North) is mainly due to the displaced persons from the war areas and better public services rather than the rural states [2]. According to United Nations High Commissioner for Refugees (UNHCR) statistics, more than 1.1 million refugees lived in Sudan in August 2019 [3].

The identity of any community is the collection of cultural aspects, including mainly ethnicity and languages of communication. There are many ethnic types; 70% of the population is Arab (the largest ethnic group in Sudan). Others include North Sudan Nubians, Zurga (South and West Sudan), and Copts [4]. There is limited cultural integration between the Arab tribes and Arabized and indigenous tribes in west areas of Sudan, due to linguistic and genealogical variations [5].

The most generally spoken language in the country is Sudanese Arabic. There are more than 50 native languages in Sudan. Other languages such as Bedawi along

H. A. H. Maki (✉)
Associate Professor of Clinical Oncology, Ahfad University for Women, Omdurman, Sudan

General Secretary of Khartoum Integrated Oncology World Congress, Khartoum, Sudan

General Secretary of Clinical Oncology Specialization Council, Sudan Medical Specialization Board, Khartoum, Sudan

© The Author(s) 2022   251
H. O. Al-Shamsi et al. (eds.), *Cancer in the Arab World*,
https://doi.org/10.1007/978-981-16-7945-2_16

the Red Sea, several Nilo-Saharan languages, and the Niger–Congo type are represented by many of the Kordofanian languages [6]. There are many local tribal languages and Sudanese sign languages but not commonly used [7]. Arabic was the official language before 2005 [8]. The political constitution approved English and Arabic languages as the official languages of the country in 2005 [9].

The huge difference in the Sudanese community in the ethnicity, languages, and religion shape the different behaviors and practices in the society. The main identifies in the country are Arab and African [10].

16.2 Cancer Statistics in Sudan

Cancer now is a more known health problem not as in the last decay, while the communicable condition (infectious and tropical diseases) had more attention and efforts [11]. Cancer was the third leading cause of death in Sudan hospitals, about 5% of all deaths (Table 16.1) [12].

The first National Cancer Registry (NCR) in Sudan started in 1967, unfortunately it is no longer acting now due to the lack of financial and technical support. The lack of proper cancer registration systems was reflected in the type of published data as it was mainly hospital-based, descriptive, and retrospective studies [13].

Most data for cancer registries comes from hospital-based registries mainly: Radiation Isotopes Center at Khartoum (RICK), National Health Laboratories (NHL), and the National Cancer Institute at Gezira University (NCI-GU). From 2010, other centers in the public and private sectors started to be in-service effectively and developed additional data sources while expanding the network of services.

Malignant epithelial tumors in the Sudanese were the first report about cancer in Sudan, published by Hickey in 1959. At that time, the most common tumor sites

Table 16.1 Ten leading causes of death in Sudan hospitals in 2000 [12]

Disease	Number of deaths	% of total deaths
Malaria	2162	19.1
Viral pneumonia	691	6.1
Malignant neoplasms	530	4.7
Iron deficiency anemias	504	4.4
Streptococcal septicemia	434	3.8
Heart failure	403	3.6
Tuberculosis	387	3.4
Severe malnutrition	382	3.4
Meningococcal infection	362	3.2
Coronary heart disease	351	3.1
Total	6206	54.7

Data is from the Sudan Federal Ministry of Health

Table 16.2 Cancer frequencies in Sudan 1967–2010 [19]

Year	Number of cancer incidents	Cancer rate/1000 population	Year	Number of cancer incidents	Cancer rate/1000 population
1967	303	0.0234	1989	1357	0.0558
1968	448	0.0339	1990	1572	0.0629
1969	540	0.0400	1991	1494	0.0582
1970	512	0.0371	1992	2157	0.0817
1971	538	0.0382	1993	1847	0.0722
1972	500	0.0348	1994	1645	0.0625
1973	562	0.0398	1995	1733	0.0640
1974	692	0.0472	1996	1810	0.0649
1975	470	0.0308	1997	2119	0.0739
1976	565	0.0357	1998	2145	0.0727
1977	738	0.0449	1999	2102	0.0692
1978	545	0.0319	2000	2541	0.0813
1979	568	0.0320	2001	2963	0.0922
1980	704	0.0381	2002	3070	0.0928
1981	672	0.0350	2003	3185	0.0936
1982	773	0.0388	2004	3450	0.0986
1983	870	0.0422	2005	3705	0.1029
1984	913	0.0431	2006	3505	0.0946
1985	903	0.0415	2007	4813	0.1262
1986	1112	0.0497	2008	5156	0.1317
1987	927	0.0403	2009	5739	0.1425
1988	1308	0.0553	2010	6303	0.1522

were the skin (32.8%) followed by the breast (22.9%) [14]. From 1954 to 1961, a study from National Health Laboratories (NHL) and the Department of Pathology, University of Khartoum showed that the number of cancer cases clearly increased twice to 2234 malignant neoplasms [15]. In Khartoum hospital (which mainly serves the Khartoum population and population referred from other parts of Sudan at that time) from 1957 to 1956, about 1578 cancer cases were reported [16]. There were 8212 cases reported in a published article about gastrointestinal tract cancers in 1976 [17]. After 1984, breast cancer was at the top of the list and most of the data came up from single centers efforts [18].

There is a clear increase in the incidence of cancer cases among the Sudanese population (Table 16.2, [19]). According to GLOBOCAN estimates, the most common cancers in both sexes are breast, non-Hodgkin lymphoma, leukemia, esophagus, and colorectal cancers [20]. Officially now the authority for estimating cancer incidence in Sudan is under the umbrella of the Federal Ministry of Health depending on the different hospitals and centers statistical reports.

The record showed that breast cancer is the most common tumor in females, while in males the prostate cancer is on top of the incidence. This data is from the population in Khartoum state (Figs. 16.1 and 16.2 [21]).

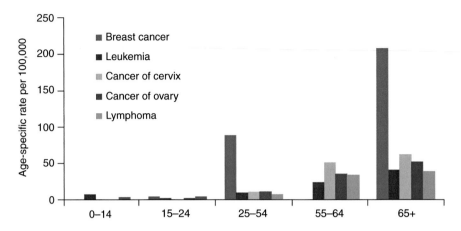

Fig. 16.1 The most common primary cancer sites among females by age group, Khartoum, Sudan (2009–2010), N = 3619 [21]

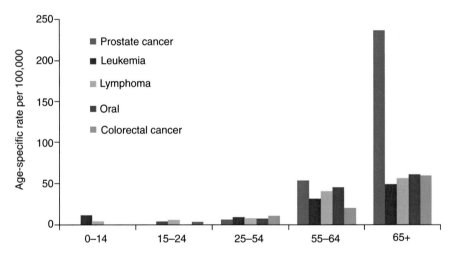

Fig. 16.2 The most common primary cancer sites among males by age group, Khartoum, Sudan (2009–2010), N = 3619 [21]

16.2.1 Breast Cancer

Breast cancer is the most frequent occurring cancer among females in Sudan, followed by gynecological tumors. In 2008, a recent study between central Sudan breast cancer records and north Italian data showed more advanced stages and negativity in the receptors in the Sudanese group [22].

Comparing data in Sudan and other African countries, the age of incidence of the disease is younger than the global data. On the other hand, Sudan is similar to

African countries in the late presentation of patients and the lack of hormonal receptor expression [23].

16.2.2   Gynecological Cancers

Cervical carcinoma is considered as the second most common malignant condition in Sudanese women seeking medical care at Khartoum Oncology Hospital and National Cancer Institute in Gezira Province over a 6-year period (2000–2006) [24]. Human Papillomavirus (HPV) is a major risk factor reported to predispose to the disease mainly type 16 or 18 [25].

16.2.3   Prostate Cancer

The most common cancer in Sudanese men is prostate cancer [26]. It is considered the second malignant condition in both sexes after the breast cancer in 2012 [20]. In the central part of Sudan (NCI), data showed that the incidence is the same among all patients regardless of their ethnic background and the presentation is usually in older ages 72 years or more with advanced clinical stages [27].

16.3   Healthcare System in Sudan

The Sudanese healthcare system is built to implement the approved strategic plans and policies. There is a need to increase the financial budget for healthcare and proper administrative efforts to achieve the goals both currently and in the future. Besides that, there is a great need for improving the health technical information systems, collaboration with international agents working in supporting medical services in the developing countries and more training for professionals [28].

16.4   Oncology Care in Sudan

In Table 16.3, there are limited radiation therapy and nuclear medicine services in the centers if compared with medical oncology services. There are good efforts in the National Cancer Department in the Federal Ministry of Health regarding supporting the governmental centers in the form of total free medications in chemotherapy and radiotherapy, including some expensive drugs according to the approved protocol in each center.

Some services are not available inside a few of these centers, such as diagnostic—interventional radiology and molecular—histopathological services.

Table 16.3 Treatment facilities in Sudan in the governmental and private sectors

No.	Name of the facility	Established	Location	Sector	Services
1	Khartoum Oncology Hospital (RICK)	1964	Khartoum state Capital of Sudan	Governmental	Radiation Nuclear medicine medical oncology services
2	National Cancer Institute	1992	Gezira state Second city of Sudan Middle Sudan	Governmental	Radiation Nuclear medicine medical oncology services
3	Tumor Therapy and Cancer Research—Shendi	2008	Nile Valley state North Sudan	Governmental	Radiation Nuclear medicine medical oncology services
4	Khartoum Oncology Specialized Center	2010	Khartoum state Capital of Sudan	Private	Medical oncology services
5	Khartoum Breast Care Center	2010	Khartoum state Capital of Sudan	Private	Medical oncology services
6	Dongla Cancer Center	2012	North state North Sudan	Governmental	Medical oncology services
7	Taiba Cancer Center	2013	Khartoum state Capital of Sudan	Private	Medical oncology services
8	Shafi Specialized Oncology Center	2015	Khartoum state Capital of Sudan	Private	Medical oncology services
9	East Oncology Center	2015	Gadarif state East Sudan	Governmental	Medical oncology services
10	Port Sudan Oncology Center	2015	Red Sea state East Sudan	Governmental	Medical oncology services
11	Kordfan Cancer Center	2015	North Kordofan state West Sudan	Governmental	Medical oncology services
12	Merowe Oncology Center	2017	North state North Sudan	Governmental with Private	Radiation Nuclear medicine medical oncology services
13	Nyala Cancer Center	2019	South Darfur state West Sudan	Governmental	Medical oncology services
14	AlFashir Cancer Center	2020	North Darfur state West Sudan	Governmental	Medical oncology services

Data is from the Sudan Federal Ministry of Health and Khartoum State Ministry of Health

16.5 Cancer Risk Factors

In general, the risk factors for cancer in Sudan are not different from the well-known globally on this issue. In Gezira state, where the Gezira agriculture scheme is located, more fertilizers and pesticides were extensively used and proposed to be associated with cancer incidence in this area [29].

The appearance of malignant conditions in young ages in both males and females in recent years has been mostly associated with risk factors such as smoking, chemical cosmetics, and environmental pollution.

16.6 Cancer Screening Programs

Sudan first started a National Cancer Control Programme (NCCP) in 1982. The plan includes three main components: preventive initiatives, early detection and screening initiatives, improved diagnosis, and treatment with special attention to the palliative care services [30].

There are many excellent efforts regarding breast cancer screening at all levels, whether government, private, or voluntary throughout the year and many campaigns in October as it is an annual month of breast cancer. On the other hand, there is a clear shortage in the screening of cervical carcinoma and not much attention to the screening programs has been given. Only two centers are working on this issue. It needs effort, especially from the gynecologists to take over this mission. The same issue is for other malignant conditions like oral cancer or prostate cancer.

16.7 Cancer Prevention Programs

The cancer prevention programs and activities in Sudan mainly include early detection campaigns, awareness activities, health education sessions, and professional training of the healthcare teams. It is a mission of collaboration with governmental strategies, private sector, voluntary organizations, and media with community activists. Although there is a lack of prevention programs, there is still a great change in the community about the cancer stigma and related issues compared with the last 10 years. In Figs. 16.3 and 16.4, are the educational materials used in awareness activities in prevention programs and health education for the community.

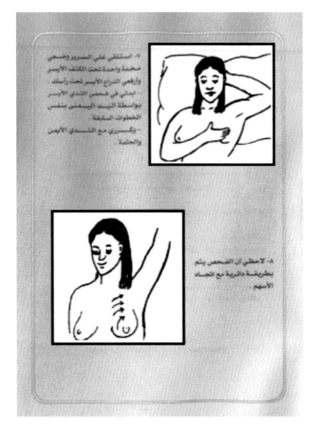

Fig. 16.3 Page from a brochure on breast self-examination that was part of a breast cancer public awareness campaign [12]

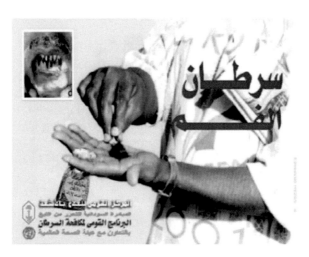

Fig. 16.4 Toombak, a moist oral tobacco extensively used in Sudan, was the subject of a public awareness campaign (in poster). Inset: Toombak ingestion causes severe leukoplakia on the gingiva and lower lip, as well as tooth weakening and loosening. Malignant changes are mostly seen when the toombak is placed into the mouth [12]

16.8   Cancer Diagnosis

The services for cancer diagnosis at the basic level are excellent. There are many departments for endoscopies, imaging such as U/S, mammographic image, Computed Tomography [CT scan], bone scan, and Magnetic Resonance Imaging [MRI], biopsies (surgical or imaging guided), and histopathological with immuno-histochemical services are widely available in the country.

There is a lack of molecular biology services which leads to personalized treatment approaches such as BRCA tests or tests that detect the sensitivity of chemotherapy. There is only one lab in the private sector that provides flow-cytometer tests for hematological malignancies.

16.9   Treatment

16.9.1   Medical Oncology

Medical oncology services are widely available in all centers across the country. It almost covers all the needs for the patients. There are excellent stores and supply chains in the country that cover tons of needs for the public sector as well as the private sector. Regarding advanced medical oncology services, there is an unavailability of services such as Bone Marrow Transplant (BMT).

16.9.2   Radiation Therapy

Radiation therapy services are distributed among four centers along with covering the external beam therapy and brachytherapy. Most of the techniques used are two-dimensional (2D) skills rather than the three-dimensional (3D) or other high etch radiation approaches.

16.9.3   Surgery

There are many surgical departments in different hospitals with excellent practice in breast surgeries and gastrointestinal tract operations. However, there are no robotic surgeries for cancer or Hyperthermic Intraperitoneal Chemotherapy (HIPEC) procedures available.

16.9.4 Pediatric Oncology

There is a lack of services for pediatric cancer treatment facilities with limited epidemiological data in Sudan. There are only two centers providing comprehensive pediatric cancer treatment, Khartoum Oncology Hospital and the National Cancer Institute. Hematological malignancies (Leukemia and Lymphomas) more than 50% of the pediatric cancer cases with limited Central Nervous System (CNS) tumors [31].

16.9.5 Survivorship Track

This picture is, to some extent, like the pattern of cancer treatment outcome and survivorship in the developing countries rather than the developed countries. With careful attention to the estimation of the outcome, unfortunately it can be counted as a poor survivorship track. This is justified by the diagnosis of the cases in the late stages, among other factors about the challenges of cancer treatment in Sudan (mentioned under Challenges and Advantages).

Factors that affect cancer patients' survivorship in Sudan include:

1. Financial difficulties and lack of insurance coverage
2. Lack of drugs through the approved system
3. Interruption of treatment and follow-up protocol post-treatment
4. No survival care plan approved either institutional or Federal at the Ministry of Health.

16.9.6 Palliative Care Track

The palliative care services in Sudan started in 2010 in the Radiation Isotopes Center at Khartoum (RICK). Now the palliative care services are distributed in many centers and hospitals such as the National Cancer Institute at Gezira University (NCI-GU) and Soba University Hospital (SUH).

16.10 Research and Education

The Sudan Medical Specialization Board (SMSB) is the main national body for postgraduate medical training and specialization for health care professionals. It was established in 1995 and has many health specialization councils.

Clinical oncology training started in 1998 with five medical residents. Now in 2020, there are more than 60 medical residents in the program.

Many scientific activities are usually in the field and aim to maximize skills and professional development. The first cancer conference organized by Khartoum Oncology Hospital in 2010, the second edition in 2011, unfortunately discontinued due to many changes in the head directors and affected by the budget which directed to maintain the supply of the drugs, while inside the hospital's scientific activities are running regularly. In 2015, the Khartoum Integrated Oncology World Congress organized by Khartoum Oncology Specialized Center (KOSC) started and continued annually as the biggest professional oncology gathering in Sudan and outside Sudan. Another impressive scientific activity is the annual East Oncology Center (EOC) Workshop in Gadarif state. There are still limited publications and research projects mainly due to the lack of funds to run such programs. On the other hand, there are many postgraduate researches not published in the field of cancer and related branches.

16.11 Cost-Effective Cancer Care

In the public sector, the government through the Federal Ministry of Health and the National Cancer Authority supports all the centers with free drugs, even the expensive medicines and other services (such as radiation therapy) for all the patients, even foreigners (non-Sudanese). However, there are some shortages in supply from time to time due to the lack of budget. Only one disadvantage is that the huge numbers of patients compared to the facilities need medical services, which causes overcrowding and exhaustion to the medical teams.

On the other hand, the private sector has a real impact on providing the services and the cost is a little high for drugs and other services and is affected by the economic situations in the country.

There are a significant number of patients traveling abroad seeking consultations, second opinion, revaluation especially by Positron Emission Tomography-Computed Tomography (PET-CT) scan and treatment, especially the sophisticated modalities which are not available in Sudan in the surgical and radiation therapy departments.

16.12 Challenges and Advantages

16.12.1 Challenges for Cancer Treatment in Sudan

A considerable challenge to the cancer treatment in Sudan is that most patients have late presentations in clinical stage III or IV disease. This will reflect mainly on the treatment outcome and overall survival [12].

Other challenges, such as illiteracy, the lack of health education and awareness programs, limited screening services, limited treatment facilities, lack of institutional collaboration, limited research grants on cancer, many populations living far away in rural areas and that is mainly due to the main work for them is agriculture and grazing animals and the social stigma of cancer in the community.

16.13 The Future of Cancer Care in Sudan

Many plans have been developed by the Federal Ministry of Health to face oncology issues and their burden on the economy and community. The policy is directed towards helping the centers in the public sector to upgrade and have new radiation therapy devices to overcome the lack of radiotherapy machines, which is the main obstacle in cancer treatment services for patients in Sudan, as well as encouraging the private sector to invest in the same issue by facilitating funds from the banks and encouraging international collaboration.

Another aim is to complete additional medical services related to cancer management, such as advanced diagnostic tools and modern laboratory techniques. Moreover, establishing main protocols at least for the common malignant tumors such as breast, ovarian, prostate, lung, and colorectal cancers, to help in the improvement of anticancer therapies supply for the whole country and evaluate the responses in other emerging scientific facts in the Sudanese population.

Encouragement for researchers and professionals to do prospective studies from the local data will support the plans for tackling different scientific issues in cancer patients as well as more activation for the Sudanese National Cancer Council in the Federal Ministry of Health to implement the different approved strategies.

16.14 Conclusion

Sudan has inadequate resources for healthcare services, including cancer prevention and treatment. There is inadequate data about cancer incidence and mortality in Sudan. Cancer in Sudan occurs at a young age and with advanced late manifestations. Cancer is emerging as a public health problem with more efforts done by the Ministry of Health and cancer centers. Measures for cancer prevention at the community level are inadequate. Much attention towards improvement of palliative care services is needed. There is a need to establish National Comprehensive Strategic Plans that include therapeutic services as well as early detection and screening programs. Establishing an effective National Cancer Registry system will help in providing the data of the cases and the data to the real consumers of drugs and other services for cancer patients and how to use the different utilities in the right way. Many efforts have been made by the National Cancer Center Authority in the Federal Ministry of Health to establish rural centers to provide care for cancer patients, but still need more support to handle the different cases.

Conflict of Interest Authors have no conflict of interest to declare.

References

1. The World Fact book—Central Intelligence Agency. https://www.cia.gov/the-world-factbook/.
2. World Population Prospects—Population Division. Population.un.org. United Nations Department of Economic and Social Affairs, Population Division. Retrieved 9 Nov 2019.
3. Sudan | Global Focus. Reportingunhcrorg Retrieved 13 Dec 2019.
4. World Directory of Minorities and Indigenous Peoples—Sudan: Copts. Minority Rights Group International 2008. Retrieved 21 Dec 2010.
5. Suliman O. The Darfur conflict: geography or institutions? Taylor & Francis; 2019. p. 115. isbn:978-0-203-83616-3.
6. Gordon RG Jr, editor. Ethnologue: languages of the world. 16th ed. Dallas: SIL International; 2009. Languages of Sudan
7. Karen Andrae (2009) Language for inclusion (Sign language in Sudan) on YouTube.
8. Leclerc J. L'aménagement linguistique dans le monde, "Soudan" (in French). Trésor de la langue française au Québec. Archived from the original on 23 October 2012. Retrieved 31 May 2013.
9. "2005 constitution in English" (PDF). Archived from the original (PDF) on 9 June 2007. Retrieved 31 May 2013.
10. Hamilton A, Hudson J. Bribery and identity: evidence from Sudan. Bath Economic Research Papers. 2014. No. 21/14.
11. Strong K, Mathers C, Leeder S, Beaglehole R. Preventing chronic diseases: how many lives can we save? Lancet. 2005;366:1578–82.
12. Hamad HMA. Cancer initiatives in Sudan. Ann Oncol. 2006;17(Suppl 8):viii32–6. https://doi.org/10.1093/annonc/mdl985.
13. Saeed IE, Elmustafa AD, Mohamed KEH, Mohammed SI. Cancer registry in Sudan: a brief overview. Int J Epidemiol. 2013;2(2) Available at http://ispub.com/IJE/11/2/14574 (Accessed 15 Jan 2014) [Google Scholar] [Ref list]
14. Hickey BB. Malignant epithelial tumours in the Sudanese. Ann R Coll Surg Engl. 1959 May;24(5):303–22.
15. Lynch JBHA, Omar A. Cancer in the Sudan. Sudan Med J. 1963;2:29–37.
16. Daoud EHHA, Zak F, Zakova N. Aspects of malignant disease in the Sudan. In: Clifford P, Linsell CA, Timms GL, editors. Cancer in Africa. Nairobi: East African Publishing House; 1968. p. 43–50.
17. Malik MO, Zaki EL, Elmasri SH. Cancer of the alimentary tract in the Sudan. Cancer. 1976;37:2533–42.
18. Mukhtar BI. The Sudan cancer registry. In: Parkin DM, editor. Cancer occurrence in developing countries. Lyon: IARC; 1978. p. 81–5. IARC Scientific Publication No. 57.
19. Mohammed EA, Alagib A, Babiker AI. Incidents of cancer in Sudan: past trends and future forecasts. Afr J Math. 2013;8:136–42.
20. Ferlay J, Soerjomataram I, Ervik M, Dikshit R, Eser S, Mathers C, et al. GLOBOCAN 2012 v1.0. Cancer Incidence Mortality Worldwide [Internet]. 2014 3/13/2014; IARC Cancer Base.
21. Saeed IE, Weng HY, Mohamed KH, Mohammed SI. Cancer incidence in Khartoum, Sudan: first results from the Cancer Registry, 2009–2010. Cancer Med. 2014;3(4):1075–85.
22. Awadelkarim KD, Arizzi C, Elamin EO, Hamad HM, De Blasio P, Mekki SO, et al. Pathological, clinical and prognostic characteristics of breast cancer in Central Sudan versus northern Italy: implications for breast cancer in Africa. Histopathology. 2008;52(4):445–56.
23. Elamin A, Ibrahim ME, Abuidris D, Mohamed MEH, Mohammed SI. Part I: cancer in Sudan—burden, distribution, and trends breast, gynecological, and prostate cancers. Cancer Med. 2015;4(3):447–56.
24. Husain N, Helali T, Domi M, Bedri S. Cervical cancer in women diagnosed at the National Health Laboratory, Sudan: a call for screening. Sudan J Med Sci. 2011;2011:183–90.
25. World Health Organization. WHO/ICO information centre on human papilloma virus (HPV) and cervical cancer. WHO/ICO Information Center on HPV and Cervical Cancer (HPV

Information Center). Human Papillomavirus and Related Cancers in the World. Summary Report 2010. 2009. http://www.who.int.hpvcentre. Accessed 15 Jan 2014. [Ref list].

26. Khalid KE, Brair AI, Elhaj AM, Ali KE. Prostate-specific antigen level and risk of bone metastasis in Sudanese patients with prostate cancer. Saudi J Kidney Dis Transpl. 2011 Sep;22(5):1041–3.

27. Hamad FA. Risk factors for prostate cancer patients among Gezira state-central of Sudan. IIUM Eng J. 2011;12(4):203–11.

28. Ebrahim EMA, Ghebrehiwot L, Abdalgfar T, Juni MH. Health care system in Sudan: review and analysis of strength, weakness, opportunity, and threats (SWOT analysis). Sudan J Med Sci. 2017;12(3):133–50. https://doi.org/10.18502/sjms.v12i3.924.

29. Elebead FM, Hamid A, Hilmi HS, Galal H. Mapping cancer disease using geographical information system (GIS) in Gezira state-Sudan. J Community Health. 2012;37(4):830–9.

30. World Health Organization. National cancer control programmes: policies and managerial guidelines. Geneva: WHO; 2002.

31. Abuidres DO, et al. Epidemiological review of childhood cancers in Central Sudan. S Afr J Oncol. 2018;2:a37. https://doi.org/10.4102/sajo.v2i0.37.

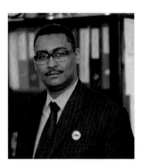

Hussein AwadElkarim Hussein Maki is an Associate Professor of Clinical Oncology at Ahfad University for Women. He is also a consultant Clinical Oncologist and a General Director of Khartoum Oncology Specialized Center (KOSC). Maki General Secretary and Founder of Khartoum Integrated Oncology World Congress. He has an MBBS from the University of Gezira—Sudan, MSc Clinical oncology—Alkasr Aliny—Cairo University and Fellowship Medical Oncology—Vehbi Koç foundation and University—Turkey. He is a member and an examiner of the Sudanese Medical Specialization Board, Clinical Oncology Department and a member of the Sudanese Oncology Society Executive Council. He is the Representative of Sudan at the AMAAC (Arab Medical Association Aganist Cancer) Executive Council.

Chapter 17
General Oncology Care in Syria

Maha Manachi, Eyad Chatty, Seham Sulaiman, and Zahera Fahed

17.1   Syria Demography

Syria is a country in the Middle East located at the eastern end of the Mediterranean Sea. Historically, it has been home to some of the world's oldest civilizations, with a rich scientific, artistic, and cultural heritage. The capital city, Damascus, is thought to be the oldest continuously inhabited city in the world. As such, Syria has often been described as the largest small country in the world owing to the depth of its history and wealth of culture [1].

The modern Syrian state was officially established as a parliamentary republic on 24 October 1945. It became a founding member of the United Nations. It has a total area of 185,180 km² consisting of 14 governorates including Damascus (~1.7 million inhabitants; Greater Damascus: four million inhabitants) [2], Aleppo (also one of the oldest continuously inhabited cities), Damascus, Rif Dimashq, Homs, Hama, Latakia, Deir ez-Zor, Ar Raqqah, Idlib, Hasakah, As-Suwayda, Daraa, Quneitra, and Tartus. The population of Syria in 2020 was estimated at 17,500,658 people.

M. Manachi (✉)
Division of Hematology/Oncology, Al Bairouni University Hospital, St Louis Hospital, Damascus, Syria
e-mail: Manachi-cancer@albairouni.net

E. Chatty
School of Medicine, Damascus University, Damascus, Syria

Department of Pathology, Alasad University Hospital, Damascus, Syria

Almwassat University. Hospital, Damascus, Syria

S. Sulaiman
Damascus University, Al Assad Hospital, Damascus, Syria

Z. Fahed
Dar Al Shifaa Hospital, St Louis Hospital, Damascus, Syria

© The Author(s) 2022   265
H. O. Al-Shamsi et al. (eds.), *Cancer in the Arab World*,
https://doi.org/10.1007/978-981-16-7945-2_17

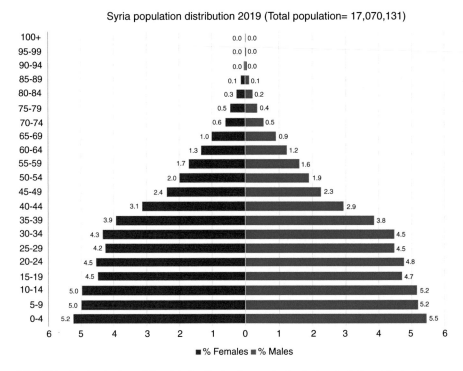

Fig. 17.1 Gender (male and female) distribution by age in the Syrian Arab Republic in the year 2019 [36]. Reproduced from the source "PopulationPyramid.net" (accessed on 09/08/2021; URL link: https://www.populationpyramid.net/syrian-arab-republic/2019/)

The population density is 95 per km^2 (247 people per mi^2) and 60% of the population is urban. Total Fertility Rate (TFR) is 2.8 (Live Births per Woman, 2020). Life expectancy at birth is 76.06 years, female 79.1 years, male 73.1 years. Infant Mortality Rate is 11.3 (infant deaths per 1000 live births) [34], while gender ratio is 50.1% male and 49.9% female (Fig. 17.1) [35, 36].

In the early 2000s, Syria embarked on a gradual economic liberalization to spur growth. However, 10 years of tragic conflict has set the country back in terms of economic, social, and human development. The economy has contracted by more than 50% in real terms since 2011 such that Syria's Gross Domestic Product (GDP) is less than half of what it was before the war started [3, 37]. During the conflict, five to six million people, out of a pre-war population of 22 million, were displaced from Syria [4, 5].

17.2 Cancer Statistics in Syria

The Syrian National Cancer Registry (SNCR) is a hospital-based registry that was established in 2001 to define the population-based incidence in Syria and provide knowledge about the extent of cancer burden, epidemiology, early detection, and cancer screening. The SNCR has been awarded associate membership to the International Association of Cancer Registries (IACR). CanReg 5 was introduced by the World Health Organization (WHO) in 2020 as an open source tool to input, store, check, and analyse cancer registry data.

According to the SNCR, the estimated cancer statistics before the beginning of the conflict in 2011, were 17,599 new cases in 2009 (total population = 21,092,000). Of those, 9213 (52%) were males and 8386 (48%) were females. The 2009 Cancer Registry shows that in males, the most frequent cancer site was the lungs (17%), followed by colon and rectum (12%) and leukaemia (10%). While in females, the most frequent cancer sites were breast (30%), colon and rectum (11%), and leukaemia (8%) (Fig. 17.2). The Age Standardized Rate (ASR) for all cancer cases combined was 128 per 100,000 for males and 117 per 100,000 for females. The cure rate is approximately 40%. Estimated mortality rate for cancer was 52 and 76 per 100,000 for females and males in 2009 [12, 38]. With about 1700 new paediatric cases, the most common types of cancer among children (0–15 years old), for boys and girls, respectively, are: leukaemia (37–34%), brain and CNS (20–22%), lymphoma (17–14%), bones and soft tissue (12–13%), kidney and other endocrine (7–6%), and all other sites (7–11%). Cancer is the third most common cause of death in Syria [12, 38].

The post-war statistical data is suboptimal for a number of reasons including the displacement of five million people outside the country. However, it was noted that cancer cases have been increasing in Syria according to the Al Bairouni 2020

2009 Estimated Syrian Cancer Cases*

		Men 9213	Women 8386		
Lung & bronchus	17%			30%	**Breast**
Colon & rectum	12%			11%	Colon & rectum
Leukemia	10 %			8%	Leukemia
Lymphoma	8%			7 %	Thyroid
C.N.S	7%			5%	Uterine Corpus
Urinary bladder	6%			5%	Lymphoma
Prostate	5%			4%	Ovary
Bone&ST	5%			4%	C.N.S
Stomach	4%			3%	Bone&ST
Larynx	3%			3%	Lung & bronchus
Liver	3%			3%	Stomach
Skin	3%			2%	Cervix
Thyroid	2%			2%	Liver
All Other Sites	15%			13%	All Other Sites

Fig. 17.2 Cancer incidence rate between male and female in Syria with most common cancers in 2009 [12, 38]. Source: Syrian National Cancer Registry, 2009 (Partially developed). Used with permission from Firas AL Jerf

Table 17.1 Percentage of each site of adult cancers in both genders at Al Bairouni University Hospital, 2020. Used with permission from Al Bairouni University Hospital

Coding (IARC.WHO) ICD-10	Percentage (%)	Total	Topography	Rank
C50	24.36	2067	Breast	1
C34	9.75	827	Lung, bronchus, trachea	3
C73	8.31	705	Thyroid	2
C18-C20	7.42	630	Colon and rectum	4
C85	4.68	397	Lymphoma	7
C40-C49	4.53	384	Bone and soft tissue	6
C53 + C55	4.17	354	Cervix and uterus	18
C71	3.92	333	Brain and CNS	8
C67	3.32	282	Bladder	9
C56	2.83	240	Ovary	14
C16	2.75	233	Stomach	13
C61	2.59	220	Prostate	10
C42	2.42	205	Leukaemia	5
C32	1.81	154	Larynx	12
C25	1.36	115	Pancreas	17
C22	1.20	102	Liver	21
C64	1.18	100	Kidney	15
C62	0.95	81	Testis	19

hospital-based registry data, the hospital sees more than 60% of Syrian cancer patients. The detailed cancer sites are shown in Table 17.1, which refers to the most common cancers at Al Bairouni, i.e. breast 24%, lung 10%, thyroid 8%, colorectal 7%, lymphoma 5%. The high number of thyroid cancers is because Al Bairouni Hospital is the only treatment centre that manages thyroid cancers in all of Syria.

There were about 9000 annual new cases in Al Bairouni University Hospital in the year 2020, of which 3960 were male (44%) and 5040 were female patients (56%). The most frequent cancer sites in both genders are breast 24%, head and neck 22%, genitourinary tract 15%, GI 15%, haematological malignancies 10%, and lung cancers 10% (Fig. 17.3).

The GLOBOCAN statistics for 2020 described the number of new cases in both sexes, all ages, where breast (20.9%), lung (9.4%), colorectal (8.4%), prostate (5.2%), and NHL (4.8%) are at the top [39].

The most frequent paediatric cancers prevalent at Al Bairouni University Hospital are CNS, leukaemia, lymphoma, bone and soft tissue sarcoma, and kidney.

Estimated cancer incidences among Syrian refugees is shown by a study written in Lancet 2020 with R4HC-MENA collaboration, describing the cancer incidence, cost of treatment among Syrian refugees in Lebanon [13].

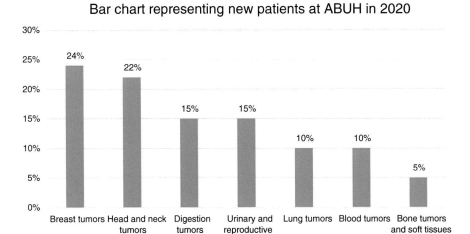

Fig. 17.3 Most common adult cancers in both genders at Al Bairouni University Hospital in 2020. Used with permission from Al Bairouni University Hospital

17.3   Healthcare System in Syria

Healthcare system is based on a collaboration between public and private sectors. Health and social services are the responsibilities of the government with Ministry of Health coverage in collaboration with partners of medical corps to provide quality health care with equity (rural populations achieving better equity than before) and sustainability [6]. The role played by the private sector has increased in many ways including patients' own pocket, Social Health Insurance (SHI) schemes, and Public–Private Partnership (PPP). Additionally, civil societies and WHO support play an important role. Health expenditures accounted for 3.3% of GDP in 2014, while the total pharmaceutical expenditure accounts for 1.11% of the GDP [7].

The top three diseases that cause mortality in Syria are: cardiovascular diseases (44.72%), respiratory diseases (16.2%), and tumours (7.0%). While diseases causing morbidity are digestive, respiratory and cardiovascular diseases, poisoning, injuries, infections, and parasitic diseases followed by cancer and kidney diseases (Table 17.2) [9].

In the early 2000s, Syria could credit itself with improved living standards, awareness of health issues, strengthened by improvements to infrastructure, access to clean water, expanding public healthcare systems and local production of >90% of medicines (despite past economic pressures and isolation). The integration of healthcare has been a significant factor for the country to be on target with health Millennium Development Goals (MDGs) [8].

Table 17.2 Top ten causes of mortality and morbidity in the Republic of Syria—2009 [9]

Rank mortality	Morbidity/disability	
1	Cardiovascular diseases	Digestive diseases
2	Respiratory diseases	Respiratory diseases
3	Cancer	Cardiovascular diseases
4	Injuries	Poisoning
5	Certain conditions originating in the P-natal period	Injuries
6	Genitourinary diseases	Infectious and parasitic diseases
7	Congenital malformations, deformations, and chromosomal abnormalities	Cancer
8	Nervous diseases	Kidney diseases
9	Digestive diseases	Blood diseases
10	Endocrine, nutritional, and metabolic diseases	Certain conditions originating in the prenatal period

Source: MOH Syrian Arab Republic 2010. Used with permission from Rajwa Jubaili

Human resources for health in Syria described according to 2010 Ministry of Health (MOH) data, there are 17,300 (8.1/10,000) licensed pharmacists, 31,194 (14.6/10,000) physicians, and 40,053 (18.8/10,000) nursing and midwifery personnel. The ratio of doctors to pharmacists is 1.8 and the ratio of doctors to nurses and midwifery personnel is 0.8. The average of total hospitals according to 2010 data was 482 with 30,206 beds, 117 public hospitals (21,849 bed) covering 65% of the country's capacity. There are 70 licensed pharmaceutical manufacturers in Syria, domestic manufacturers hold 91% of the market share by value produced [9].

Since the 2011 conflict, Syria faced inhumane economic sanctions with severe consequences on health care. Sanctions have prevented the entry of essential medical supplies into the country, including those for cancer treatment which are not produced locally, as well as preventing spare parts for medical machines hence preventing repair of essential hospital equipment. The pharmaceutical sector which suffered significant destruction is now rebuilding and gearing up to reach its pre-conflict productivity. A survey conducted by HRAMS WHO about war destruction for health services showed that 47% of public health centres were reported fully functioning, 22% partially functioning, and 31% non-functioning (completely out of service) [10].

17.4   Oncology Care in Syria

Despite war strain, COVID-19 pandemic, and global cancer burden, the Syrian government continues to provide free cancer services to all patients with less than 10% involvement of private sector, insurance companies, and charitable civil societies.

Al Bairouni University Hospital (ABUH) for cancer treatment in Damascus is a comprehensive specialized referral hospital (550 beds) that recruits about 60% of cancer patients (annual new cases 11,000). All types of cancer treatments including chemotherapy, targeted therapy as well as radiation oncology are provided as standard of care. The exception is bone marrow transplant. For the time being, cancer registry statistics are ABUH-based.

At least 15 more oncology centres provide cancer treatment in different governorates. Tishreen University Hospital in Latakia is the second most comprehensive centre with 3000 new cancer cases annually. Whereas Al Kindi University Hospital in Aleppo is currently being re-established aiming to deliver a high standard of care in the north of Syria.

Figure 17.4 shows the distribution of public hospitals that provide cancer care services in Syria [11].

The rapid progress and promising developments in oncology care in Syria were interrupted by the conflict with effects including shortage of drugs and availability of specialized medical equipment. Collaborating with WHO and allied countries, alongside starting local cancer drugs production in near future will hopefully enhance the country's cancer care services.

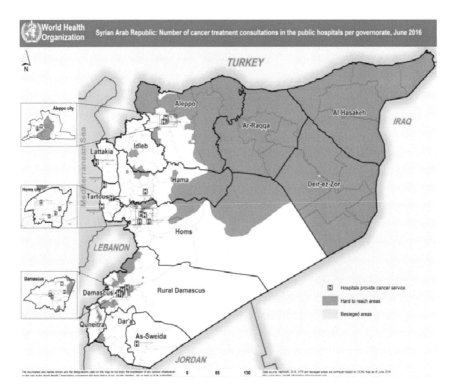

Fig. 17.4 Distribution of public hospitals that provide cancer treatment services [11]. Used with permission from Firas AL Jerf

The Syrian National Cancer Control Committee (NCCC) was established in June 2019, with the objective of coordinating cancer care between all oncology services and hence significantly improving oncology care across all of Syria. Ultimately, the aim is to build more comprehensive centres covering the middle, east, and north part of the country in order to deliver satisfactory cancer care with unified oncology practice guidelines that will diminish heterogeneity in oncology practice.

17.5 Cancer Risk Factors

Syria is undergoing an epidemiological transition in healthcare burden from communicable to non-communicable diseases (NCDs) [14]. NCDs were estimated to account for 45% of causes of death [15]. Overall, the three primary health risk factors are dietary, high blood pressure, and high Body-Mass Index (BMI).

Obesity represents a major public health concern; with a prevalence of about 34% for women and 20.9% for men (higher than surrounding countries) [17]. Tobacco consumption is responsible for approximately 22% of all cancer deaths. Estimated tobacco smoking among university students (18–26 years) was 24.73% for cigarettes (39.82% male, 5.54% female) and 30.4% for water pipe (33.2% male, 26.8% female) [18]. The Aleppo Household Survey involved a representative sample of 2038 adults. The prevalence of cigarette smoking was 56.9% among men and 17.0% among women, while the prevalence of waterpipe smoking was 20.2% among men and 4.8% in women [19].

Syria's Presidential Decree no. 62, in 2009 banned smoking including the waterpipe inside cafes, restaurants, and other public spaces. This law went into effect in April 2010 [29]. Syria was the first Arab country to introduce such a ban. The decree also outlaws smoking in educational institutions, health centres, sports halls, cinemas, theatres, and on public transport. A previous decree in 1996 banned tobacco advertising. People under the age of 18 are not allowed to buy tobacco in Syria.

Other risk factors include alcohol consumption, viral infections (especially HBV, HCV, HPV, and EBV), exposure to ultraviolet light or ionizing radiation, and increased exposure to industrial and agricultural carcinogens. Furthermore, postwar environmental pollution is an added risk factor for cancer in Syria [16].

According to the global review of hepatitis B and C in 2013, the Syrian Arab Republic is classified as having a high prevalence of hepatitis C virus (HCV) and low–intermediate prevalence of hepatitis B virus (HBV). The decreasing trend in HBV positivity may be linked to the continuous HBV vaccination programmes. The highest positivity for HBV and HCV was seen in the northern and eastern regions according to a 2004 survey by the Syrian MoH in cooperation with the Central Bureau of Statistics. The seroprevalence of HCV was found to be 2.8% as indicated by HCV antibodies and 5.6% for HBV as indicated by HBV surface antigen (HBsAg) [22]. HPV-related cancer incidence in Syria (estimates for 2012) is 2.8, 0.5, 0.1 per 100,000 for cervix uteri, other anogenital, and head and neck cancer, respectively [23].

17.6 Cancer Screening Programmes

The cancer screening and prevention programmes initiated in Syria under MOH coverage along with partners, namely the Ministry of Social Affairs and Labour (MOSAL), civil societies, and the WHO. Many of these programmes were established following 2018–2019. These programmes play an important role in raising awareness through educating the general population about cancer prevention, screening, counselling programmes, and epidemiology studies. Recently, the Syrian government has developed several national cancer awareness and screening programmes, particularly focusing on breast cancer, cervical cancer, prostate cancer, and colon cancer.

The Syrian Society of Breast Cancer, established in 2006, by the MOSAL, played an important role in breast cancer early detection campaign collaborating with civil societies like the Syrian Family Planning Society, Red Crescent, and others, offering counselling, educational programmes, breast ultrasound and mammogram to all women aged 35–70. The first major national early detection and screening programme was done in October 2019, guided by the Syrian National Committee for cancer control. This screened a total of 380,000 women aged 35–70 by mammogram and with guided biopsy for those with suspected lesions. Several national screening programmes were interrupted by the conflict in the country and by the COVID-19 pandemic.

17.7 Cancer Prevention Programmes

Human Papillomavirus (HPV) vaccine was supported by the government but not routinely used before the crisis. Cervical cancer ranks as the 12th most frequent cancer among women in Syria and ninth most frequent cancer among women between 15 and 44 years of age. Around 2.5% of women in the general population are estimated to carry cervical HPV 16/18 infection at a given time, and 72.4% of invasive cervical cancers are attributed to HPVs 16 or 18 [26]. The fact that cervical cancer is preventable necessitates the 2021 national campaign programme by the NCCC and MOH with WHO partnership for cervical cancer screening.

The MOH in partnership with the WHO conducts a programme with the aim of eliminating new hepatitis B and C infections in Syria by 2030 and reduction of chronic hepatitis cases and hence hepatocellular carcinoma (HCC) liver cancer.

In addition to breast cancer screening and prevention programmes, the Tobacco Control Law (174/2011) was also introduced in August 2011 for tobacco control and regulation of tobacco products' manufacturing, packaging, and advertising that forbid smoking indoors, at workplace and in public transportation [18].

17.8 Cancer Diagnosis

17.8.1 Imaging

Radiation therapy was established in Syria at the Nuclear Medicine Centre (the oldest radiotherapy centre in Syria) in the 1970s. Since then, the role of diagnostic radiology has rapidly expanded in both the public and private sectors. Many challenges facing this field in terms of equipment, devices, and expertise have arisen during the crisis. Sanctions and financial difficulties prevented new devices from replacing damaged ones. Current active nuclear medicine centres are mostly located in big cities like Damascus, Aleppo, Latakia, Swayda, and Tartouse. The radiation doses delivered to patients are monitored with accurate radiation dosimeters to save patients from radiation injuries. These dosimeters are calibrated at the Secondary Standards Dosimetry Laboratory (SSDL). In addition, a dedicated Quality Audit programme (QA) of the radiation doses delivered to patients in the radiotherapy centres around the country has been established. A recent survey showed that active imaging includes about 351 Computed Tomography (CT) scans, 170 Magnetic Resonance Imaging (MRI) machines, 4 Positron Emission Tomography (PET-CT) devices (located in Damascus), 7 Gamma cameras (including Single Photon Emission Computed Tomography (SPECT) System), and one clinical cyclotron. Few other facilities include 1100 general X-ray systems, 314 fluoroscopy and angiography systems, 185 mammography machines, 769 panoramic and cephalometric X-ray equipment, 69 bone-densitometry systems, 74 interventional radiology systems for cardiology, neuroradiology, and peripheral vascular. According to the Syrian Radiologist Society, there are more than 400 radiologists in Syria.

According to the Atomic Energy Commission of Syria (AECS), a list of available diagnostic tracers is 131I, 99mTc, 67Ga citrate, 123I-NaI, 123I-Datscan, 201TICI, 123I-MIBG, 18F-FDG, 18F-NaF, 11C-radiotracers and therapeutic agents (186RE, 64CU, 64 Cu-DOTATATE, 90Y, 89 Sr) [20]. Based on the latest data from MOH (AECS), there are about 8 nuclear medicine physicians, in addition to 25 medical physicists available in the country.

17.8.2 Laboratory

Histopathology plays an essential role in oncology, both in the initial tissue diagnosis of the tumour and later in the detailed examination of the surgical specimen. Immunohistochemistry has revolutionized histopathology over the last 20–30 years and a number of tumours now require immunohistochemistry for their accurate diagnosis or sub-classification. Molecular genetic analysis has significantly changed the physician's treatment decisions to more precise personalized management. Pathology in Syria is expanding and integrating these advanced techniques into daily practice for patients' benefit. The main public diagnostic cancer lab is at the Al Bairouni University Hospital and Atomic Energy Commission of Syria.

17.8.3 Cytogenetics and Molecular Genetics

Cytogenetic (karyotype, cytogenetic for both constitutional and non-constitutional defects) and molecular genetic techniques are available in Syria. These are provided by both the government and private sectors. University hospitals and Atomic Energy Commission of Syria are the main providers and perform tests of high standards by highly trained and dedicated staff. These advanced tests include a wide range of molecular techniques from conventional Fluorescence in Situ Hybridization (FISH) and Polymerase Chain Reaction (PCR, e.g. Reverse Transcription (RT-PCR) and quantitative (qPCR)) for diagnosis and monitoring residual disease activity for haematological and non-haematological cancers. Mutation driven studies aimed at adopting certain targeted therapy including EGFR, KRAS, and BRAF are routinely done. Liquid biopsy/Next Generation Sequencing (NGS) is funded by the government for research purposes.

17.9 Treatment

17.9.1 Medical Oncology

17.9.1.1 Advanced Treatments

All essentials cancer care outlined by the WHO cancer care in addition to advanced services such as mutation guided and targeted therapy (i.e. first to third generation of anti-Her2, anti-CD20 for Lymphoma, TKIs for CML or CLL for HCC, RCC, mutations guided treatment in lung, colon, etc.) are provided by the Syrian MOH. The oncology committee in each institution sets the indicators and guidelines for each disease. The Syrian National Cancer committee with the Syrian Association of Oncology and Scientific boards is processing a national guideline based on overall survival rate, progression free survival, national burden of disease, and financial considerations. This aims to parallel global guidelines such as those by the WHO, NICE, European Society for Medical Oncology, National Comprehensive Cancer Network.

17.9.1.2 Bone Marrow Transplantation

Syria first started bone marrow transplantation (BMT) in 2008, at Tishreen Military Hospital, Ministry of Defence (MOD), Damascus. This was followed by the Syrian Stem Cell Transplant Group (SSCTG) in 2012, Damascus. These offer both autologous and allogeneic transplant types. To date, approximately 150 cases have been transplanted. Among them, 85% of the cases are autologous transplant and 15% are allogeneic. Transplants slowed down during the crisis for many reasons [27].

A standard of care paediatric transplant centre is currently being established at the Children University Hospital. This centre is fully supported by the government and will run a free service for all Syrian children.

17.9.2 Radiation Therapy

Radiation oncology is mostly provided by the Ministry of Higher Education (MOHE). All governmental radiation services within MOHE and MOH are free of charge. Private radiotherapy services are limited. Radiation oncology is located mainly in two cities, Damascus and Latakia with tremendous efforts to renovate Aleppo and Homs post-war. There are five modern active linear accelerators delivering standard safe External Beam Radiotherapy (EBRT) treatment that includes traditional 2D/3D conformal radiation therapy, Intensity Modulated Radiation Therapy (IMRT), Image Guided Radiotherapy (IGRT), and brachytherapy system. Also, there are five cobalt-60 machines that support these services. About 30 devoted radiation oncologists collaborate with highly qualified technicians and physicists to provide successful advanced radiation treatment options to the patients. Close cooperation between the AECS and University of Damascus exists to provide education and training related to nuclear science and technology including radiation protection and medical physics. The Nuclear Science and Technology Training Centre (NSTTC), opened in February 2010, has one of the most important strategic solutions to meet the country's needs.

Currently, it is a big task to fulfil treatment requirements in time for all patients, with one linear accelerator per three million, a delay in appointments is expected. A rapid assessment survey conducted by the WHO in 2016 showed a 30-day waiting period for radiotherapy treatment (Fig. 17.5). Sanctions imposed on Syria prevent the maintenance and repair of the damaged parts of the machines which contributes to these delays [11].

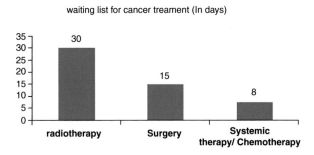

Fig. 17.5 Waiting list for each cancer treatment type (systemic therapy/chemotherapy, surgery, and radiotherapy) [11]. Used with permission from Maha Manachi

The National Cancer Committee Plan in collaboration with AECS aims to provide more advanced linear accelerators from the year 2021. These particularly aim to target the north, middle, and east of Syria to deliver the necessary cancer treatment to all patients. Nonetheless, radiation oncology is associated with significant costs especially with regard to the purchase and maintenance of expensive complex machinery required as well as the required international licensing.

17.9.3   Surgery

With the recognition of surgical oncology as a separate speciality, the training programmes in this field were first accredited by the MOH about 15 years ago. Nearly 25 surgical oncologists have registered in Syria. Limb sparing and breast saving surgery are the most commonly performed surgeries up to date [30].

17.9.4   Paediatric Oncology

Paediatric cancers account for 10% of the total number of cases. The estimated annual new paediatric cancer cases are about 1200. Most five common cancers according to 2019 data are Central Nervous System (CNS), leukaemia, lymphoma, bone and soft tissue sarcoma, and kidney followed by eye cancers.

A few paediatric oncology centres in Syria deliver cancer care as a part of paediatric general hospitals. The national referral centre is in Damascus at Children University Hospital which handles most cases up to age 13. All radiotherapy cases are referred to the Al Bairouni University Hospital.

Most facilities are available at Children University Hospital, i.e. diagnostic labs, Computed Tomography (CT) scans, Magnetic Resonance Imaging (MRI), pathology lab, and flow cytometry as well as specialized adequate blood bank with full blood component support. Treatment guidelines are according to the International Society of Paediatric Oncology (SIOP), St Jude, and other global guidelines for paediatric cancer. A paediatric bone marrow transplant unit is going to be established in 2021.

Other governmental paediatric centres are at Al Bairouni University Hospital (ABUH), Tishreen Military Hospital in Damascus, Tishreen University Hospital in Latakia, Aleppo National Hospital, and Al Kendi University Hospital [31].

BASMA society is a non-governmental organization (NGO) in Syria that supports children with cancer including the provision of all treatment types free of charge. About 200 new annual cases were added to the BASMA registry in 2019 (Fig. 17.6).

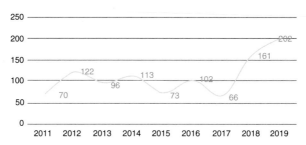

Fig. 17.6 Number of paediatric new cancer cases registered at BASMA per year (Ghanem et al., manuscript in press) [32]. Used with permission from Khaled Ghanem (BASMA)

17.9.5   Survivorship Track

The clinical outcome of patients enrolled between 2009 and 2018 was difficult to measure due to a high percentage (18%) of lost follow-up cases because of war. We are sure that at least 50% of patients diagnosed between 2009 and 2018 survived the disease. Between June 2018 and May 2020, the short-term 2-year overall survival rate of the 363 enrolled patients exceeded 90% with a very low treatment-related mortality rate of 2%. Multiple research and quality improvement projects are currently ongoing in the unit, including data management and infection control programmes. The unit has very good ties with regional and international tertiary care paediatric oncology hospitals [31].

17.9.6   Palliative Care Track

The need for Palliative Care (PC) is increasing due to the ageing population and increased incidence of cancer and other NCDs. About 30% of NCDs are cancers with end-of-life complications and pain [21]. Despite this need, palliative care is underdeveloped and limited in Syria and has worsened after the crisis. The MoH acknowledges Palliative Care (PC) as a part of the healthcare system and defines the national clinical guidelines and protocols that aim to enhance patients' quality of life and improve patient outcomes. MOH provides legal medical access to opioids when available and mostly in injection forms. Other slow-release oral morphine types are not available at the current time.

The WHO rapid assessment data in 2016 showed that 88% of inpatient settings had palliative care, while the mentioned service was available in 75% of outpatients and in 63% of community or home based [9]. The highest primary barriers to palliative care services were inadequate financial resources and limited human resources expertise (88%), while low health priority accounts for (50%) among primary barriers and the lowest barriers were related to lack of referral mechanisms [11].

17.10   Research and Education

The School of Medicine was founded in Damascus in 1901 but officially opened in 1903 and consisted of the faculties of Medicine and Pharmacy. The University of Damascus is the largest and oldest university in Syria, founded in 1923 through the merger of the School of Medicine and the Institute of Law. In Syria, 7 out of 8 public universities teach medicine, whereas 3 out of 23 private universities do. Medicine is primarily taught in Arabic [28]. During the recent decades, a significant amount of research has been conducted in Syria, particularly the University of Damascus. Annually, over hundreds of research papers have been published in Syria. However, a smaller number of papers are published in peer review journals. The collaboration between Faculty of Medicine, Oncology Division at ABUH, and the Faculty of Pharmacy is well established with the main focus being at the molecular level in cancer cell biology. Moreover, there is a profound research collaboration between the AECS and ABUH. The cross-region universities have a curriculum in accordance with the University of Saint Joseph (USJ) in Beirut, which has been considered a good example of fruitful collaboration.

17.11   Challenges and Advantages

17.11.1   Oncology Physicians

The Syrian Association of Oncology (SAO) was established in 1997 and has been a part of the Syrian Medical Association since then [32]. About 150 active consultants are registered as oncologist, haematologist, and radiotherapist. Most of them received their speciality training in Syria, 60–70% of consultants have experience or higher degrees from abroad such as Russia, UK, France, Spain, and the USA. All are registered under the Syrian MOH with accreditation from the Syrian Board in haematology, oncology, radiation oncology as well as paediatric oncology [33].

The SAO has a good scientific relationship and collaborates extensively with similar societies in the Middle East and North-Africa and Gulf regions. As such, the SAO has played an important role in the establishment of the Arab Medical Association Against Cancer (AMAAC).

17.12   The Future of Cancer Care in Syria

Cancer care in Syria is progressing rapidly, hence a new era has begun in cancer management with different modalities that give better treatment options to patients. These include the advancement of molecular pathology techniques with the ability to detect targetable mutations and immunotherapies. The responsibilities are extremely high on medical bodies to raise and maintain different oncology domains up to standards. There are major difficulties that both the government and medical professionals have experienced especially with over a decade of war, destruction of healthcare facilities, harsh economic sanctions, people displacements, and loss of human resources.

The National Cancer Control Committee, MoH, and MoHE, in collaboration with allied medical bodies both governmental and non-governmental, are working on five objectives (outlined below). In addition, they also constantly reinforce strategic regional partnerships, with the aim for fruitful and effective communication with other countries and centres which support the country's national plan and aid in improving the country's institutions, as well as adopting clear standards and systematic policies.

- Reducing cancer incidence rates through primary prevention.
- Ensuring the implementation of effective early screening and detection programmes in order to reduce mortality rates especially for breast, cervical, colon, and prostate cancers. This also includes increasing population awareness and participation in these programmes.
- Ensuring effective diagnosis and treatment to reduce cancer morbidity and mortality rates. This also involves the development of national treatment protocols in accordance with international standards for cancer management but specifically tailored to Syria's demographics, needs, and capabilities.
- Improving the quality of life for cancer patients via rehabilitation and palliative care.
- Improving cancer research.

17.13   Conclusion

Since 1969, oncology, both in Syria and internationally, has been advancing rapidly as reflected in significantly improved survival rates. These improvements in Syria's oncology care were largely attributable to government efforts in providing advanced centres equipped with the necessary resources to handle the rising incidence of cancer such as Al Bairouni University Hospital. Medical societies, the private sector, and civil societies also played an important role. Unfortunately, as with most other aspects of Syrian healthcare, the progress in cancer care was radically interrupted by over a decade of crisis involving a violent conflict and harsh economic sanctions. These destroyed previously developed resources and institutions, limited the import of new equipment and technologies, and led to the loss of human resources. Despite all of this, healthcare professionals continue to work tirelessly, overcoming unimaginable obstacles and often working under extremely difficult conditions to provide the best care they can for their patients. For this we would like to recognize Syrian doctors, particularly our fellow oncologists, and all other allied healthcare workers as the unsung heroes they truly are. Nonetheless, recent improvements including a significant decrease in the violence make us hopeful of a new era in Syrian healthcare but especially oncology. We particularly aim to keep up, implement, and contribute to the immense improvements and research in cancer care globally. For this purpose, a multitude of medical bodies collaborate but importantly the National Committee for Cancer Control is responsible for coordinating these efforts. The National Cancer Registry has been re-established and progressing to give a solid cancer registry data that is crucial to develop a national strategy with clear research objectives and comprehensive centres. Currently, our focus is on establishing unified guidelines, providing up-to-date national essential cancer medical list, restoring and building additional comprehensive cancer centres with the capacity for advanced management options such as radiation oncology systems, and expanding the role of palliative care.

Conflict of Interest Authors have no conflict of interest to declare.

Acknowledgements We would like to acknowledge all those who assisted and supported us in writing this book chapter. We would particularly like to acknowledge the following colleagues for their valuable contributions:

Nabeel Rajeh, MD: Professor of Medicine, Saint Louis University, programme director haematology oncology fellowship.

Rajwa Jbeily, Bachelor of Pharmacy (Damascus University), Ph.D. (Damascus University).

Khalil Saadeh, BA (Hons) Cantab, School of Clinical Medicine, University of Cambridge.

Khaled Ghanem, MD: Paediatric haematologist oncologist, medical director at BASMA Paediatric Oncology Unit.

Ousamah Anjak: Medical physicist, advisor at Atomic Energy Commission of Syria.

Feras Al Jerf, MA (Public health): director of Syrian National Cancer Registry.

Abbreviations

ABUH	Al Bairouni University Hospital
AECS	Atomic Energy Commission of Syria
EBRT	External beam radiotherapy
EML	Essentials medicine list
IAEA	International Atomic Agency Association
IARC	International Agency for Research on Cancer
IGRT	Image-guided radiotherapy
IMRT	Intensity-guided radiotherapy
LINAC	Linear accelerator
LMICs	Low- and middle-income countries
MENA	Middle East and North Africa
MOD	Ministry of Defence
MOH	Ministry of Health
MOHE	Ministry of Higher Education
MOLA	Ministry of Local Administration
MOSAL	Ministry of Social Affairs and Labour
NCCP	National Cancer Control Plan
NGO	Non-Governmental Organization
PPP	Public-private partnership
SHI	Social Health Insurance

SNCCC   Syrian National Committee for Cancer Control
SNCR   Syrian National Cancer Registry
SPECT   Single photon emission computed tomography
SRS   Syrian Radiological Society
WHO   World Health Organization

References

1. (Syria—the Cradle of Civilization and the Gateway to Historywww.sanatravelagency.com › pages › About-Syria).
2. (Syria—Wikipediaen.wikipedia.org › wiki › Syria).
3. World Population Prospects: The 2019 Revision—United Nations Population Division World Urbanization Prospects—Population Division—United Nations.
4. World Bank. The Toll of War the economic and social consequences of the conflict in Syria, in: site of The World Bank (10.7.2017). 2017. Available at: https://www.worldbank.org/en/country/ [CITATION] GROWTH AFTER WAR IN SYRIA S Devadas, I Elbadawi, NV Loayza—2019.
5. Syria/publication/the-toll-of-war-the-economicand-social-consequences-of-the-conflict-in-syria (last Accessed on 25 Feb 2019).
6. http://www.moh.gov.sy/ Syria Ministry of Health.
7. Syria Neoliberal Reforms in Health Sector Financing Syria: Embedding Unequal Access Kasturi Sen and Waleed al Faisal...https://www.researchgate.net. 21 Apr 2012—Health Sector Modernization Program 2009, Damascus: Ministry of Health; 2009. Available from: http://www.hsmp.moh.gov.sy/.
8. Sen K, Al-Faisal W, AlSaleh Y. Syria: effects of conflict and sanctions on public health. J Public Health. 2013;35(2):195–9. https://doi.org/10.1093/pubmed/fds090. Published: 23 Nov 2012
9. http://digicollection.org/hss/documents/s19144en/s19144en.pdf. Syrian Arab Republic Pharmaceutical Country Profile Published by the Damascus Ministry of Health in collaboration with the World Health Organization.
10. https://www.ecoi.net/en/file/local/2039609/syria_health_sector_bulletin_september_2020.pdf
11. Rapid Assessment of Cancer Management Care in Syria. December- 2016.
12. Simaan S, Jerf FA. Cancer in Syria (magnitude of the problem). Int J Cancer Tremnt. 2018;1(1):10–5.
13. A http://gco.iarc.fr/today/data/factsheets/populations/760-syrian-arab-republic-fact-sheets.pdf
14. World Health Organization. Towards a strategy for cancer control in the Eastern Mediterranean Region. 2009.
15. World Health Organization—noncommunicable diseases (NCD) Country Profiles, 2018.
16. 10-GBD Profile: Syria—Institute for Health Metrics and ...www.healthdata.org › country_profiles › GBD. Global Burden Of Diseases, Injuries, And Risk Factors Study 2010.
17. https://globalnutritionreport.org/resources/nutrition-profiles/asia/western-asia/syrian-arab-republic/.
18. WHO EMRO. Smoking behaviour and patterns among university students during the Syrian crisis. EMHJ. 2018;24(2)
19. Ward KD, Eissenberg T, Rastam S, Asfar T, Mzayek F, Fouad MF, Hammal F, Mock J, Maziak W. The tobacco epidemic in Syria. https://doi.org/10.1136/tc.2005.014860.
20. http://www.aec.org.sy/dep.php.
21. Global Atlas of Palliative Care at the End of Life Stephen R. Connor, PhD, Senior Fellow to the Worldwide Palliative Care Alliance (WPCA). Maria Cecilia Sepulveda Bermedo, MD, Senior Adviser Cancer Control, Chronic Diseases. Prevention and Management, Chronic Diseases and Health Promotion, World Health Organization.

22. Bashour H, Muhjazi G, WHO EMRO. Hepatitis B and C in the Syrian Arab Republic: a review. East Mediterr Health J. 2016;22(4)
23. Human Papillomavirus and Related Diseases Report. Syrian Arab Republic www.hpvcentre. net on 17 June 2019.
24. http://siopyi.blogspot.com/2020/06/how-non-governmental-organization.html?m=1 How a Non-Governmental Organization Changed the Face of Childhood Cancer Care in Syria.
25. https://www.globalhep.org/country-progress/syrian-arab-republic
26. https://hpvcentre.net/statistics/reports/SYR_FS.pdf. ICO/IARC Information Centre on HPV and Cancer, Syria Human Papillomavirus and Related Cancers, Fact Sheet 2018 (2019-06-17).
27. How Did the War Affect Organ Transplantation in Syria? Exp Clin Transplant. 2020;18(Suppl 1):19–21. https://doi.org/10.6002/ect.TOND-TDTD2019.L23.
28. https://archive.unescwa.org/sites/www.unescwa.org/files/page_attachments/syria-ntto-innovation-landscape-study-ar_0.pdf
29. https://www.fctc.org/wp-content/uploads/2018/05/FCTC-implementation-Syria-2010.pdf
30. https://sboms.org/en/general-surgery/. Syrian Board of Medical Specialties.
31. http://siopyi.blogspot.com/2020/06/how-non-governmental-organization.html?m=1
32. www.syrma.org
33. https://syrianoncology.net/
34. https://www.worldometers.info/world-population/syria-population/
35. https://data.worldbank.org/indicator/SP.POP.TOTL.FE.ZS?locations=SY
36. Syrian Arab Republic. 2019. https://www.populationpyramid.net/syrian-arab-republic/2019/
37. Syria's Conflict Economy https://doi.org/10.5089/9781498336826.001.A001
38. WHO—Cancer Country Profiles Syrian Arab Republic 2020.
39. The economic burden of cancer care for Syrian refugees: a population-based modelling study. https://doi.org/10.1016/S1470-2045(20)30067-X

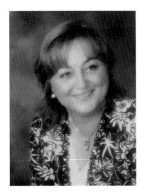

Maha Manachi is a Hemato-Oncologist who trained in both Syria and the UK. She is head of the Hematological Malignancy Division at Al Bairouni University Hospital, the largest cancer centre in Syria. She is a member of the hospital's Breast Cancer Committee. As a member of the Syrian National Committee for Cancer Control, she develops the national screening program, supports the Cancer Registry program, and establishes national treatment guidelines. Manachi contributed significantly to the Syrian Stem Cell Transplantation Group, pioneering the bone marrow transplant field in the region. Her regional and international roles include participation in various WHO cancer programs, as well as regional oncology meetings. She is an active member of cancer societies such as ASCO, ESMO, EHA, and AMAAC.

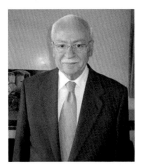

Eyad Chatty studied medicine at Damascus University and later completed his training in the USA: Cleveland Clinic, Case Western Reserve University and AFIP: he earned his Board in Pathology and DPL in Cytology and Neuropathology. He established and chaired the Oncology Department at Damascus University from 1974 to 1987. He became Dean of the Medical School and then Minister of Health from 1987 to 2004. He was elected Chairman of the Executive Committee, WHO. He is now a Professor of Pathology and a Head of Departments of Pathology in both University Hospitals. He published many books and articles. The last: Synovial sarcoma of the maxillary sinus, 2021, https://doi.org/10.1016/j.amsu.2021.102538.

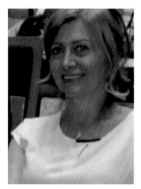

Seham Sulaiman studied medicine at the University of Tishreen and later completed her Ph.D. in 1991 on a scholarship to Russia. She is currently a professor of haematology and oncology at the University of Damascus and the Syrian Private University. In addition to her role as a lecturer, she supervises masters and Ph.D. students. Furthermore, Sulaiman is an active researcher who has published research articles and contributed to medical book chapters. She has also held several prestigious academic and administrative positions as well as being a member of many medical societies (e.g. ESMO) and a participant on a variety of regional pharmaceutical advisory boards.

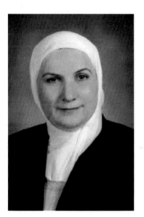

Zahera Fahed is a consultant in haematology, oncology, and Bone Marrow Transplantation. She was the Head of breast cancer at Al Bairouni University Hospital and the general secretary of the Syrian Association of Oncology. Zahera also served as a secretary of the Syrian Society of Breast cancer.

Chapter 18
General Oncology Care in Tunisia

Nesrine Mejri, Haifa Rachdi, Lotfi Kochbati, and Hamouda Boussen

18.1 Tunisia Demographics

With 155,360 km^2 (59,985 square miles), Tunisia is the smallest country in North Africa with a population density of 75 people per km^2 (195 people per m^2) and a Gross Domestic Product (GDP) per capita is at \$4341, in 2017 [1]. The country is currently divided into 24 governorates. The most important is Tunis (with more than one million inhabitants), followed by major cities like Sfax and Sousse [1, 2]. Unlike many other North African and Arab countries, Tunisia has led a modern governmental strategy promoting family planning and birth control by Habib Bourguiba, the first President of the country, in the early 1970s. A recent data report indicates a population of about 11.818.61 with a yearly change of +1.06% and a global world rank of 78 [1]. The fertility rate is probably the lowest within Arab countries at 2.2 live births per woman in 2020. In conjunction with a health policy covering the whole country, the famous strategy of family planning revealed a 77.4-year life expectancy (79.3 for females and 75.4 for males) but also an age distribution of 25.2% from 0 to 14 years, 65.8% from 15 to 64 and 8.8% aged 65 years or more. The population median age is 32.7 years old (2020) being 32 in males and 33.3 in females and gender equality is observed between both sexes [1, 2].

N. Mejri · H. Rachdi · H. Boussen (✉)
Department of Medical Oncology, University Hospital Abderrahman Mami, Ariana, Tunis, Tunisia

Faculty of Medicine of Tunis, University Tunis El Manar, Tunis, Tunisia

L. Kochbati
Faculty of Medicine of Tunis, University Tunis El Manar, Tunis, Tunisia

Department of Radiotherapy, Abderrahman Mami Hospital 2090, El Manar University, Tunis, Tunisia

© The Author(s) 2022
H. O. Al-Shamsi et al. (eds.), *Cancer in the Arab World*,
https://doi.org/10.1007/978-981-16-7945-2_18

18.2   Cancer Statistics in Tunisia

The latest cancer incidence estimates for 2018 are about 15,894 new cases vs 12,189 in 2012, with a standardized incidence of 115/100,000 for the sexes, 131.7 in males and 102 in females [2]. The five most common cancers for both sexes in Tunisia are breast (2305 cases), lung (1909), colorectal (1657), bladder (1323), and prostate with 829 cases. We observed an epidemiologic transition, especially in females with a top position of breast cancer followed by colorectal cancer, while cervical cancer dropped to the third position, probably due to a policy of cervical extended pap smears tests in the primary healthcare centers in parallel with the policy of birth control. In 2018, cancer was responsible for 16.1% of deaths in Tunisia (Figs. 18.1, 18.2, and 18.3) [2].

As in the Arab world, breast cancer in Tunisia remains by far the most common among females [1, 3]. In a recent series of 1262 Tunisian patients treated for breast cancer, the 5-year overall survival was 72%, while poor-risk factors in the multivariate study were negative HR ($P < 0.001$) and number of involved axillary lymph nodes were $P = 0.023$ [4]. A particular kind recognized locally in the country is Inflammatory Breast Cancer (IBC) with Tunisian and North African experience in its diagnosis and management [5]. A study has evaluated breast cancer burden in Tunisia and its impact in terms of adjusted life years (DALY) in 2017 and projections for 2030. The incidence and mortality rate among females in Tunisia was 50.17/100,000 persons per year and 14.04/100,000 persons per year, while breast cancer DALY was at 25,145 (438/100,000 persons per year). Projections for 2030 were at 40071 in 2030 with a standardized rate of 507/100,000 persons per year [6]. Breast cancer in young women, particularly in Tunisia, showed a retrospective study of 83 patients younger than 35 years, treated in Sfax observed a mean age of 31.7 years. They have mostly T2 tumor stage, high histologic grade, and positive axillary node tumors [7]. Overall Survival (OS) at 5 years was 66.8% and poor prognostic factors were CT T3-T4 stages, and several lymph nodes were involved [7].

Lung cancer remains diagnosed at an advanced and/or metastatic stage. In a recent study of 118 Non-Small Cell Lung Cancer (NSCLC) patients, the median age was 43.8 years and 79, 7% of the patients were at an advanced or metastatic stage. Median overall survival was 8 ± 0.72 months [8]. A significant change has been observed in the histological types of lung cancer with an increase of adenocarcinoma over squamous cell carcinoma forms in the last two decades in Tunisia, smoking being responsible for 90% of all lung cancer cases in Tunisia. The evaluation of one study shows tobacco use prevalence was about 25% in the Tunisian population according to a meta-analysis [9]. Tunisia has a higher prevalence of tobacco use, almost 35%, the highest in Arab countries and smokers use cigarettes while traditional sniffed or mouth tobacco has become rare. The number of smokers from 10 to 70 years is estimated at 1.7 million and tobacco is responsible for 7000 deaths per year in Tunisia [9]. Tunisian authorities applied regulatory measures in 2012 prohibiting tobacco advertising on national/international television and radio, local/international magazines and newspapers, billboards, and the outdoors. Nevertheless, there was no toll-free Quitline with a live person to discuss smoking cessation in Tunisia. Nicotine replacement therapy is legally available in the market and could

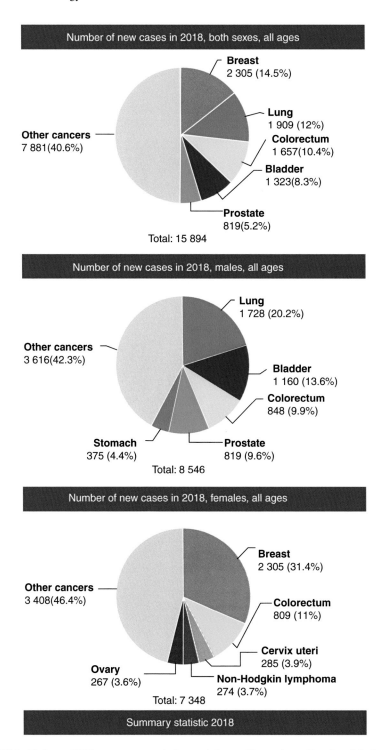

Fig. 18.1 Globocan 2018 cancer cases, whole population and by sex https://gco.iarc.fr/today/data/factsheets/populations/788-tunisia-fact-sheets.pdf [2]

Incidence, Mortality and Prevalence by cancer site								
	New cases			Deaths			5-year prevalence (all ages)	
Cancer	Number	Rank	(%)	Cum.risk	Number	Rank	(%)	Cum.risk	Number	Prop.
Breast	3 092	1	15.9	4.28	986	2	8.3	1.28	9 749	0
Lung	2 929	2	15.1	2.18	2 634	1	22.2	1.95	2 941	0
Bladder	1 406	3	7.2	1.08	822	3	6.9	0.51	3 777	0
Prostate	1 186	4	6.1	1.68	541	6	4.6	0.13	4.044	0
Colon	988	5	5.1	0.80	542	5	4.6	0.41	2 337	0
Rectum	787	6	4.0	0.62	379	11	3.2	0.26	2 044	0
Non-Hodgkin lymphoma	738	7	3.8	0.56	364	12	3.1	0.26	2 029	0
Liver	634	8	3.3	0.47	599	4	5.1	0.43	665	0
Leukaemia	617	9	3.2	0.43	442	8	3.7	0.29	1 673	0
Pancreas	524	10	2.7	0.38	517	7	4.4	0.37	416	0
Brain central nervous system	480	11	2.5	0.36	413	9	3.5	0.31	1 235	0
Stomach	466	12	2.4	0.37	383	10	3.2	0.30	658	0
Thyroid	416	13	2.1	0.28	70	22	0.59	0.02	1 293	0
Larynx	413	14	2.1	0.35	259	13	2.2	0.21	1 131	0
Cervix uteri	342	15	1.8	0.53	185	16	1.6	0.30	897	0
Nasopharynx	342	16	1.8	0.24	218	14	1.8	0.17	963	0
Kidney	325	17	1.7	0.25	173	17	1.5	0.12	848	0
Corpus uteri	306	18	1.6	0.50	66	24	0.56	0.10	940	0
Ovary	284	19	1.5	0.41	186	15	1.6	0.28	726	0
Hodgkin lymphoma	271	20	1.4	0.18	68	23	0.57	0.05	885	0
Lip, oral cavity	246	21	1.3	0.18	116	20	0.98	0.08	656	0
Multiple myeloma	187	22	0.96	0.14	155	18	1.3	0.11	443	0
Gallbladder	153	23	0.79	0.13	118	19	1.00	0.09	192	0
Oesophagus	102	24	0.52	0.08	97	21	0.82	0.08	110	0
Anus	90	25	0.46	0.07	44	25	0.37	0.03	237	0
Melanoma of skin	81	26	0.42	0.05	32	26	0.27	0.02	228	0
Kaposi sarcoma	57	27	0.29	0.05	16	29	0.13	0.01	154	0
Hypopharynx	44	28	0.23	0.04	19	27	0.16	0.02	73	0
Vulva	41	29	0.21	0.04	19	28	0.16	0.01	112	0
Salivary glands	36	30	0.19	0.03	14	32	0.12	0.01	104	0
Testis	35	31	0.18	0.04	8	33	0.07	0.00	122	0
Oropharynx	30	32	0.15	0.03	14	31	0.12	0.01	74	0
Mesothelioma	16	33	0.08	0.01	15	30	0.13	0.01	17	0
Vagina	13	34	0.07	0.03	6	34	0.05	0.01	33	0
Penis	6	35	0.03	0.02	2	35	0.02	0.01	18	0
All cancer sites	19 446			13.54	11 855			7.90	45 541	0

Fig. 18.2 Cancer incidence, mortality and prevalence in Tunisia in 2020 https://gco.iarc.fr/today/data/factsheets/populations/788-tunisia-fact-sheets.pdf [2]

	Males	Females	Both Sexes
Population	5 760 714	5 898 461	11 659 175
Number of new cancer cases	8 546	7 348	15 894
Age-standardized incidence rate (World)	131.7	102.0	115.4
Risk of developing cancer before the age of 75 years (%)	13.8	10.2	11.9
Number of cancer deaths	6 075	4 017	10 092
Age-standardized mortality rate (World)	92.2	53.2	71.3
Risk of dying from cancer before the age of 75 years (%)	9.4	5.5	7.4
5-year prevalent cases	16 906	18 053	34 959
Top 5 most frequent cancers excluding non-melanoma skin cancer (ranked by cases)	Lung Bladder Colorectum Prostate Stomach	Breast Colorectum Cervix uteri Non-Hodgkin lymphoma Ovary	Breast Lung Colorectum Bladder Prostate

Fig. 18.3 Epidemiologic data of cancer in Tunisia https://gco.iarc.fr/today/data/factsheets/populations/788-tunisia-fact-sheets.pdf [2]

be purchased in a pharmacy with a prescription, but it is not cost covered and is not on Tunisia's essential drug list. Certainly, informational, and educational campaigns relating to tobacco control should be intensified.

Data from the North Tunisia cancer registry showed 6909 colorectal cancers during the period 1994–2009 with an Age-Standardized Incidence Rate (ASR) raising from 6.4/100,000 in 1994 to 12.4/100,000 in 2009 and a trend in CRC with an Annual Percentage Change (APC) of +3,9%. Projections for 2024 are predicting an ASR of 39.3/100,000 [10]. CRC is rapidly growing but a lot of cases remain diagnosed at advanced stages and even stage II is discussed for an adjuvant medical therapy according to their anatomo-clinical features [11].

18.3   Cancer Risk Factors

The prevalence of Tunisia's smoking rate in 2016 was 32.70%, a 0.1% increase from 2015 and the rates increased slowly since 2012 [11]. Within a population of 3643 cases of Non-Communicable Diseases, active smoking was found in 1076 cases, accounting for 29.5% of cases [12]. Among the NCD groups, CVD was the most common (65%). Tobacco was significantly associated with CVD ($P < 0.001$), CRD ($P = 0.002$), bronchopulmonary CS ($P < 0.001$), hematological malignancy ($P = 0.023$), and DM ($P < 0.001$) in uni and multivariate analyses [12]. Most Arab countries, so as Tunisia, have the common habit of Shisha consumption and, according to a study from Saudi Royal University, based on atomic absorption methods, out of 14.685 mg (heavy) metals present in 1 g of the Jurak paste, only 3.075 μg was transferred to the smoker [13].

Cervical cancer is ranked 15th among females in the country, with a slight decrease probably related to the extensive campaigns of pap smears launched in the primary care structures in the 1970s [14]. Within a screened population of 391 patients from the grand Tunis, overall HPV prevalence was 13.2% and the most prevalent HPV genotypes were HPV6 (40%), HPV40 (14%), HPV16 (12%), HPV52 (9%), HPV31 and HPV59 (7%), and HPV68 (4%), their mean age being 40.7 years. Associated risk factors of HPV infection were smoking (OR: 2.8), low income (OR: 9.6), bad socioeconomic level (OR:2.5), and single woman [15].

18.4   Cancer Screening Programs

In Tunisia, an extensive effort at cervical cancer screening with pap smears based on primary health structures, since the 1970s, led to a down staging of the diagnosed cases [15]. Despite this elementary care effort, there is no primary prevention program like systematic HPV vaccine [16]. There is no structured mammography screening for breast cancer, excluding pilot studies performed in Ariana state in Tunis by the Family Planification Office and another in Sfax [17, 18].

A cancer plan is now running with four axes: training for professionals, clinical and basic research besides the improvement of the quality of care. Biological studies are also concerned with the predisposing factors for breast cancer and nasopharyngeal carcinoma [19, 20].

18.5   Cancer Prevention Programs

Hepatitis B vaccination started in Tunisia in 1995, leading to a slight risk reduction of hepatocellular carcinoma [21]. Multiple units of smoking cessation have been available at university hospitals and pulmonology departments for 20 years [22]. A strict regulation concerning smoking is available in Tunisia, but unfortunately not applied, especially concerning prohibition of smoking in public spaces, and very high taxation concerning tobacco in Tunisia and, currently, Tunisia exerts taxes at a level of 70% on the retail prices of cigarettes [23, 24].

18.6 Cancer Diagnosis

Data from 2014 showed levels for one million inhabitants of MRI at 2, CT scans 8,91, gamma cameras 1.18, Pet-scan, 0, mammography facilities 22. 58, radiotherapy machines 1.64, and Linear Accelerator (LINAC) at 0.64 [25]. However, during the last 2 years, five PET-scans have been available and six LINAC available for stereotactic radiotherapy. Every big Tunisian city has a department of nuclear medicine inside university hospitals (Tunis, Sousse, Sfax, Monastir, Gabes) as well as private centers of nuclear medicine. Translational research is available due to the close collaboration between the researchers from the faculties of sciences and clinicians and the faculties of medicine of Tunis, Sousse, Sfax, and Monastir. Molecular testing is available for leukemia by cytogenetics, BRCA1 and BRCA2, HER2, ALK, EGFR, and ROS1 in both universities and faculties of sciences, as well as private laboratories.

18.7 Treatment

18.7.1 Medical Oncology

Public academic oncology structures are represented by a comprehensive cancer center (Institut Salah Azaiez), oncology and radiotherapy units in university hospitals in Tunis, Sousse, Sfax, Monastir, Jendouba, and medical oncology units in general hospitals in Gafsa, Gabes, Beja, Bizerte, and Sidi Bouzid [1, 3]. Salah Azaiez Institute has the highest recruitment rate with more than 10,000 new patients per year and a structured Multidisciplinary Tumor Boards (MDT) that has disseminated to all the satellite oncology structures created since the year 2000 in Tunis state and other regions. The Medical Oncology Department at Abderrahman Mami hospital in Ariana (SOMA), is inside an oncology center located in a pulmonology hospital. It started initially with only a medical oncology department in 2010, then a radiation oncology department with one Linear Accelerator in 2017. The center recruits about 2000 patients per year, mainly for breast, lung, and colorectal cancers. This oncology hub administers 18,000 ambulatory treatments, a specific Friday devoted to Trastuzumab and other anti-HER2 treatments, other targeted therapies like Beva or Ceuximab, Immunotherapy, 100,000 emergencies, and 15,000 outpatients on average per year. This oncology center coordinated for 3 years, an extended program of translational research combines researchers from the faculty of science of Tunis, Institut Pasteur, and clinicians from university hospitals Charles Nicolle, Abderrahman Mami, Military hospital, and Salah Azaiez, within a program of breast and ovarian family cancers. Medical oncology center in Ariana, Tunisia (the SOMA center) also conducts various social and artistic activities with a program of musicotherapy with and for the patients, with scheduled activities during Pink October. Paramedical and medical staff are around 40 and 20. They are trained with programmed sessions inside the department and at the national level as well as international level, in North Africa and Europe.

18.7.2   Radiation Therapy

There is a need for radiotherapy infrastructure expansion since there are only 21 radiotherapy units in the country (15 Linear Accelerators LINAC, and six Cobalt 60 machines in 5 public hospitals and 7 private clinics) covering less than 46% of the total need [25, 26]. More than 8000 patients undergo radiation therapy on an annual basis with a focus on hypofractionated regimens for breast and rectum cancers to reduce waiting lists. This gap is painfully expressed in very long waiting lists in public hospitals while it remains expensive in the private sector. Therefore, limiting access to the treatment. New RT techniques such as IMRT and Steretacticc radiotherapy (SRT/SBRT) are developed in university hospitals and in private clinics. There is a strategy to stop using Cobalt Units by 2023 which will be replaced with linear accelerators. University departments of radiotherapy are involved in research programms with IAEA and participate in training programms for african countries.

18.7.3   Surgery

Surgical oncology is available at Salah Azaiez Institute, with the highest concentration of surgical oncologists (around 30), having a high experience with breast and gynecologic oncology.

18.7.4   Pediatric Oncology

The facility of pediatric oncology has been available since 1988 at the Salah Azaiez Institute, then in 1995 at Tunis children's hospital and Sousse and Sfax university hospitals [27]. Most of the oncology teams apply the protocols of the International Society of Pediatric Oncology (SIOP).

18.7.5 Survivorship Track

The available associations that have "on the field" activities of education and patient training for socio-economic sustainability, like housing during treatment. The ATAMCS, devoted to breast cancer and AMC to all cancers, organizes charity and annual events with patients and treating teams (https://jamaity.org/association/association-tunisienne-dassistance-aux-malades-du-cancer-du-sein/ and https://www.facebook.com/AMCTun). There is no specific action concerning cancer survivors.

18.7.6 Palliative Care Track

The palliative cancer treatment initiatives were started in 1988 with the creation of the Tunisian Association for study of pain, which trained in collaboration with Gustave Roussy Institute, medical oncologists for cancer pain diagnosis and management. Since then, 4 units of ambulatory palliative care have been created at Salah Azaiez institute and Sousse and Sfax university hospitals [28].

18.8 Research and Education

In Tunisia, basic research is mostly performed at the faculties of sciences or the biotechnology centers located in the big cities, Tunis, Sousse, Sfax, and Monastir [29, 30]. An effort is needed to increase the collaboration with clinicians in the cancer treatment centers and units as well as recruitment of researchers inside the clinical areas. Cancer education has started for students at the faculties of medicine with hematology-oncology devoted modules and for residents and confirmed physicians, devoted certificates, and masters in thoracic, gastrointestinal, breast, and dermatology oncology.

18.8.1 Breast Cancer Features and Therapeutic Results in Arab Countries

Breast cancer remains late detected due to the absence of mammography screening programs in Arab countries. Anatomo-clinical features are characterized by a younger age at diagnosis (around 50 years, compared to the Western countries, 10% of patients younger than 35 years, 10–13% of initial metastases, and around 17–20% of triple-negative cases and 5% of inflammatory breast cancer (Table 18.1). Five-year overall survival is varying from 70 to 80%.

Table 18.1 Anatomo-clinical characteristics and therapeutic results of breast cancer in Arab countries

Author/C/ Ref.	Period	Number	MA	less 35 years	HR+	Her 2+	TN	MTS	Overall survey
Belaid/ TN/[4]	2007–12	1262	50	7%	57%	23%	19%	12%	5 year 80%
Manai/TN/ [40]	2008–13	210(5%) IBC	42	15%	41%	32%	25%	12%	5 year 55%
Kallel/TN/ [7]	2002–8	83/781(10.6%)	31.7	All	55%	29%	NA	12%	5 year 75%
Bendardaf/ UAE/[41]	2016–18	98	51	13%	61%	25%	13%	NA	NA
Slaoui/ Mo/[42]	2005–10	219(4%) IBC	47	16%	45%	28%	21%	30%	3 year 70%
Smaili/ Alg/[43]	2016	1437	48	17%	NA	NA	NA	12%	NA
Chaher/ Alg/[44]	2005–9	117 IBC	48	NA	71%	20%	17%	NA	25.1 months
Zeineldin/ Eg/[45]	1999–07	5459	49	10%	66%	7%	NA	13%	5 year 81.2%
Darwish/ Eg/[46]	2008–10	458(9.2%)	32	All	62%	30%	NA	10%	3 year DFS 70%

18.9   Cost-Effective Cancer Care

In Tunisia, since 1998, legislation has guaranteed free healthcare for the low-income/unemployed population. Hence, cancer patients with low-income are provided with free healthcare coverage (indigent). Such patients receive treatment in the public sector exclusively. On the other hand, the National Health Insurance Fund (Caisse Nationale d'Assurance Maladie, CNAM) offers insurance for workers and taxpayers treated in the private and public sectors. In Tunisia, there is a universal public healthcare system. Ninety-five percent of the population has governmental coverage to free healthcare access and 80% of the population is treated in the public sector [31]. The private healthcare system in Tunisia has significantly expanded in terms of infrastructure as well as human resources. This sector offers, for example, high-quality cosmetic surgery, spas, and thalassotherapy to attract foreigners, but unfortunately, few patients remain fully covered and mostly must pay their expenses. Every big city has private clinics devoted to cancer treatment, two clinics in Tunis, one in Sousse and two in Sfax. Most of the oncologists have been trained at the Salah Azaiez Institute with the spirit of a multidisciplinary approach and an organ devoted committee for diagnosis and treatment. Globally, patients having social insurance have access to public and private cancer centers, while indigents are covered by the Ministry of Health and Social Affairs. The available patient's association for cancer in general and breast cancer, provide hospitalizations if needed and help to access therapeutic innovations within donations of administrative sustain.

18.10 Challenges and Advantages

Cytotoxic drugs and targeted therapies are provided to patients covered by social insurance in 55% of cases, while indigent patients (35%) with needs are covered by the Ministry of Health [31]. Usual cytotoxic drugs are covered by the social insurance and for indigents, while targeted therapies like trastuzumab, rituximab, bevacizumab, cetuximab, sunitinib, imatinib, crizotinib, and erlotinib are available only for social insured, with difficulty for indigents, excluding an access program. The entry to therapeutic innovations remains limited due to the high cost of drugs, especially in the absence of approval by ministerial authorities for immunotherapy. Drug prescriptions outlasted slowed by a heavy administrative circuit, installed to reduce, and control the costs of cancer therapies like trastuzumab, bevacizumab erlotinib, erlotinib, and imatinib. The SOMA Oncology Centre adopted a legal approach based on compassionate grounds. This mixed view offers the opportunity to facilitate access to these drugs mainly to Crizotinib, Palbocilib, Ribociclib, and subsequent lines in ALK and EGFR+ lung cancers. Molecular tests are available in public and private structures for ALK, EGFR, ROS1, PD1, BRAF, and RAS and are performed at diagnosis according to the local and international existing guidelines [32].

An effort is being made by the National Agency for accreditation and guidelines (INEAS) to publish guidelines for diagnosis and management of cancer, applicable in both public and private clinics [33, 34]. These efforts were made in collaboration with the Tunisian Society of Medical Oncology (STOM), Radiation Oncology (STOR), and Surgical Oncology (STCO) [33]. There are now almost 100 medical oncologists, 50 radiation oncologists, and 45 surgical oncologists in the public and private sectors.

Tunisian oncologists have robust experience in clinical trials, regulated by a detailed and adapted procedure for more than 20 years [35–37]. They have also recognized expertise in specific North African cancers, like Inflammatory Breast Cancer (IBC) and nasopharyngeal cancer [5, 37]. Cancer diagnosis and management requires to be adapted and devoted structures, platforms of histopathology, molecular biology as well as artificial intelligence tools. Tunisian centers remain under-equipped, notably at the molecular biology level. The SOMA oncology center had the opportunity to host a multisite and multidisciplinary study group on breast and family cancer. The group performed huge work on clinical but also translational research with Next Generation Sequencing (NGS), by familiarizing clinical oncologists with basic sciences and translational research [20, 29].

Patients with cancer are at higher risk of being infected with COVID-19 and of developing a more severe form. In China, 1.7% of COVID-19 patients with severe symptoms were found to be cancer patients [38]. The SOMA Oncology Centre is in a university hospital with the most important recruitment of COVID-19 patients, hospitalized in the pulmonology units and the intensive care department. This orientation made the oncologists involved in COVID-19 patient care at the emergency department and the pulmonology units. The oncologists from this unit acquired experience in COVID-19 cases' detection and management. The oncologists from SOMA cancer center observed more than 20 COVID-19 plus cancer cases, mostly breast cancer, lung, and gynecologic cancers, with two deaths in lung cancer patients. COVID-19 diagnosis was facilitated by easy access to radiologic (chest X-ray and CT-scan) and biologic access with a very close availability of hospitalization beds at Mami Hospital. Strict measures were implemented such as stringent instructions to medical staff and patients about personal hygiene and usage of Personal Protective Equipment (PPE) amongst the clinical staff. All staff and patients have their temperature checked and answer COVID-19 related clinical questions before entering for consultation or treatment administration [39].

18.11   The Future of Cancer Care in Tunisia

The future of cancer care in Tunisia will need important efforts to increase the number of platforms of molecular biology and translational research toward a more innovative and personalized therapeutic approach. The multidisciplinary spirit and approach, following strict national and international guidelines, may warrant better therapeutic results (Fig. 18.4). A structured effort in continuous medical education, at the national, regional, and Arab levels may improve oncologists in terms of Good Clinical Practice (GCP). At the social level, an effort is mandatory to sustain patients and their families, due to the induced "financial toxicity" [47].

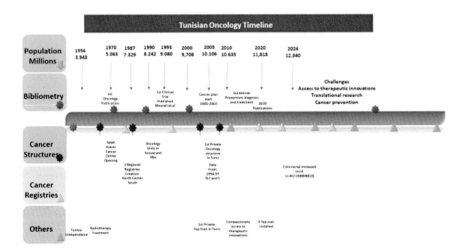

Fig. 18.4 Development of oncology in Tunisia

18.12 Conclusion

In comparison with other Arab countries, Tunisia is living in a difficult socio-economic and political situation, which combined with the COVID-19 pandemic, increased health expenses, especially for cancer patients. Oncologists are encountering some difficulties in offering their patients modern diagnoses, therapeutic methods, and access to treatment innovations. A regional and international collaboration, especially at the Arab level, could help to perform multicentric epidemiologic and therapeutic studies.

Conflict of Interest Authors have no conflict of interest to declare.

References

1. https://www.worldometers.info/demographics/tunisia-demographics/. Accessed on 26 Oct 2020.
2. https://gco.iarc.fr/today/data/factsheets/populations/788-tunisia-fact-sheets.pdf. Accessed on 26 Oct 2020.
3. Chouchane L, Boussen H, Sastry KS. Breast cancer in Arab populations: molecular characteristics and disease management implications. Lancet Oncol. 2013 Sep;14(10):e417–24.
4. Belaid I, Ben Fatma L, Ezzairi F, Hochlaf M, Chabchoub I, Gharbi O, et al. Trends and current challenges of breast cancer in Tunisia: a retrospective study of 1262 cases with survival analysis. Breast J. 2018;24(5):846–8.
5. Boussen H, Bouzaiene H, Ben Hassouna J, Dhiab T, Khomsi F, Benna F, et al. Inflammatory breast cancer in Tunisia: epidemiological and clinical trends. Cancer. 2010;116(11 Suppl):2730–5.
6. Cherif A, Dhaouadi S, Osman M, Hsairi M. Breast cancer burden in Tunisia: situation in 2017 and projections by 2030. Eur J Public Health. 2019;2019(Supplement_4)
7. Kallel M, Elloumi F, Ghorbal L, Chaabouni S, Frikha M, Daoud J. Breast cancer in young women in southern Tunisia: anatomical study and clinical prognostic factors: about a series of 83 patients. Rep Practic Oncol Radiother. 2015;20(3):155–60.
8. Joobeur S, Ben Saad A, Migaou M, Fahem N, Cheikh S, Rouatbi N. Survival and prognostic factors of non-small-cell lung cancer among young people in central Tunisia. Pan Afr Med J. 2020 Jan;23(35):19.
9. Serhier Z, Bendahhou K, Soulimane A, Bennani Othmani M, Ben AA. Tobacco prevalence in Tunisia: literature systematic review and meta-analysis. Tunis Med. 2018;96(10):545–56.
10. Khiari H, Ben Ayoub-Hizem W, Ben Khadhra H, Hsairi M. Colorectal cancer incidence trend and projections in Tunisia (1994–2024). Asian Pac J Cancer Prev. 2017;18(10):2733–9.
11. https://www.macrotrends.net/countries/TUN/tunisia/smoking-rate-statistics Accessed on 25 Jan 2021.
12. Ben Ayed H, Ben Hmida M, Nen Jemaa M, Trigui M, Jedidi J, Karray R, Mejdoub Y, Kassis M, Feki H, Yaich S, Damak J. Active smoking: a major risk factor for human non-communicable diseases in a hospital survey. Rev Mal Respir. 2019 Feb;36(2):171–8.
13. Chaouachi K. Shisha smoking, nickel and chromium levels in Tunisia. Environ Sci Pollut Res. https://doi.org/10.1007/s11356-013-1935.
14. Sancho-Garnier H, Chami Khazraji Y, Hamdi Cherif M, Mahnane A, Hsairi M, et al. Cervical cancer screening practices in the extended Middle East and North Africa countries. Vaccine. 2013 Dec;30(31 Suppl 6):G51–7.
15. Ardhaoui M, Ennaifer E, Letaief H, Rejaibi S, Lassili T, Chahed K, Bougatef S, Bahrini A, El Fehri E, Kaouther Ouerhani K, Paez Jimenez A, Guizani I, Boubaker MS, Alaya NBB. Prevalence, Genotype distribution and risk factors for cervical human papillomavirus infection in the Grand Tunis Region, Tunisia. PLoS One. 2016;11(6):e0157432.

16. Yazghich I, Berraho M. Cervical cancer in the Maghreb country (Morocco–Algeria–Tunisia): epidemiological, clinical profile and control policy. Tunis Med. 2018;96(10–11):647–57.
17. Zaanouni E, Ben Abdallah M, Bouchlaka A, Ben Aissa R, Kribi L, M'barek F, Ben Hamida A, Boussen H, Gueddana N. Preliminary results and analysis of the feasibility of mammographic breast cancer screening in women younger than 50 years of the Ariana area in Tunisia. Tunis Med. 2009;87(7):443–9.
18. Frikha M, Yaiche O, Elloumi F, Mnejja W, Slimi L, Kassis M, Daoud J. Results of a pilot study for breast cancer screening by mammography in Sfax region, Tunisia. J Gynecol Obstet Biol Reprod (Paris). 2013;42(3):252–61.
19. Hamdi Y, Ben Rekaya M, Jingxuan S, Nagara M, Messaoud O, Benammar Elgaaied A, Mrad R, Chouchane L, Boubaker MS, Abdelhak S, Boussen H, Romdhane L. A genome wide SNP genotyping study in the Tunisian population: specific reporting on a subset of common breast cancer risk loci. BMC Cancer. 2018;18(1):1295.
20. Hamdi Y, Boujemaa M, Ben Rekaya M, Ben Hamda C, Mighri N, El Benna H, PEC Consortium, et al. Family specific genetic predisposition to breast cancer: results from Tunisian whole exome sequenced breast cancer cases. J Transl Med. 2018;16(1):158.
21. Ben Hadj M, Bouguerra H, Saffar F, Chelly S, Hechaichi A, Talmoudi K, Bahrini A, Chouki T, Hazgui O, Hannachi N, Letaief H, Bellali H, Bahri O, Ben-Alaya-Bouafif N. Observational study of vaccine effectiveness 20 years after the introduction of universal hepatitis B vaccination in Tunisia. Vaccine. 2018;36(39):5858–64.
22. El Mhamdi S, Sriha A, Bouanene I, Ben Salah A, Ben Salem K, Soussi-Soltani M. Predictors of smoking relapse in a cohort of adolescents and young adults in Monastir, Tunisia. Tob Induc Dis. 2013;11:12
23. WHO Tunisia Country Report. http://www.who.int/tobacco/surveillance/policy/country_profile/tun.pdf. Accessed on 18 Jan 2021.
24. Harizi C, El-Awa F, Ghedira H, Audera-Lopez C, Fakhfakh R. Implementation of the WHO framework convention on tobacco control in Tunisia: progress and challenges. Tob Prev Cessat. 2020;6:72.
25. Rosenblatt E, Fidarova E, Zubizarreta EH, Barton MB, Jones GW, Mackillop WJ, et al. Radiotherapy utilization in developing countries: an IAEA study. Radiother Oncol. 2018 Sep;128(3):400–5.
26. https://apps.who.int/gho/data/node.main.510. Accessed on 24 Jan 2021.
27. Letaief F, Khrouf S, Yahiaoui Y, Hamdi A, Gabsi A, Ayadi M, Mezlini A. Prognostic factors in high-grade localized osteosarcoma of the extremities: the Tunisian experience. J Orthop Surg (Hong Kong). 2020;28(3):2309499020974501.
28. Chatti I, Woillard JB, Mili A, Creveaux I, Ben Charfeddine I, Feki J, Langlais S, Ben Fatma L, Ali Saad A, Moez Gribaa M, Libert F. Genetic analysis of mu and kappa opioid receptor and COMT enzyme in cancer pain Tunisian patients under opioid treatment. Iran J Public Health. 2017;46(12):1704–11.
29. Mighri N, Hamdi Y, Boujemaa M, Othman H, Ben Nasr S, El Benna H, Mejri N, Labidi S, Ayari J, Jaidene O, Bouaziz H, Ben Rekaya M, M'rad R, Haddaoui A, Rahal K, Boussen H, Boubaker S, Abdelhak S. Identification of Novel BRCA1 and RAD50 mutations associated with breast cancer predisposition in Tunisian patients. Front Genet. 2020;11:552971.
30. Mahfoudh W, Bettaieb I, Ghedira R, Snoussi K, Bouzid N, Klayech Z, Gabbouj S, Remadi Y, Hassen E, Bouaouina N, Zakhama A. Contribution of BRCA1 5382insC mutation in triple negative breast cancer in Tunisia. J Transl Med. 2019;17(1):123.
31. https://fr.april-international.com/en/healthcare-travellers/healthcare-system-tunisia. Accessed on 26 Oct 2020.
32. Toumi A, Blel A, Aloui R, Zaibi H, Ksentinini M, Boudaya MS, et al. Assessment of EGFR mutation status in Tunisian patients with pulmonary adenocarcinoma. Curr Res Transl Med. 2018;66(3):65–70.
33. http://www.ineas.tn/fr/rapport-et-publication/le-depistage-du-cancer-du-sein. Accessed on 26 Oct 2020.
34. http://www.santetunisie.rns.tn/fr/prestations/tarifications-des-prestations-hospitalieres. Accessed on 26 Oct 2020.
35. http://www.dpm.tn/essai-clinique/liste-des-essais-cliniques. Consulted on 26 October 2020.

36. Boussen H, Cristofanilli M, Zaks T, De Silvio M, Salazar V, Spector N. Phase II study to evaluate the efficacy and safety of neoadjuvant lapatinib plus paclitaxel in patients with inflammatory breast cancer. J Clin Oncol. 2010;28(20):3248–55.
37. Frikha M, Auperin A, Tao Y, Elloumi F, Toumi N, Blanchard P, Lang P, Sun S, Racadot S, Thariat T, Alfonsi M, Tuchais C, Cornely A, Moussa A, Guigay J, Daoud J. A randomized trial of induction docetaxel-cisplatin-5FU followed by concomitant cisplatin-RT versus concomitant cisplatin-RT in nasopharyngeal carcinoma (GORTEC 2006-02). Ann Oncol. 2018;29(3):731–6.
38. Yang K, Sheng Y, Huang C, Jin Y, et al. Clinical characteristics, outcomes, and risk factors for mortality in patients with cancer and COVID-19 in Hubei, China: a multicentre, retrospective, cohort study. Lancet Oncol. 2020;21(7):904–13.
39. Belkacemi Y, Grellier N, Ghith S, Debbi K, Coraggio G, et al. A review of the international early recommendations for departments organization and cancer management priorities during the global COVID-19 pandemic: applicability in low- and middle-income countries. Eur J Cancer. 2020;135:130–46.
40. Manai M, Finetti P, Mejri N, Athimni S, Birnbaum D, Bertucci F, Boussen H. Inflammatory breast cancer in 210 patients: a retrospective study on epidemiological, anatomo-clinical features and therapeutic results. Mol Clin Oncol. 2018;2019(10):23–230.
41. Bendardaf R, Saheb-Sahrif FS, Saheb-Sharif N, Guraya SY, AlMadhi SA, Abusnana S. Incidence and clinicopathological features of breast cancer in the northern emirates: experience from Sharjah breast care center. Int J Womens Health. 2020;12:893–9.
42. Slaoui M, Azaque Zoure A, Mouh FZ, Bensouda Y, El Mzibri M, Bakri Y, Amran M. Outcome of inflammatory breast cancer in Moroccan patients: clinical, molecular and pathological characteristics of 219 cases from the National Oncology Institute (INO). BMC Cancer. 2018;18:713. https://doi.org/10.1186/s12885-018-4634-9.
43. Smaili F, Boudjella A, Dib A, Braikia S, Zidane H, Reggad R, et al. Epidemiology of breast cancer in women based on diagnosis data from oncologists and senologists in Algeria. Cancer Treat Res Commun. 2020;25:100220.
44. Chaher N, Arias-Pulido H, Terki N, Qualls C, Bouzid K, Verschraegen C, Wallace AM, Royce M. Molecular and epidemiological characteristics of inflammatory breast cancer in Algerian patients. Breast Cancer Res Treat. 2012;131(2):437–44.
45. Zeeneldin AA, Ramadan M, Elmashad N, Fakhr I, Diaa A, Mosaad E. Breast cancer laterality among Egyptian patients and its association with treatments and survival. J Egypt Natl Canc Inst. 2013;25(4):199–207.
46. Darwish AD, Helal AM, Aly El-din NH, Solaiman LL, Amin A. Breast cancer in women aging 35 years old and younger: the Egyptian National Cancer Institute (NCI) experience. Breast. 2017;31:1–8.
47. Mejri N, Berrazega Y, Boujnah R, Rachdi H, El Benna H, Labidi S, Boussen H. Assessing the financial toxicity in Tunisian cancer patients using the comprehensive score for financial toxicity (COST). Support Care Cancer. 2021; https://doi.org/10.1007/s00520-020-05944-6.

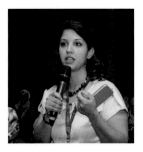

Nesrine Mejri is an assistant professor in medical oncology at the University Hospital, Abderrahmen Mami, Tunisia. She is affiliated with the University of medicine, University Tunis El Manar, Tunisia. Dr. Nesrine Mejri participated in several research projects on breast cancer in collaboration with Institute Pasteur Tunisia and co-authored several research articles on inflammatory breast cancer and genetic alterations of breast cancer. She was a member of the working group that elaborated "Tunisia guidelines of breast cancer individual screening" and is a previous member of the Tunisian Society of Medical Oncology.

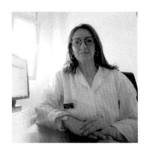

Haifa Rachdi is an assistant professor in medical oncology at the University Hospital, Abderrahmen Mami, Tunisia. She is affiliated with the University of medicine, University Tunis El Manar, Tunisia. She was a member of the working group that elaborated "Tunisian guidelines of medical oncology" 2020–2021 and is actually the vice president of the Tunisian Society of Medical Oncology. Dr. Haifa Rachdi is actually participating in several research projects on breast cancer in collaboration with the Institute Pasteur Tunisia, especially BRCA mutation.

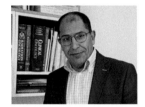

Lotfi Kochbati is a professor in Radiation Oncology at the El Manar University, School of Medicine, Tunis, Tunisia. He is the Head of the Radiotherapy Department, Abderrahmen Mami teaching Hospital, Ariana Tunisia. He is currently the President of the Tunisian Society of Radiation Oncology and the Immediate Past President of the African Radiation Oncology Group (AFROG). Dr. Kochbati is the Project Scientific Consultant for the AFRA/IAEA program and a Course Director of many Regional Training courses on pediatric and GU cancers. He is also the author and co-author of many articles in peer-review journals and chapters in Oncology manuals.

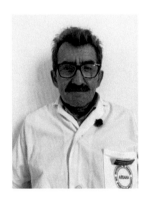

Hamouda Boussen is an MD from the faculty of medicine of Tunis, Training in Tunisia (Salah Azaiez Institute) and Institut Gustave Roussy, Villejuif, France in pediatric and adult medical oncology. He is a professor in medical oncology and the Head of the Department of medical oncology, University Hospital Abderrahman Mami, Ariana, Tunis, Tunisia. Dr. Boussen also served as the president of the Tunisian Society of medical oncology (ST0M) and currently is the president of Association de Formation et de Sensibilisation à l'Oncologie Multidiscciplinaire de l'Ariana. Board member of AROME (Association de recherche en oncologie de la Méditerranée) and IBC (Inflammatory Breast Cancer Consortium). He is an ESMO and ASCO member. He has 216 indexed publications, peer review for Bulletin du Cancer, Clinical Care Reports, Radiotherapy Oncology, Ther Adv Oncol, Oncotarget.

Chapter 19
General Oncology Care in the UAE

Ibrahim H. Abu-Gheida, Neil Nijhawan, Aydah Al-Awadhi ⓘ**,
and Humaid O. Al-Shamsi** ⓘ

19.1 Demographics

Located in the Southeast of the Arabian Peninsula, The United Arab Emirates
(UAE) is a member of the Gulf Cooperation Council (GCC) in the Arab world.
Established in 1971, the UAE is a comparably young country yet with abundant
development potential. The UAE has a well-established distinct presence at the
regional and international stages. Seven Emirates constitute the UAE including,
Dubai, Sharjah, Ajman, Fujairah, Ras-Al-Khaimah, Umm Al-Quwain, and the capital: Abu Dhabi. Over the past two decades, the UAE's population has surged at

I. H. Abu-Gheida
Emirates Oncology Society, Dubai, United Arab Emirates

Burjeel Medical City, Abu Dhabi, United Arab Emirates

College of Medicine and Health Sciences, United Arab Emirates University,
Abu Dhabi, United Arab Emirates

N. Nijhawan
Emirates Oncology Society, Dubai, United Arab Emirates

Burjeel Medical City, Abu Dhabi, United Arab Emirates
e-mail: neil.nijhawan@burjeelmedicalcity.com

A. Al-Awadhi
Emirates Oncology Society, Dubai, United Arab Emirates

H. O. Al-Shamsi (✉)
Emirates Oncology Society, Dubai, United Arab Emirates

Burjeel Medical City, Abu Dhabi, United Arab Emirates

University of Sharjah, Sharjah, United Arab Emirates
e-mail: humaid.al-shamsi@medportal.ca

almost triple the rate (www.worldpopulationreview.com). The estimate of the current population is around 10 million. Most of the country's population consists of expatriates. Most of them are South Asians that make up 58% of expatriates in the UAE.

The UAE has the third and fifth largest conventional oil and natural gas reserves, respectively, in the world. In 2015, the Gross Domestic Product (GDP) per capita was ranked at 95th percentile, globally. This makes the UAE a famous destination for employment opportunities and hence, the country has a relatively young population and a median age of 30.3 years. Moreover, male/female ratio remains high reaching 2.2 and 2.75 for the 15–65 age groups [1].

19.2 Cancer Statistics in the UAE

In 2002, the first official cancer incidence report was published [2] and the regional GCC cancer registry incorporated this report [3]. The central cancer registry was launched by the Department of Health, Abu Dhabi in 2012. One Thousand seven hundred twenty-nine new cancer cases were reported in the first published comprehensive cancer incidence report in Abu Dhabi; of which, UAE citizens accounted for 28% and expatriates accounted for the remainder. Breast cancer in females and hematological malignancies in males were the most common cancers among them [4]. Although the Emirate of Dubai has various hospital-based tumor registries, the results of the combined tumor registry are yet to be released. A common tumor registry, established in 2014 by the government, has been shared by all private and public hospitals of the Northern Emirates. It is mandatory for these Emirates to register all cancer diagnosis in this registry [5]. An updated incidence report from the Department of Health in the Emirates of Abu Dhabi from 2016 is summarized in Table 19.1 [6].

Table 19.1 Cancer incidence in the Emirate of Abu Dhabi (2016) [6]

	Total	National	Expatriates
Breast	300	73	227
Thyroid gland	212	76	136
Colorectum	159	48	111
Leukemia	108	23	85
Prostate gland	86	28	58
Non-Hodgkin's lymphoma	80	19	61
Bronchus and lung	79	20	59
Uterus	59	16	43
Kidney and renal pelvis	57	15	42
Skin	50	6	44
Stomach	50	17	33
Liver	47	14	33

Table 19.1 (continued)

	Total	National	Expatriates
Cervix uteri	45	14	31
Brain and other CNS	41	12	29
Bladder	39	11	28
Pancreas	39	11	28
Hodgkin's lymphoma	34	16	18
Connective and soft tissue	27	5	22
Multiple myeloma	26	9	17
Unknown and ill-defined sites	24	11	13
Mouth	23	6	17
Ovary	23	6	17
Testis	23	1	22
Pharynx	22	4	18
Gall bladder and other unspecified parts of biliary tract	18	3	15
Larynx	17	4	13
Tongue	17	3	14
Bone and cartilage	12	1	11
Esophagus	10	2	8
Small intestine	7	3	4
Melanoma of skin	6	1	5
Retroperitoneum and peritoneum	6	1	5
Salivary gland	6		6
Parotid gland	5		5
Eye	4	1	3
Heart, mediastinum, and pleura (including mesothelioma)	3		3
Other and ill-defined digestive organs	3	2	1
Myelodysplastic syndrome	2	1	1
Other endocrine glands	2	1	1
Placenta	2	1	1
Vagina	2	1	1
Kaposi sarcoma	1		1
Lip	1		1
Nasal cavity, middle ear, accessory sinus	1	1	
Tonsil	1		1
Ureter	1		1

Source: Department of Health, Abu Dhabi, UAE

The UAE cabinet has established a comprehensive population-based registry, the UAE National Cancer Registry (UAE-NCR). This registry is used for collecting, storing, summarizing, and analysis of information on patients who are diagnosed and/or treated for cancer within the UAE. Data is consolidated from all relevant entities including Department of Health Registry Abu Dhabi, Dubai Health Authority Cancer Registry, Northern Emirates Registries, all public and private based hospitals record on malignancies that were certified by medical professionals, pathology laboratories' reports, and mortality data. This data is utilized for guiding cancer care services plans, oncology research programs, future developments, and advancing screening programs. Annually, a report is published on the data collected on malignant neoplasms by this registry according to international standards.

The UAE-NCR's recent data (for the year January 1–December 31, 2017) [7] indicates a total of 4299 newly diagnosed cancer cases in the country. Malignant cancer accounted for 4123 (95.91%), while in situ cancer accounted for 176 (4.09%) cases. Out of the total newly diagnosed cancer cases (4299), just over a quarter 1160 (26.9%) were diagnosed among UAE citizens, while 3149 cases were diagnosed in non-UAE citizens. More females 2370 (55.1%) were affected than males 1929 (44.9%) and the overall crude incidence rate of cancer was 46.2/100,000 for both genders. According to the cancer mortality data, there were a total of 955 deaths from cancer (517 in males and 438 in females), which accounted for 10.82% of all deaths regardless of nationality, type of cancer, or gender.

Table 19.2 has illustrated the summary of demographics and most common cancer types among the UAE population from 2017 data [7]. By 2040, the number of new cancer cases is anticipated to increase in the UAE. This highlights the important role of government-established national cancer registries to meet the demand for this projected increase in cancer cases [9].

Table 19.2 Cancer Prevalence in the UAE (2017) stratified by site, gender, and citizenship status [8]

Primary site ICD-10	Non-UAE citizens			UAE citizens			Grand total
	Female	Male	Total	Female	Male	Total	
(C00-C96) All invasive cancers (malignant cases)	1570	1448	3018	680	425	1105	4123
C00-C14 Lip, oral cavity, and pharynx	24	96	120	15	16	31	151
C16 Esophagus	4	14	18	6	6	12	30
C16 Stomach	17	51	68	19	8	27	95
C17 Small intestine	6	12	18	3	1	4	22
C18-C21 Colorectal	108	197	305	58	59	117	422
C22 Liver and intrahepatic bile ducts	17	27	44	8	20	28	72
C23-C24 Gallbladder, other, and unspecified part of biliary tract	7	17	24	4	3	7	31
C25 Pancreas	15	30	45	11	13	24	69
C30, C31 Nasal cavity, middle ear, accessory sinuses	2	6	8	2	0	2	10
C32 Larynx	2	11	13	0	7	7	20
C34 Bronchus and lung	30	70	100	7	33	40	140
C40-C41 Bone and articular cartilage	7	12	19	5	2	7	26
C43 Skin melanoma	9	15	24	0	2	2	26
C44 Skin	55	119	174	19	15	34	208
C45 Mesothelioma	0	2	2	0	1	1	3
C45 Kaposi sarcoma	0	2	2	0	2	2	4
C48 Retroperitoneum and peritoneum	5	8	13	2	4	6	19

Table 19.2   (continued)

Primary site ICD-10	Non-UAE citizens			UAE citizens			Grand total
	Female	Male	Total	Female	Male	Total	
C49 Connective and soft tissue	17	29	46	4	8	12	58
C50 Breast	609	8	617	216	1	217	834
C53 Cervix uteri	66	0	66	16	0	16	82
C54-C55 Uterus	63	0	63	48	0	48	111
C56 Ovary	55	0	55	15	0	15	70
C61 Prostate	0	109	109	0	46	46	155
C62 Testis	0	35	35	0	8	8	43
C64-C65 Kidney and renal pelvis	21	40	61	8	15	23	84
C66, C68 Ureter and other urinary organs	0	6	6	0	1	1	7
C67 Urinary bladder	10	68	78	11	23	34	112
C63 Eye	0	2	2	2	0	2	4
C70-C72 Brain and CNS	23	44	67	5	4	9	76
C73 Thyroid	203	86	289	99	24	123	412
C74-C75 Other endocrine glands	3	5	8	1	1	2	10
C80 Unknown primary site	25	23	48	6	8	14	62
C81 Hodgkin's lymphoma	23	29	52	9	14	23	75
C82-C85, C96 Non-Hodgkin lymphoma	42	84	126	23	23	46	172
C88, C90 Multiple myeloma	10	25	35	4	11	15	50
C91-C95 Leukemia	71	152	223	47	44	91	314
Other malignancy	21	14	35	7	2	9	44
(D00-D09) Non-invasive cancers (in situ cases)	91	40	131	29	16	45	176
D00 Carcinoma in situ of oral cavity, esophagus, and stomach	0	1	1	0	0	0	1
D01 Carcinoma in situ of other and unspecified digestive organs	1	3	4	2	0	2	6
D02 Carcinoma in situ of middle ear and respiratory system	0	2	2	0	1	1	3
D03 Melanoma in situ	8	10	18	1	2	3	21
D04 Carcinoma in situ of skin	4	2	6	1	0	1	7
D05 Carcinoma in situ of breast	43	1	44	14	0	14	58
D06 Carcinoma in situ of cervix uteri	29	0	29	9	0	9	38
D07 Carcinoma in situ of other and unspecified genital organs	1	0	1	0	0	0	1
D09 Carcinoma in situ of other and unspecified sites	5	21	26	2	13	15	41
Grand total	1661	1488	3149	709	441	1150	4299

Source: Ministry of Health and Prevention, Statistics and Research Center, National Disease Registry—UAE National Cancer Registry Report 2017

19.3   Healthcare System in UAE

The UAE's healthcare system has been ranked 27th worldwide by the World Health Organization (WHO) due to its rapid growth and development [10]. Sincere efforts made by the government to provide full coverage for its citizens, along with mandating health insurance for expatriates along with their families. Moreover, direct payment to health care facilities by patients can be made to any service they receive. Finally, several charities are active in aiding UAE residents for expensive oncology treatments if diagnosed with cancer.

Within the UAE, there are several health governing organizations closely working together in harmony to ensure a smooth and well-being of the residents. The Ministry of Health and Prevention (MOHAP) is the prime federal regulatory health authority for the whole UAE healthcare system working closely with the Department of Health in Abu Dhabi, the Dubai Health Authority, and the Sharjah Health Authority.

Despite the relatively young average age within the UAE residents, cancer is the third leading cause of death in the UAE after accidents/injuries and cardiovascular disease. Data reported from the UAE capital, Emirates of Abu Dhabi shows that 16% of mortality is cancer related in the Emirates [11]. A national agenda by the UAE federal government has initiated plans to reduce the tally of cancer-related deaths [12].

19.4   UAE Oncology Care

The first published document of oncology care from the UAE dates back to 1981 addressing five cases of hepatocellular carcinoma [13]. The first and largest cancer care facility was established in one of Abu Dhabi's main cities, Al-Ain. Established in 1979, the first hospital to deliver comprehensive cancer care services in the UAE was Tawam Hospital. By 1983, Tawam Hospital was designated as UAE's cancer referral hospital [14]. In order to allow cancer patients to reach closer-to-home health care facilities, several general oncology care services began across the country. Until 2007, the entire oncology treatment cost was covered by the UAE government for all UAE citizens and residents living in the country. The UAE government continues to cover the cost of cancer treatment for all UAE citizens. While noncitizens, as previously mentioned, are covered by insurance plans. Sometimes, expatriates are forced to leave for their home countries to continue medical treatment due to insurance plans that are subject to expiration dates. This scenario has led to a recent collaborative publication from the prestigious Emirates Oncology Society (EOS), providing alternative solutions for adjustments in cancer insurance packages across the country [15].

Due to the involvement of high capital expenditure, oncology care in the private healthcare sector is uncommon. A very successful model has been shown in the

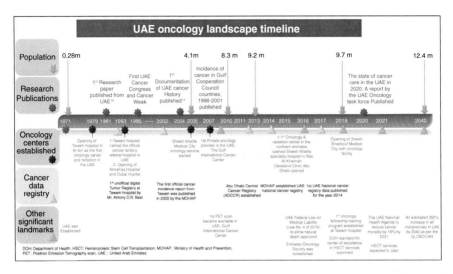

Fig. 19.1 Progress of oncology in the United Arab Emirates [15]. Used with permission from Gulf Journal of Oncology

UAE by integrating the public and private sectors for oncology services. Many hospitals and healthcare entities are now adapting to this model. Moreover, basic and comprehensive cancer care services are now available in private hospitals. Figure 19.1 shows the timeline summarizing the stages of oncology development in the UAE.

19.5   Cancer Risk Factors

There are several identified modifiable risk factors for cancers. For example, obesity is well known to be related to several types of cancer such as colorectal, esophageal, breast, etc. [16]. The UAE has a comparable obesity rate with the USA [3]. Moreover, the UAE has a high childhood obesity rate, which usually transcribes into an estimated high obesity rate [17].

Another risk factor for cancers is smoking [18]. The gender-wise distribution of UAE smokers is estimated to be 0.8% females and 24.3% males [18]. A variety of ways have been offered in different parts of the world for inhaling smoke, yet cigarette smoking (77.4%) remains the prevalent form of smoking in the UAE, following that midwakh, shisha, and cigars [18, 19]. Seven percent and 3 percent of males and females are reported to smoke Shisha/Hubble Bubble or Hookah. Having a significant carcinogenic effect, one Shisha consumption has been estimated to be comparable to 100 cigarettes consumption [20]. A midwakh has an Arabian origin, it is a small pipe in which aromatic leaf and bark herbs are mixed with dokha and smoked [21]. The traditional western tobacco pipe has a larger bowl than midwakh pipe, which is usually smaller. A bowl is dipped into dokha flakes container for loading purpose [22]. Iran and the UAE are the primary producers of Midwakh. Dokha has the same effects as other forms of smoking, i.e., acute effects on blood pressure and respiratory rates. However, given the use of tobacco mixture, it is suspected to contain a significantly high content of carcinogen [18].

19.6   Cancer Screening Programs

The UAE leadership has led the efforts in establishing solid cancer screening programs. In 2009, a screening program was started which advised all UAE national women aged 40 years and above to undergo annual mammography screening. Subsequently, in July 2010, a nationwide colorectal cancer screening program was launched, by 2014, three screening programs were established for breast, colorectal, and cervical cancers [23]. Finally, and after the release of lung cancer data in 2017, lung cancer screening with low dose CT scans was implemented [8]. Moreover, various initiatives for cancer screening and awareness have been made, such as the "Pink Caravan" event. This awareness campaign used to raise breast cancer awareness and encourage screening, now occurs on an annual basis, and reaches more than 45,000 women annually across the UAE [24].

19.7   Cancer Prevention Programs

As previously mentioned, cancer incidence has been related to several risk factors that can be modified on a nationwide scale. The UAE has increased awareness of obesity linked to malignancies, also fighting childhood and adult obesity [25]. The government has taken an initiative related to this and in December 2019, increased the tax on sweetened beverages [26]. Other preventive measures are also in effect, such as the offering of counseling services and programs and implementation of healthy lifestyles in the UAE.

Smoking cessation programs have also been established on a nationwide scale. In the UAE, the prohibition of smoking in indoor public spaces and an increased tax on all tobacco products have been implemented [27]. As early as 2014, the government has banned all advertisements for tobacco products, all cigarette packages have mandated warning labels, and lastly, the restriction to selling any tobacco products to an individual who is less than 18 years of age. Moreover, the government also introduced a law that bans smoking inside personal vehicles in the presence of a child who is less than 12 years of age [28]. In public areas of some Emirates, smoking shisha is banned [29].

Another very important step in the cancer prevention programs includes the vaccination efforts. The UAE leadership has also led the efforts in promoting vaccination for cancer prevention. As in 1991, the hepatitis B vaccine was mandated [30], in large part because hepatocellular carcinoma is linked with hepatitis B virus infection [31]. Moreover, the government has now started screening hepatitis B and C for all new immigrants in the UAE, also analyzing hepatitis B immunity and vaccination profiles from 2006 [32]. Moreover, since 2008, all public and private schools have been provided with an optional Human Papillomavirus (HPV) vaccination for girls aged 11–12 years. The vaccine is strongly associated with a decline in cancer rate [33]. More efforts are being made by educating the public on HPV vaccinations for cancers like cervical and head and neck in the UAE, in part because HPV vaccinations might have few misconceptions [34].

19.8   Cancer Diagnosis

19.8.1   Cytogenetics and Molecular Genetics

A fundamental part in cancer diagnosis and follow-up response assessment is liquid biopsy for assessing serum circulating tumor DNA (ct-DNA) components [35]. A momentum has gained in the UAE by access to specialized laboratories which are equipped for either ct-DNA or molecular testing on cancer specimens. This will determine the most suitable target for therapy in the near and distant future, consequently individualized cancer treatment will be given. All practicing oncologists in the UAE can access different types of molecular and genetic testing summarized by the recently established Emirates Oncology Society. They are currently available at www.eos.ae.

19.9   Treatment

19.9.1   Oncology Physicians

The UAE cancer-treating physicians are active, coming from different backgrounds of training and expertise and are working in an effective and efficient harmony in order to provide the best care available for patients. In the currently available published databases, The Department of Health, Abu Dhabi has 34 registered medical and radiation oncologists, Dubai Health Authority has 26 and the Northern Emirates has six, hence a total of 66 oncologists are registered within the UAE [36]. However, there has been a significant influx of talent and highly specialized physicians in multiple aspects, including oncology care into the UAE allowing more expertise and knowledge sharing among rapidly growing oncology societies such as the Emirates Oncology Society.

19.9.2   Specialized Oncology Services

19.9.2.1   Advanced Treatments

The UAE health care authorities have facilitated adequate access to all approved medications, including the new and novel drugs for the treatment of cancer. These medications are usually made available to patients as they have passed rigorous assessment and approved by the Food and Drug Administration (FDA). The UAE implements very strict packaging and storing guidelines to ensure safety of those medications along with best practice to ensure safe delivery of those. The hospitals normally request it directly from the pharmaceutical companies that supply certain drugs, and the drug costs are covered if indicated. As a suggestion by the EOS consensus group, bulk ordering of medications through the government rather than directly by hospitals is an approach to reducing the cost of such drugs [15].

19.9.2.2   Stem Cell Transplantation

Up until recently, adult and pediatric patients from the UAE had to travel abroad to receive Hematopoietic Stem Cell Transplant (HSCT), putting a significant distress and expenditure on the patients, their families, and to the healthcare authorities. However, very successful recent developments have been happening in this field, including the first successful bone marrow transplant (BMT) by Abu Dhabi Stem Cell transplant cell, operated by the government, and the opening of the bone marrow transplant unit in Burjeel Medical City in Abu Dhabi as well. Further optimistic and more bone marrow programs are being launched within the UAE to cover all aspects of HSCT and advanced CAR-T cell therapy.

19.9.3   Radiation Oncology

Radiation Oncology/or Radiation Therapy is also becoming more available and accessible to patients within the UAE and international patients travel to the UAE for their treatment. Despite its significant expense, complexity and high caliber and unique training required, the UAE has had a very successful start and growth of radiotherapy departments offering the most complex and comprehensive form of treatments. Tawam Hospital had the first radiotherapy department in Abu Dhabi. Currently, there are three operational radiotherapy departments in Abu Dhabi, three in Dubai, one in Ras-Al Khaimah (Northern Emirates). Several new private and government hospitals have announced the plans to start radiotherapy departments, allowing patients for adequate access to high-quality well-maintained radiotherapy departments for both local UAE residents and international patients flying from abroad to receive radiotherapy in the UAE [15].

19.9.4 Pediatric Oncology

Pediatric hematology and oncology cases are in the expected range, despite the UAE consisting of a mostly young population. According to 2015 data, a total of 165 children, aged 0–14 years, were diagnosed with cancer. The public and private healthcare sectors of the UAE have many pediatric oncology centers. Such entities have an appropriate number of nursing staff, pediatric oncologists, therapists, and radiation therapy facilities. However, the lack of HSCT centers remains the most significant limitation of pediatric oncology in the UAE. Many established cancer centers and facilities are trying to address this concern [15].

19.9.5 Palliative Care Track

A strong call to promote palliative and support care in the UAE has been urged since early access to palliative care can improve the patients' outcomes and quality of life [37]. Tawam Hospital as well as other private oncology providers in the UAE has a dedicated palliative care service. The palliative care medications that are frequently used are available in the country. The UAE Federal Law No. 4 on Medical Liability [38] has validated the permissibility of natural death of terminally ill patients since 2016. This new law refrains healthcare professionals from performing cardiopulmonary resuscitation (CPR) and allowing natural death of terminally ill or dying patients who are suffering from incurable illnesses, provided the following conditions are met:

- Irremediable condition of the patient
- Exhaustion of all treatment methods
- A medical condition where the treatment has proven to be useless
- The provision of CPR has been refrained to the patient on the advice of treating doctor; and
- Three consulting doctors, at minimum, decide that natural death is allowed as per requirement of patients' interest, and that CPR should be avoided. (In this case, the patients', his guardian/custodians' consent is not required.)

In the National Cancer Control Plan, multiple locations in the UAE should establish a national palliative and supportive care program, as recommended by EOS [15].

19.10   Research and Education

19.10.1   Research

UAE oncology societies have research activities too. Recent publications led by UAE investigators are appearing in premiere medical journals, despite comparable limited research capacity [39–41]. UAE population specific research should be evaluated in the light of distinct epigenetic and biological variables in the UAE, which are most likely to be contrasted in other societies. The earlier onset of breast cancer in the UAE compared with Western countries is an example of this phenomenon [42]. Hence, Western based treatment protocols might have to be altered according to the unique patient population in the UAE.

19.10.2   Education and Training

The UAE has increased the number of dedicated oncology training programs in the country. Tawam Hospital has launched a first medical oncology fellowship program, in November 2019. Other public and private hospitals also have few oncology training programs. As the scope of medical practice increases, the UAE has planned for more advanced training programs, empowering medical professionals from the region to train and practice in the UAE [15].

19.11   Cost-Effective Cancer Care

Individuals and the government are always burdened by the cost of cancer care services. The anticipation of an increase in cancer cases poses a special challenge in the UAE to requiring diagnostic and treatment services. Cancer has become a chronic disease, leading to the advancements in cancer therapy (new and costly drugs such as immunotherapies). EOS has recently tried to address the cost issue by suggesting the bulk purchase of drugs from pharmaceutical companies rather than individual purchase by hospitals or institutions [15].

Another way of improving efficiency and reducing cost on the health care system would be to adopt more innovative models for reimbursement; for example, a "per-site" rather than a "per-fraction" radiation model [43]. This means more cost-effective cancer treatment, and reducing the number of treatments, hence patients and their caregivers, who often accompany their patients, can have a reduced number of potential days off to the radiotherapy facilities.

Guidelines relating to the utilization of cutting-edge imaging modalities, for example, Positron Emission Tomography (PET/CT) scans have been carried out and this has diminished the follow-up expenses that oncology patients often need.

Additionally, unimportant X-ray or CT scans have likewise been controlled to prevent unnecessary and potentially hazardous scans for the patient [44].

Finally, and probably most importantly, screening and early detection of common cancers is crucial. Nationwide cancer screening programs have been implemented by the UAE health authorities. However, such screening programs still have a low compliance rate. Despite this, the number of patients diagnosed with advanced, stage IV breast cancer has been significantly reduced from 20% to 6%.

19.12 Challenges and Advantages

19.12.1 Medical Tourism in the UAE

The process of traveling internationally outside the resident's country aimed at receiving medical care is termed as "Medical Tourism" [45]. The UAE government has financially supported a significant number of patients who seek cancer treatment abroad [46]. Every case is assessed at the individual level, and a decision to provide medical treatment abroad is made. The UAE official health authorities, Armed Forces, Presidential Affairs, Police, and charitable organizations are a few sponsoring agencies. Moreover, patients can also pay directly through self-payment mode. The highest percentage of medical tourism undertaken by UAE citizens is attributed to oncology and orthopedic surgery, while cancer treatment comprises the highest number of trips and expenditure (Salim et al., 2008). USA, South Korea, Germany, Singapore, and Thailand are some treatment destinations for cancer patients [47].

However, on the opposite hand, there has been a recent other-way-around medical tourism. That is, patients from abroad are coming to the UAE to seek medical support. This has been mostly related to the recent government led and supported state-of-the-art health care facilities, along with leading private sector health care providers attracting international talent to come and practice in the UAE.

19.13 The Future of Cancer Care in the UAE

Since the UAE is moving towards improved cancer care services, the alliance of the public and private sector has led to the establishment of organizations such as Emirates Oncology Society (EOS), with the purpose to regularize oncology care services in the UAE [15]. The UAE has almost all cancer modalities and therapies available, yet the government continues to support those who need and seek treatment abroad. Cancer patients have continuous support from the UAE government within the UAE. Patients have been advised by the Federal Cancer Care Agency on cancer care. Additionally, an important role is being played by the Federal National

Cancer Registry to plan oncology care across the country and designate population need based resources.

The UAE Oncology Society established the cancer system quality index. This will administer various variables to measure the quality of cancer care including waiting times from diagnosis to treatment, chemotherapy utilization, radiation treatment timelines and treatment delivery, monitoring of complications related to chemotherapy, radiotherapy, and surgery. The Quality Measurement Advisory Council in Ontario (Canada) has created this model to establish an independent advisory cancer care quality council that aims to standardize and unifies treatments of oncology patients [48, 49]. The UAE has adapted the same model. However, it is critical for UAE cancer care entities to collaboratively work with leading oncology institutions to monitor outcomes regularly.

The UAE has announced various public and private new cancer care tertiary centers. Such hospitals commonly cooperate with other world-leading oncology care facilities, for instance, the collaboration between the Mayo Clinic and Sheikh Shakhbout Medical City, or Johns Hopkins Hospital collaboration with Tawam Hospital, Burjeel Medical City along with its 2021 European Society of Medical Oncology (ESMO) accreditation and so on. The increased number of highly trained physicians in the UAE is the result of such collaborative efforts, offering complex as well as comprehensive cancer treatment services. Although Tawam Hospital remains the prime comprehensive cancer care facility in the UAE, its location, which is at the far east end of the country, makes the conveyance to and from the facility extra challenging. Therefore, comprehensive cancer care facilities elsewhere that are more accessible to patients in the UAE can help cancer care facilities to grow.

As the economy and population of the UAE is growing, the number of cancer patients is also increasing, regardless of the relatively small population. This predicts an increase in the number of cancer patients that will have better clinical outcomes, if treated in specialized cancer care facilities [50]. The best solution has been presented by EOS to equip the cancer care facilities with multiple satellites for a centralized cancer care with approachable clinics across the country [15].

Nationwide establishment of the cancer electronic health record system is another useful recommendation by EOS [15]. Oncologists can request all the genetic workup platforms, which are currently available at the website (www.eos.ae). Such platforms can be utilized in Unified treatment protocols with various institutions and the establishment of a national ordering system for chemotherapy/immunotherapy, aiming to optimize resource allocation in the UAE in the future.

Finally, a multidisciplinary approach is involved in cancer care, hence a centralized virtual multidisciplinary tumor board across the UAE governing different health facilities can be a good resource to take cancer care forward. The diagnosis and management of newly diagnosed cancer cases is guided by this group in the UAE.

19.14   Conclusion

Despite a comparatively young population, the healthcare system of the United Arab Emirates is one of the leading health systems in the world. Various public and private healthcare facilities are providing comprehensive cancer care services. Developmental programs are planned to make the UAE a central part of inflowing medical tourism soon. Complex cancer care in the UAE has improved due to highly trained healthcare providers, in addition with governmental funding and logistic support. More advancements are required to enhance collaborative efforts with other cancer centers at national and international level including those in the Arab world.

Conflict of Interest Authors have no conflict of interest to declare.

References

1. https://worldpopulationreview.com/countries/united-arab-emirates-population/. Accessed 1 July 2020.
2. UAE Ministry of Health. Cancer Incidence Report: UAE (1998–2002). Abu Dhabi: UAE Ministry of Health. Cancer Incidence Report: UAE (1998–2002). Abu Dhabi, 2002.
3. Al-Hamdan N, Ravichandran K, Al-Sayyad J, Al-Lawati J, Khazal Z, Al-Khateeb F, Abdulwahab A, Al-Asfour A. Incidence of cancer in Gulf Cooperation Council countries, 1998-2001. East Mediterr Health J. 2009;15(3):600–11.
4. Health Statistics 2012, Department of Health Abu Dhabi. https://www.scad.ae/Release%20 Documents/Health%202012%20English.pdf. Accessed 1 July 2020.
5. MCCR-01-344 Cancer Notification Policy—United Arab Emirates Ministry of Health Central Cancer Registry (MCCR) June 2014, https://www.mohap.gov.ae/en/OpenData/Pages/default. aspx. Accessed 1 July 2020.
6. Workbook: non-communicable diseases. Cancer Incidence 2016. Department of Health. https://tableau.doh.gov.ae/views/NonCommunicableDiseases/CancerIncidence?%3AisGuest RedirectFromVizportal=y&%3Aembed=y&%3Atoolbar=no. Accessed 7 Aug 2021.
7. https://www.mohap.gov.ae/Files/MOH_OpenData/1585/CANCER%20INCIDENCE%20 IN%20UNITED%20ARAB%20EMIRATES%20ANNUAL%20REPORT%20OF%20 THE%20UAE%20-%20NATIONAL%20CANCER%20REGISTRY%20-%202017.pdf
8. Department of Health Abu Dhabi. https://www.haad.ae/simplycheck/tabid/112/Default.aspx. Accessed 1 July 2020.
9. GLOBOCAN database (September 2018)—https://gco.iarc.fr/today/home a--: GLOBOCAN database (September 2018)—https://gco.iarc.fr/today/home. Accessed 1 July 2020.
10. Blair I, Sharif A. Health and health systems performance in the United Arab Emirates. World Hosp Health Serv. 2013;49(4):12–7.
11. Health Statistics 2011, Health Authority Abu Dhabi. https://www.haad.ae/HAAD/LinkClick. aspx?fileticket=clGoRRszqc. Accessed 1 July 2020.
12. The Official Portal of the UAE Government, Cancer. https://government.ae/en/information- and-services/healthand-fitness/special-health-issues/cancer. Accessed 1 July 2020.

13. Tadmouri GO, Al-Sharhan M. Cancers in the United Arab Emirates, genetic disorders in the Arab World, p. 59–61.
14. https://gulfnews.com/uae/health/741-bed-hospital-toopen-in-abu-dhabi-1.66698698. Accessed 1 July 2020.
15. Al-Shamsi H, Darr H, Abu-Gheida I, Ansari J, McManus MC, Jaafar H, Tirmazy SH, Elkhoury M, Azribi F, Jelovac D, et al. The state of cancer Care in the United Arab Emirates in 2020: challenges and recommendations, a report by the United Arab Emirates oncology task force. Gulf J Oncolog. 2020;1(32):71–87.
16. Wolin KY, Carson K, Colditz GA. Obesity and cancer. Oncologist. 2010;15(6):556–65.
17. Al Junaibi A, Abdulle A, Sabri S, Hag-Ali M, Nagelkerke N. The prevalence and potential determinants of obesity among school children and adolescents in Abu Dhabi, United Arab Emirates. Int J Obes (Lond). 2013;37(1):68–74.
18. Al-Houqani M, Ali R, Hajat C. Tobacco smoking using Midwakh is an emerging health problem—evidence from a large cross-sectional survey in the United Arab Emirates. PLoS One. 2012;7(6):e39189.
19. Aden B, Karrar S, Shafey O, Al Hosni F. Cigarette, water-pipe, and Medwakh smoking prevalence among applicants to Abu Dhabi's pre-marital screening program, 2011. Int J Prev Med. 2013;4(11):1290–5.
20. British Heart Foundation, Shisha. https://www.bhf.org.uk/heart-health/risk-factors/smoking/shisha. Accessed 1 July 2020.
21. Vupputuri S, Hajat C, Al-Houqani M, Osman O, Sreedharan J, Ali R, Crookes AE, Zhou S, Sherman SE, Weitzman M, et al. Midwakh/dokha tobacco use in the Middle East: much to learn. Tob Control. 2016;25(2):236–41.
22. Jayakumary M, Jayadevan S, Ranade AV, Mathew E. Prevalence and pattern of Dokha use among medical and allied health students in Ajman, United Arab Emirates. Asian Pac J Cancer Prev. 2010;11(6):1547–9.
23. The Dubai Health Authority (DHA). https://www.dha.gov.ae/en/Pages/AboutUs.aspx. Accessed 1 July 2020.
24. The U.A.E. Healthcare Sector: An Update, U.S.-U.A.E. Business Council. http://usuaebusiness.org/wp-content/uploads/2017/05/Healthcare-Report-Final-1.pdf. Accessed 1 July 2020.
25. Malik M, Bakir A. Prevalence of overweight and obesity among children in the United Arab Emirates. Obes Rev. 2007;8(1):15–20.
26. https://gulfnews.com/uae/from-december-1-payextra-for-sweetened-drinks-juices-1.1575109321210. Accessed 1 July 2020.
27. Gulf News hgcuf-d--d-t-b-c-a-e-t-o-i-cs-i-u-A--: Gulf News, https://gulfnews.com/uae/from-december-1-dh040-to-be-charged-asexcise-tax-on-individual-cigarettes-sold-in-uae-1.1571744782489. Accessed 1 July 2020.
28. UAE Anti-tobacco Law in effect: rules and fines. http://www.emirates247.com/news/emirates/uae-anti-tobaccolaw-in-effect-rules-and-fines-2014-01-21-1.535551. 2014. Accessed 1 July 2020.
29. Shisha smoking will invite Dh500 fine in Sharjah. http://www.khaleejtimes.com/nation/sharjah/shisha-smokingwill-invite-dh500-fine-in-sharjah. Accessed 1 July 2020.
30. Four per cent rise in hepatitis B, C; http://www.khaleejtimes.com/nation/uae-health/four-per-centrise-in-hepatitis-b-c; 2012, Accessed 1 July 2020.
31. Xu C, Zhou W, Wang Y, Qiao L. Hepatitis B virus-induced hepatocellular carcinoma. Cancer Lett. 2014;345(2):216–22.

32. Screening for hepatitis for newly employed health care workers. https://www.haad.ae/haad/Portals/0/Policies_Docs/Screening-for-Hepatitis-for-newly-employed-Health-Care-Workers.pdf; 2006, Accessed 1 July 2020.
33. Immunization Guidelines—Dubai Health Authority. https://www.dha.gov.ae/Documents/HRD/Immunization%20Guidelines.pdf, Accessed 1 July 2020.
34. Elbarazi I, Raheel H, Cummings K, Loney T. A content analysis of Arabic and English newspapers before, during, and after the human papillomavirus vaccination campaign in the United Arab Emirates. Front Public Health. 2016;4:176.
35. Sokolenko AP, Imyanitov EN. Molecular diagnostics in clinical oncology. Front Mol Biosci. 2018;5:76.
36. Ministry of Health UAE Wide Physician Census 2016, 2016.
37. Ambroggi M, Biasini C, Toscani I, Orlandi E, Berte R, Mazzari M, Cavanna L. Can early palliative care with anticancer treatment improve overall survival and patient-related outcomes in advanced lung cancer patients? A review of the literature. Support Care Cancer. 2018;26(9):2945–53.
38. https://www.dha.gov.ae/Asset%20Library/MarketingAssets/20180611/(E)%20Federal%20Decree%20no.%204%20of%202016.pdf
39. Al-Shamsi HO, Alhazzani W, Alhuraiji A, Coomes EA, Chemaly RF, Almuhanna M, Wolff RA, Ibrahim NK, Chua MLK, Hotte SJ, et al. A practical approach to the management of cancer patients during the novel coronavirus disease 2019 (COVID-19) pandemic: an international collaborative group. Oncologist. 2020;25(6):e936–45.
40. Abu-Gheida I, Bathala TK, Maldonado JA, Khan M, Anscher MS, Frank SJ, Choi S, Nguyen QN, Hoffman KE, McGuire SE, et al. Increased frequency of mesorectal and perirectal LN involvement in T4 prostate cancers. Int J Radiat Oncol Biol Phys. 2020;107(5):982–5.
41. Al-Shamsi HO, Coomes EA, Alrawi S. Screening for COVID-19 in asymptomatic patients with cancer in a Hospital in the United Arab Emirates. JAMA Oncol. 2020;
42. Humaid O, Al S, Sadir A. Breast cancer screening in the United Arab Emirates: is it time to call for a screening at an earlier age? Open Acc J Oncol Med. 2018;2(1) https://doi.org/10.32474/OAJOM.2018.02.000131.
43. Proposed Radiation Oncology (RO) Model. https://www.cms.gov/newsroom/fact-sheets/proposed-radiation-oncology-ro-model. Accessed 1 July 2020.
44. Martinuk SD. The use of positron emission tomography (PET) for cancer care across Canada, Time for a National Strategy. https://www.triumf.ca/sites/default/files/TRIUMF-AAPS-Martinuk-PET-Across-Canada-REPORT.pdf. 2011. Accessed 1 July 2020.
45. Connell J. Contemporary medical tourism: conceptualisation, culture and commodification. Tour Manag. 2013;34:1–13. https://doi.org/10.1016/j.tourman.2012.05.009.
46. 600 million UAE Dirhams spent on cancer care medical tourism. 16 June 2014. http://www.alittihad.ae/details.php?id=90507&y=2014.
47. Sahoo S. Rising numbers in outbound medical tourism, http://www.thenational.ae/business/industry-insights/tourism/rising-numbers-in-outbound-medical-tourism.
48. Wild C, Patera N. Measuring quality in cancer care: overview of initiatives in selected countries. Eur J Cancer Care. 2013;22(6):773–81.
49. Anas R, Stiff J, Speller B, Foster N, Bell R, McLaughlin V, Evans WK. Raising the bar: using program evaluation for quality improvement. Healthc Manage Forum. 2013;26(4):191–5.
50. Pfister DG, Rubin DM, Elkin EB, Neill US, Duck E, Radzyner M, Bach PB. Risk adjusting survival outcomes in hospitals that treat patients with cancer without information on cancer stage. JAMA Oncol. 2015;1(9):1303–10.

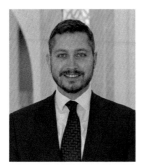

Ibrahim H. Abu-Gheida is the founding head of the Department of Radiation Oncology in Burjeel Medical City and an adjunct assistant professor at the United Arab Emirates University. Abu-Gheida completed his undergraduate training where he earned a Bachelor of Science with honors degree from the American University of Beirut. Following which Abu-Gheida completed his Medical School training at the American University of Beirut Medical Center. He continued and joined the Department of Internal Medicine at the American University of Beirut. Then did his training in the Department of Radiation Oncology at the American University of Beirut Medical Center, where he also served as the chief resident. During his training, Abu-Gheida completed a Harvard-affiliated NIH-funded research program as well. After his residency, Ibrahim went to the Cleveland Clinic/Ohio, where he was appointed as an Advanced Clinical Radiation Oncology Fellow. Abu-Gheida went and joined the University of Texas MD Anderson Cancer Center. Abu-Gheida has many publications in prestigious medical journals including the American Society of Radiation Oncology official journal—International Journal of Radiation Oncology Biology and Physics, Nature, Journal of Clinical Oncology, and several others. He is also the primary author of several book chapters published in prestigious books. He also has been granted research awards during his residency.

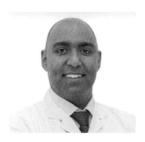

Neil Nijhawan is a UK-trained Consultant in Palliative Medicine working at Burjeel Medical City. After medical school at Kings College London, he pursued specialty training in Palliative Medicine in London and previously worked as a Consultant in Palliative Medicine at Imperial College Healthcare NHS Trust in London, where he was a Clinical Lead for palliative medicine. He has experience in all aspects of Palliative and Supportive Care and has worked in the UK, the West Indies, and the UAE. Nijhawan's ethos is to treat every patient like family and firmly believes that there is always something that we can do to help make people feel better.

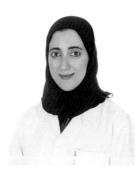

Aydah Al-Awadhi is a consultant medical oncologist, graduated medical school from the United Arab Emirates University in 2012, then completed her internal medicine residency in the United States and completed her Medical Oncology and Hematology fellowship from the University of Texas MD Anderson Cancer Center in 2019 and is American Board Certified in Hematology and Medical Oncology. She was awarded the Emirates Oncology Society (EOS) Member of the Year award, 2021. Al-Awadhi has published many articles and book chapters on breast cancer and oncology.

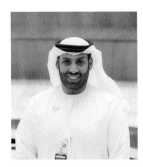

Humaid O. Al-Shamsi is the director of VPS oncology services in the United Arab Emirates which is the largest cancer care provider network in the UAE. He is also the President of the Emirates Oncology Society and an adjunct professor at the College of Medicine—University of Sharjah. Prof. Al-Shamsi holds triple specialty board certifications in medical oncology from the UK, the USA, and Canada. He completed his Bachelor of Science and Bachelor of Medicine from Cork University, the National University of Ireland with honors in 2005. He then completed his internal medicine residency followed by a medical oncology fellowship, he then completed a subspecialty combined fellowship in gastrointestinal and palliative oncology at McMaster University in Canada in 2013. He then joined MD Anderson Cancer Center, The University of Texas Houston, USA as an assistant professor from 2014 to 2017. Prof. Al-Shamsi is the founder of Burjeel Cancer Institute at Burjeel Medical City in Abu Dhabi, UAE which is the most comprehensive cancer center in the UAE. He has more than 70 peer reviewed articles and book chapters. His research focus is on precision medicine and health policies related to cancer care in the UAE and the Arab region. He was awarded the researcher of the year in 2020 and 2021 by the Emirates Oncology Society.

Chapter 20
General Oncology Care in the Republic of Yemen

Amen Bawazir, Huda Basaleem, Ahmed Badheeb, and Gamal Abdul Hamid

20.1 Yemen Demographics

The Republic of Yemen is situated at the southwestern corner of the Arabian Peninsula, at the entrance to the Bab-el-Mandeb Strait, which links the Red Sea to the Indian Ocean (via the Gulf of Aden) and is one of the most active and strategic shipping lanes in the world. Yemen is bordered by the North with Saudi Arabia and from the East by Oman and it occupies around 527,970 km^2 [1]. Administratively, 22 governorates were declared in the year 2014 [2]. The total population of Yemen is nearly 29,826,305 people (15,271,909 males and 14,973,391 females) at mid-year, and 61.6% of population residing in the rural area of the country [3–5] The population pyramid show a very young population, with a median age of 20.2 years and around 39.2% of the population were under 15 years of age, and only 2.6% are

A. Bawazir (✉)
Faculty of Medicine and Health Sciences, University of Aden, Aden, Yemen

College of Public Health and Health Informatics, King Saud Bin Abdulaziz University of Health Sciences, Riyadh, Saudi Arabia
e-mail: bawazira@ksau-hs.edu.sa

H. Basaleem
Department of Community Medicine and Public Health, Faculty of Medicine and Health Sciences, Aden Cancer Registry and Research Center, University of Aden, Aden, Yemen

A. Badheeb
Medicine and Medical Oncology, National Oncology Center (NOC), Hadhramout and Hadhramout Cancer Registry (HCR), Hadhramout University College of Medicine, Mukalla, Yemen

Oncology Center, King Khalid Hospital, Najran, Saudi Arabia

G. Abdul Hamid
Hematology and Laboratory Department, Faculty of Medicine and Health Sciences, University of Aden, Aden, Yemen

© The Author(s) 2022
H. O. Al-Shamsi et al. (eds.), *Cancer in the Arab World*,
https://doi.org/10.1007/978-981-16-7945-2_20

65 years [6]. According to the revised population estimates or the life expectancy at birth, both sexes combined for the Yemeni population rose from 58.2 years in the year 1990 to 66.4 in the year 2020 with around 4 years differences for the favor of females (64.7 years and 68.2 years, respectively) [3]. However, the projected data for the year 2030 showed a very slow increase in the life expectancy of the Yemeni population to only 67.8 years [7].

20.2 Cancer Statistics in Yemen

Accurate cancer incidence in Yemen is unknown due to many reasons, such as limited diagnostic and clinical resources, as well as the poor quality of medical records. Furthermore, ongoing civil conflict has recently contributed to the ambiguity of the burden of cancer at national level.

20.2.1 Current Status

According to the GLOBOCAN estimation of the overall Age-Standardized Rate (ASR) of cancer in Yemen (2020) of 97/100,000 population, with 92.7/100,000 in males and 102.2 in females [8]. These rates showed Yemen with lower rates of cancer in comparison to other countries in the region, which ranged from 108.7/100,000 in Oman to 170.9/100,000 in the United Arab Emirates [8], which is probably due to underreporting of cancer cases in Yemen. On the other hand, the Aden Cancer Registry (ACR) showed an ASR of 38.2/100,000 in males and 36.1/100,000 in females, respectively, for the period 1997–2011 [9]. However, the National Oncology Center (NOC) in Yemen reported for the year 2007, illustrated an ASR ranged from 17 to 28 per 100,000 population [10].

20.2.2 Cancer Mortality Rate

Deaths by cancer in Yemen for the year 2020 were estimated with a total of 12,103 cases with 76.5 ASR (world) per 100,000. Males showed a slightly higher rate than females (77.9 vs. 76.1 ASR (world) per 100,000, respectively) [8]. Among the sites of cancer, breast cancer ranked in the top of the death rates (12.1%), followed by colorectum (10.0%), stomach (9.7%), leukemia (8.6%), esophagus (8.3%), liver (6.5%), lung (6.2%), brain, CNS (6.0%), and non-Hodgkin lymphoma (3.2%) [11].Precise mortality and survival rate from cancer is not easy to count, particularly for those coming from remote areas of Yemen, and thus, it becomes difficult for them to access back the health care centers located in the main cities of the country [12].

20.2.3 Top Ten Cancers in Yemen

The rank of cancer types in Yemen is probably not like what exists in the neighboring Gulf countries. According to the GLOBOCAN, estimated age-standardized incidence rates (World) in the year 2020 for both sexes and all ages shows breast cancer was ranked number one in Yemen with ASR 30.5 per 100,000 population, followed by colorectum (10.7), stomach (7.1), esophagus (6.4), lung (5.8), liver (5.1), leukemia (4.2), Non-Hodgkin Lymphoma (4.0), brain/Central Nervous System (3.8), and ovary (3.4 per 100,000 population), as shown in Table 20.1 [13]. However, the reported data from ACR counted leukemia the first (10.5%), Non-Hodgkin Lymphoma (NHL) (10.1%), colorectal (7.5%), Hodgkin diseases (6.1%), and stomach (5.1%) among male cases, while breast cancer ranking the top (30.0%), followed by leukemia (7.6%), NHL (6.6%), colorectal (4.9%), and ovarian cancer (4.5%) among females [9]. Another previous study from ACR (1997–2001) showed that head and neck cancers occupy the fourth position among all registered cancers (1734 cases) in a 5 year period [14]. Some differences in the reported data on cancer from the NOC was breast cancer at the top, however, followed with Non-Hodgkin's Lymphoma, leukemia, liver, and stomach cancers. Among children below 15 years, the most common types were leukemia, Non-Hodgkin's lymphoma, Hodgkin's lymphoma, and CNS tumors [10].

20.2.4 Age-Specific Related Cancer

Figure 20.1 illustrated the increasing trend in cancer cases as age increases with the peak of the ASR per 100,000 population incidence was seen to be higher among females, predominantly in the young and middle age groups (30–59 years), which could be explained as due to the higher rate of breast cancer in this female age group, but was then surpassed by higher incidences in males, particularly in those 60 years and older according to the data reported from GLOBOCAN 2020 [8].

For better understanding of the most common cancers by gender (Fig. 20.2), five categories of classification were used: children <15 years old; adolescents and teenagers: 15–24 years; young adults: 25–49 years; adults: 50–69 years; and elder adults: ≥70 years. Accordingly, males, for example, showed leukemia as the most common in children and teenagers <25 years of age; NHL was the most common in the cohort of 25–49 year; colorectal cancer was the most common type in the 50–69 year cohort; whereas esophageal cancer was found the most common among the elderly cohort aged ≥70 years [9].

Table 20.1 Estimated age-standardized incidence and mortality rates (World) in 2020, both sexes, all ages. Yemen [13]

All cancers	Incidence	Mortality	Male	Incidence	Mortality	Female	Incidence	Mortality
Breast	30.5	18.9	Colorectum	12.0	8.6	Breast	30.5	18.9
Colorectum	10.7	7.7	Stomach	8.9	8.0	Colorectum	9.5	6.9
Stomach	7.1	6.4	Liver	7.1	7.0	Esophagus	7.2	7.0
Esophagus	6.4	6.2	Lung	6.7	6.5	Stomach	5.7	5.1
Lung	5.8	5.5	Esophagus	5.3	5.2	Lung	5.1	4.8
Liver	5.1	5.0	NHL [a]	5.0	3.9	Leukemia	4.0	3.4
Leukemia	4.2	3.6	B/CNS [b]	4.9	4.7	Thyroid	3.9	1.3
NHL [a]	4.0	3.0	Larynx	4.4	3.8	Liver	3.5	3.4
B/CNS [b]	3.8	3.5	Leukemia	4.4	3.8	Ovary	3.4	2.9
Ovary	3.4	2.9	Bladder	4.0	2.9	NHL [a]	3.2	2.2

[a] *NHL* Non-Hodgkin lymphoma
[b] *B/CNS* Brain, central nervous system

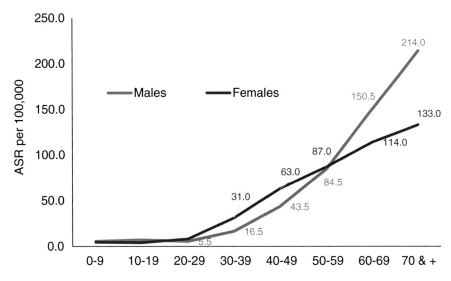

Fig. 20.1 Age-specific incidence rate per 100,000 population of cancer cases [8]. Copyrights—Cancer Today—IARC, 150 Cours Albert Thomas, 69,372 Lyon CEDEX 08, France—powered by GLOBOCAN 2020

20.2.5 Public/Private Sector

Since 1990, most of the cancer diagnosing and treatment centers were publicly located in the main hospitals in the big cities such as Sana'a and Aden. As the strategy of the health system changed to corporate the private sector in taking part of the health care load, thus many private hospitals and diagnostic laboratories were established, and oncology activities were expanded [15].

20.2.6 Cancer Registry in Yemen

Cancer surveillance plays a critical role in the development and implementation of health policy. Currently, five cancer registries were minimally functioning to collect the data on cancer patients and analyzing the findings: Aden Cancer Registry (the pioneer in the country since 1997 under the authority of Aden University), Hadhramaut cancer registry in Al-Mukalla City, Hadramout Valley and Desert Oncology Center (HVDOC), National Oncology Center in Sana'a, and the last one established was Taiz cancer registry (under the authority of the Ministry of Public Health and Population). However, all these registries often struggle with insufficient health services, transient populations, lack of finances, lack of qualified workforces, inadequate or imprecise data due to incomplete coverage, difficulty in establishing a trustworthy, reasonable cancer registry in the nation, and difficulty to obtain data on cancer mortality [9].

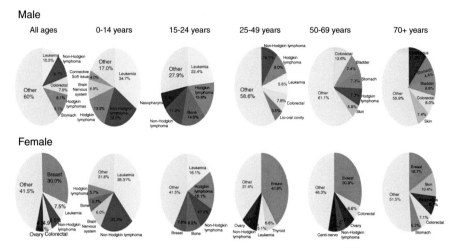

Fig. 20.2 The most common five cancer types by gender and age category from the ACR (1997–2011) [9]. Copyrights—*Bawazir AA. Cancer incidence in Yemen from 1997 to 2011: a report from the Aden cancer registry. BMC cancer 2018;18(1):540

For better understanding of the most common cancers by gender (Fig. 20.2), five categories of classification were used: children <15 years old; adolescents and teenagers: 15–24 years; young adults: 25–49 years; adults: 50–69 years; and elder adults: ≥70 years. Accordingly, males, for example, showed leukemia as the most common in children and teenagers <25 years of age; NHL was the most common in the cohort of 25–49 year; colorectal cancer was the most common type in the 50–69 year cohort; whereas esophageal cancer was found the most common among the elderly cohort aged ≥70 years [9].

20.3 Healthcare System in Yemen

Health care is guaranteed by the state as a right to all citizens under the Yemeni constitution. Historically, the Ministry of Public Health and Population (MoPHP) was responsible for the delivery of health care and overall health system governance [16]. According to the World Health Organization/Regional Office for the Eastern Mediterranean (2018), Yemen's health situation is one of the least favorable in the world, with various factors such as poverty (GNP = 7$/year), poor access to water and sanitation, low educational level mainly among women, and high fertility rates which led to worsening the health of Yemeni people. The three-tier system of primary care, based on health units, health centers, and hospitals, is insufficient to cover the health needs of the population, especially since the population growth rate is faster than the expansion rate of available health facilities. Moreover, the general government expenditure on health was only 3.9%; thus, the out-of-pocket expenditure is much higher per capita [17]. These findings illustrate the weaknesses of the health system in Yemen with insufficient functionality and provision of health services and public health programs with more disruption of the health system due to the ongoing conflict [17].

20.4 Cancer Risk Factors

The main risk factor attributed to cancer in Yemen was Tobacco use (16.3%), followed by overall infections (13.4%), including Hepatitis B infection, obesity (2.5%), and occupational risks (1.4%) [3, 18, 19].

20.4.1 Smoking Epidemiology

A study in Yemen reported that the majority (83.8%) of lung cancer cases were smokers [20]. The WHO report on the global tobacco epidemic in 2017 indicated an increased prevalence rate of smokers in Yemen by 18.7% with higher prevalence in males than females (20.7% vs. 6.0%, respectively) [18]. Despite the increase in tobacco taxes of retail price $\leq 25\%$, no tobacco control policy, strategy, or active action plan exists in the country.

20.4.2 Khat Chewing (Catha edulis)

Based on the Family Health Survey carried in 2003 in Yemen, it was estimated that 58% of males and 29% of females aged 10 years and older chewed Qat during their lifetime [21]. The evidence linking Khat use to cancer is sparse and circumstantial [22, 23], although there is some suggestion that oral leukoplakias (perhaps precancerous) are more frequent in users of Khat [24]. Smoking of cigarettes and/or Waterpipe are commonly practiced during Khat sessions and considered as a direct or indirect risk for the people in the settings [25, 26]. However, various pesticides and insecticides are known to be used by Khat growers, and they, and consumers of the leaves, are probably exposed to elevated levels of various chemicals [27, 28]. This may therefore pose a further hazard to health.

20.4.3 Diet, Physical Activity, and Obesity

There have been no studies in Yemen on the possible role of dietary intake on cancer risk. Furthermore, population surveys, providing accurate data on intake of different nutrients, on levels of physical activity, or even on the height/weight of the population are lacking. The WHO estimates the prevalence of overweight as 37.5% in women and 29.7% in men [29]. A local study from Yemen suggested that the mean BMI was significantly higher overall in females (23.9%) than in males (21.8%). However, this trend was also associated with age, mainly in the age group between 35 and 44 years of age [30].

20.5 Cancer Screening Programs

Very limited access for cervical and breast cancer screening in the main hospitals, where the facilities for performing screening tests coexist. Organized screening is known to be effective for cancers of the cervix, large bowel, and breast; however, it is difficult to establish in countries with major limitations in healthcare services [31]. Therefore, the development of a program of early detection of breast cancer through public and professional education, and establishment of diagnostic and treatment facilities to deal with cases discovered, should be a priority [32, 33].

20.6 Cancer Prevention Programs

Prevention involves minimizing or eliminating exposure of the population to the known causes of cancer and promotion of lifestyles known to protect against cancer. Prevention is the most cost-effective long-term cancer control approach and offers the greatest public health impact. Among the successful strategies to combat hepatocellular cancer, vaccination against HBV was used with a reported coverage of 88% among the Yemeni infants [34]. The Human Papillomavirus (HPV) vaccine as considered to protect against cervical cancer was not yet included in the National Vaccination Program [35].

In spite of the fact that most cancers are related to a modifiable risk factor, such as tobacco control, encouraging lifestyle, physical activity, and balanced diet, it remains a major public health problem in Yemen [36]. The involvement of primary healthcare physicians in counseling patients about smoking cessation or obtaining screening CT scan for high-risk patients is very limited. Digital mammography should be allocated in the main care centers in the main cities as the crucial first step with the training of female doctors to perform breast imaging. The same for colorectal cancer, colonoscopy units led by trained doctors in colonoscopy, is of great importance for early detection and to provide good outcomes. Educational campaigns should target tobacco control, encouraging hepatitis vaccination programs, use of mammograms, and human papilloma vaccination.

20.7   Cancer Diagnosis

Imaging diagnostic and interventional diagnostic services such as multi-slice CT scans, MRI, digital mammography also the facility of imaging guided minimally invasive biopsy, were available in many private centers in the country [37]. Similarly, the unique functional nuclear medicine departments are in Sana'a that include the PET CT scan, technical bone scan, thyroid iodine scan, other cancer type-specific scans, in addition to the radioactive iodine therapy service, which are crucial for hematological malignancies, mainly acute leukemia and aggressive lymphomas diagnosis [37].

20.7.1   Laboratory

Diagnostic pathology centers were available in Sanaa, Aden, Taiz, Hudaidah, and Hadramout. Molecular testing in addition to the other diagnostic facilities like flow cytometry, cytogenetics, and PCR machines were also available in Sanaa and Aden. However, immunohistochemistry analysis, molecular profiling to confirm the diagnosis, and hematological malignancies laboratory services were found only in Sana'a city [37].

20.8   Treatment

20.8.1   Medical Oncology

Currently, eight public centers under the umbrella of the National Cancer Control Program (NCCP) in Yemen are providing cytotoxic chemotherapy treatment free for patients with cancer. They are distributed as one in each of the following cities: Sana'a, Aden, Hudaidah, Taiz, Mukalla, Siyun, Ebb, and in Ataq [37]. Other two will be soon established in Al-Mahra and Mareb. Other chemotherapy centers are also functioning in about five more private hospitals; however, the patient must provide the medication. Although Leukemia is considered among the top cancers in the country, Stem Cell Transplantation is not available. Moreover, immunotherapy/targeted therapy/biological agents were also not available in Yemen; therefore, patients must travel to other countries with available facilities such as to India, Egypt, and Jordan.

Currently, few numbers of oncologists were known in the country based on their career of specialty, but most of them were not registered officially in the Ministry of health as a medical oncologist, and no precise number is currently available, moreover, some general practitioners due to lack of specialists, use to work by practice to prescribe chemotherapy and for some general surgeons to deal with cancer surgeries. Worldwide, the NCCN guidelines are the most widely accepted, cost-effective and evidence-based guidelines that are usually adopted in Yemen as is the case in most of the developed and developing countries.

20.8.2 Radiation Therapy

Three centers in Yemen were responsible for radiotherapy services; one in a public hospital (National Oncology Center) and the other two in private hospitals (Yemeni-German Hospital and the Azal Hospital), all in Sana'a. However, it does not satisfy the long queue of patients waiting for a long time (up to more than 4 months). The available machines in Sana'a were Cobalt Machine, Simulator (conventional old Toshiba one) at the NOC and one linear machine in Azal hospital. However, a number of the following machines in Yemen like gamma knife, cyberknife, Brachytherapy, or any other radiation services such as 3D, VMAT, SBRT, SRS, except the IMRT located in Sana'a only.

According to the registered Radiation oncologist or clinical oncologist provides Radiation and gender information were counted as 17 radiation oncologists (3 females and 14 males) in the year 2021. Programs of expanding radiotherapy facilities at NOC were planned but not started. Additional three radiotherapy units were planned to be established in Aden, Taiz, and Hadhramaut, but no action [37].

20.8.3 Surgery

Despite the large number of surgeons in Yemen who received their career from different schools of surgery in the world, centers for oncological surgery were not available. So usually, surgery is performed in any tertiary level hospital or referral hospital in the main cities. Moreover, robotic surgeries for cancer, and Hyperthermic Intraperitoneal Chemotherapy (HIPEC) procedure, were not available in the country [37].

20.8.4 Pediatric Oncology

Pediatric oncology statistics is part of the main sources for adult cancer statistics which are mainly in the main hospitals, and some were collected at the available cancer registries in Yemen. However, centers providing comprehensive pediatric cancer treatment were not available in the country, except in Sana'a (NOC) and in Aden (Al-Sadaka Teaching Hospital). Therefore, the future needs to consider pediatric oncology as part of the medical oncology services that should be provided to patients with cancer [37].

20.8.5   Survivorship Track

According to the WHO report in 2019, more investment in cancer care, such as the provision of radiation therapy equipment, is needed to guarantee a multidisciplinary approach to achieve Universal Health Coverage for this category of patients [38]. As more patients are successfully treated for cancer, a new challenge awaits navigating the physical and emotional challenges of being a survivor. No survival registry is found in the country, and no previous research work in this field to determine the survival track in the country.

20.8.6   Palliative Care Track

At present, no oncology center is dedicated for the provision of palliative care, and even those hospitals providing specialist services (radiotherapy and chemotherapy) care make no provision for supportive or terminal care once a patient is terminal and not fit for therapy. Centers for physical rehabilitation (e.g., for amputees) are present, but there are no specialized services in pain control or palliative care in Yemen. Opioids (e.g., oral morphine) are available but used with much restriction in some hospitals and require special authorization for general physicians to prescribe it [37].

20.9   Research and Education

Scientific research works on cancer have been published in regional and international peer-reviewed journals concerning cancer in Yemen [9, 10, 13, 20, 25, 26, 31, 39–47]. However, most of these publications were in concern based around clinical series from a variety of hospital departments and laboratories. There are several areas where research is clearly indicated to assist in planning and evaluation for cancer control in Yemen. It is important to establish the true cancer profile in Yemen, as well as important indicators such as stage at diagnosis and survival from common cancers. Some studies conducted on the potential carcinogenicity of Khat, focusing initially on oral or esophageal cancers. Other publications were focused on knowledge and behavior of the population in some common cancers such as breast, colorectal, leukemia, and head and neck cancers. Previous studies by Ba-Saleem et al. (2005) and Kahiry W (2011) suggest that the most common cases (generally at advanced stage) include are: breast, leukemia, lymphoma (NHL, HL) head and neck, especially nasopharynx, gastrointestinal (especially esophagus and gastric, colorectal, hepatocellular carcinoma) [39, 41, 43, 44]. Some authors recently showed that there is a significant decrease in patients presenting with advanced-stage cancers such as breast cancer, where stage IV breast cancer diagnosis decreased from 20% to 6% [41].

20.10   Cost-Effective Cancer Care

Increasing numbers of cancer cases in the country to be treated in public and private hospitals require a cost-sharing in public facilities, cost-recovery of drugs and cost exempted treatments in public facilities, which is high in country with marked population poverty. Out-of-pocket payments in times of illness are very high, and in most cases, people seek for better treatment abroad, at the same time, they try to avoid the expensive medications (such as targeted therapy and immunotherapy). In recent years, the principal drugs for cancer therapy were received as grants from some countries outside (donations mainly from King Salman Center, Kingdom of Saudi Arabia through the World Health Organization). Thanks to the generous support of the donors, all cancer centers are currently open and providing cancer care across the country [12]. Therefore, people pay for the low-cost generic drugs (mainly from India). Other NGOs donations also contribute to the treatment cost in some areas, such as the example of "Selah" Foundation in Hadhramaut.

20.11   Challenges and Advantages

20.11.1   Human Resources

Human resources are a key factor for the appropriate implementation of the program at different levels. A gap still exists between what might be and what is running. Capacity building including training programs in different disciplines technical and managerial should be established through short-term and long-term programs mainly for surgeons, medical oncologists, radiation oncologists, pediatric oncologists, histopathologists, hematologists, epidemiologists, registry clerks, nurses, and other paramedics. Moreover, the main defect in the health allied team is the qualified oncology pharmacists and nurses.

20.11.2 Role of Non-Governmental Organizations (NGOs)

Partnership between local and international organizations is an important factor for the success of a program. In Yemen, some local NGOs are already active in providing services to the patient and contributing to some educational campaigns. However, probably more actions were needed to work in cooperation with the government in some other areas, such as producing health educational materials, supporting scientific work, establishing, and funding of cancer registries, hospice/palliative/terminal care, and patient and family support. Among these NGOs are Yemen Cancer Society based in Aden, Yemeni Cancer Foundation (mainly in Sana'a), and Hadhramaut Cancer Foundation (based in Hadhramaut).

20.12 The Future of Cancer Care in Yemen

The national cancer program in Yemen is planned to improve the future care for patients with cancer. A road map was established for capacity building of principal elements through local and abroad training programs in different disciplines technical and managerial using a short-term and long-term training mainly for surgeons, medical oncologists, radiation oncologists, pediatric oncologists, histopathologists, hematologists, epidemiologists, registry clerks, nurses, and other paramedics. Establishment of reliable cancer profile in Yemen, which includes accurate data reporting of the registered cases, improve staging at diagnosis, counting the survival rate of at least the common cancers. Establish a dedicated unit in the main hospitals for provision of palliative care with the training of the oncologists in this field. Strengthening cooperation and collaboration with other oncology centers in the region as well as some international agencies to support in the training and exchange of opinions in oncology medication. Encourage local capitals to invest in the diagnosis and treatment of patients with cancer, particularly those who need specific interventions such as stem cell transplantation and HIPEC procedures [37].

20.13 Conclusion

Priority and emphasis on the burden of breast cancer among Yemeni women should be given special consideration due to the high incidence and consequently high rate of deaths. Hence, efforts are needed to increase breast cancer awareness in Yemen for early detection at all age groups and to target women living in areas that have lower access to health care services. Research is needed to study the factors related to equity in health services for diagnosis, screening, and management of cancer patients in different regions of the country, with more focus, should be given for most people residing in the rural areas. Yemen has been characterized by three decades of scattered, fragmented, and unfocused cancer research. Furthermore, much is needed to improve cancer care in Yemen through redesigned, better organized, and well-functioning cancer facilities in the country according to clear developmental programs. Moreover, the National Cancer Control Plan seeks to address the inadequacy of cancer patient care services through integrating different services and aiming for the most effective and efficient use of existing, and, hopefully, additional resources, in an equitable way, for the whole population. It is necessary to focus on some priority areas, to ensure that some concrete steps are taken and that the best does not become the enemy of the good.

Conflict of Interest Authors have no conflict of interest to declare.

References

1. UN. In: The United Nations in Yemen: sociodemographic profile. Sana'a Yemen: United Nation; 2020. https://yemen.un.org/en/about/about-the-un.
2. NIC/Yemen. In: Republic of Yemen administrative governorates. National Information Center; 2014. https://yemen-nic.info/yemen/gover/#.
3. WM. In: Yemen demographics: life expectancy in Yemen. Worldometers; 2020.https://www.worldometers.info/demographics/yemen-demographics/#life-exp.
4. WM. In: Worldmetric: Yemen population. Worldmetric; 2020. https://www.worldometers.info/world-population/yemen-population/#:~:text=Yemen%202020%20population%20is%20estimated,146%20people%20per%20mi2.
5. UN. Prospects 2019: Highlights (ST/ESA/SER.A/423): United Nations, Department of Economic and Social Affairs, Population Division (2019). World Population; 2019. https://population.un.org/wpp/Publications/Files/WPP2019_Highlights.pdf.
6. UNFPA. In: Population pyramid, Yemen. United Nations Population Fund; 2020. https://www.unfpa.org/ageing.
7. UNESCWA. In: The demographic profile of Yemen: population trend. 2020. https://www.unescwa.org/sites/www.unescwa.org/files/yemen_2017-single_pages_jan_8.pdf.
8. IARC. In: Cancer today: estimated age-standardized incidence rates (world) in 2020, all cancers, all ages (Yemen). Lyon: World Health Organization/International Agency for Research on Cancer; 2021. https://gco.iarc.fr/today/online-analysis-map?v=2020&mode=population&mode_population=continents&population=900&populations=900&key=asr&sex=2&cancer=39&type=0&statistic=5&prevalence=0&population_group=0&ages_group%5B%5D=0&ages_group%5B%5D=17&nb_items=10&group_cancer=1&include_nmsc=1&include_nmsc_other=1&projection=globe&color_palette=default&map_scale=quantile&map_nb_colors=5&continent=0&rotate=%255B10%252C0%255D.
9. Bawazir AA. Cancer incidence in Yemen from 1997 to 2011: a report from the Aden cancer registry. BMC Cancer. 2018;18(1):540. https://doi.org/10.1186/s12885-018-4411-9.
10. Afif A, Algharati AM, Hamid GA, Al-Nehmi AW, Shamlan A. Pattern of cancer in Yemen: first result from the National Oncology Center, Sana'a. Eur J Pharm Med Res. 2017;4(1):149–54. https://www.ejpmr.com/home/abstract_id/1880
11. ICCP. In: Cancer country profiles Yemen 2020: WHO-international cancer control partnership. The International Cancer Control Partnership; 2020. https://www.iccp-portal.org/who-cancer-country-profiles-yemen-2020.

12. WHO/EMRO. In: Cancer patients in Yemen face the compounded pain of disease and conflict. Cairo: The World health Organization/Eastern Meditterranean Region; 2020. http://www.emro.who.int/yemen/news/cancer-patients-in-yemen-face-the-compounded-pain-of-disease-and-conflict.html.
13. Basaleem HO, Bawazer AA, Al-Sakkaf KAZ. Head and neck cancer: is it a problem among Yemeni patients? (A five year retrospective study). J Nat Appl Sci. 2005;9(1)
14. IARC/WHO. Global Health Observatory. In: World Health Organization. 2018. Global health observatory. Geneva: International Agency for Research on Cancer/World Health Organization; 2018. https://gco.iarc.fr/today/home.
15. MOPHP. National Health Strategy: toward better health for all through developing a fair health system. Sana'a: Ministry of Public Health and Population; 2010. https://extranet.who.int/countryplanningcycles/sites/default/files/planning_cycle_repository/yemen/nat_health_strategy_-_yemen_eng.pdf
16. Qirbi N, Ismail SA. Health system functionality in a low-income country in the midst of conflict: the case of Yemen. Health Policy Plan. 2017;32(6):911–22.
17. WHO/EMRO. Yemen: Health Systems Profile; 2018. https://rho.emro.who.int/sites/default/files/Profiles-briefs-files/YEM-Health-System-Profiles-2018.pdf.
18. WHO. WHO report on the global tobacco epidemic, 2017: monitoring tobacco use and prevention policies. Geneva: World Health Organization; 2017. Report No.: 9241512822. https://apps.who.int/iris/bitstream/handle/10665/255874/97892415?sequence=1.
19. WHO. Report on the global tobacco epidemic, 2015: raising taxes for tobacco. In: EMRO. Algeria: World Health Organization; 2015. https://www.who.int/tobacco/global_report/2015/en/.
20. Abdul Hamid G, Al-Nabhi A, Baom N, Algalabi A. Lung cancer in Aden, Yemen. World J Pharm Res. 2015;4(7):324–32. www.wjpr.net
21. MOPHP. Family Health Survey 2011. Sana'a: Ministry of Public Health and Population; 2003. www.mophp-ye.org/
22. Hassan N, Gunaid A, Murray Lyon I. Khat [Catha edulis]: health aspects of khat chewing. East Mediterr Health J, 13 (3), 706–718, 2007 2007.
23. El-Zaemey S, Schüz J, Leon M. Qat chewing and risk of potentially malignant and malignant oral disorders: a systematic review. Int J Occup Environ Med. 2015;6(3):129–43.
24. Ali AA, AlSharabi AK, Aguirre JM, Nahas R. A study of 342 oral keratotic white lesions induced by qat chewing among 2500 Yemeni. J Oral Pathol Med. 2004;33(6):368–72.
25. Laswar AK, Darwish H. Prevalence of cigarette smoking and khat chewing among Aden university medical students and their relationship to BP and body mass index. Saudi J Kidney Dis Transpl. 2009;20(5):862–6. SaudiJKidneyDisTranspl_2009_20_5_862_55381 [pii]. http://www.ncbi.nlm.nih.gov/pubmed/19736493
26. Marway R. Oral health: the destructive effects of Khat. Br Dent J. 2016;221(1):2. https://doi.org/10.1038/sj.bdj.2016.468.
27. Date J, Tanida N, Hobara T. Qat chewing and pesticides: a study of adverse health effects in people of the mountainous areas of Yemen. Int J Environ Health Res. 2004;14(6):405–14.
28. Hassan AA, Abdullah SM, Khardali IA, Oraiby ME, Shaikain GA, Fageeh M, et al. Health impact of Khat chewing and pesticides: detection of 8 pesticides multi-residues in Khat leaves (Catha edulis) from Jazan region. KSA Adv Environ Biol. 2016;10:30–6.
29. Bagchi K. Nutrition in the eastern Mediterranean region of the World Health Organization. East Mediterr Health J. 2008;14:S107–13.
30. Gunaid A. Obesity, overweight and underweight among adults in an urban community in Yemen. East Mediterr Health J. 2012;18(12):1187–93.
31. Bawazir A, Bashateh N, Jradi H, Breik AB. Breast cancer screening awareness and practices among women attending primary health care centers in the Ghail Bawazir District of Yemen. Clin Breast Cancer. 2019;19(1):e20–9. https://doi.org/10.1016/j.clbc.2018.09.005.
32. Sancho-Garnier H, Khazraji YC, Cherif MH, Mahnane A, Hsairi M, El Shalakamy A, et al. Overview of cervical cancer screening practices in the extended Middle East and North Africa countries. Vaccine. 2013;31:G51–7. https://doi.org/10.1016/j.vaccine.2012.06.046.

33. Nasher AT, Al-hebshi NN, Al-Moayad EE, Suleiman AM. Viral infection and oral habits as risk factors for oral squamous cell carcinoma in Yemen: a case-control study. Oral Surg Oral Med Oral Pathol Oral Radiol. 2014;118(5):566–572.e1.
34. WHO/UNICEF. WHO and UNICEF estimates of immunization coverage: 2019 revision. Yemen: The World Health Organization and UNICEF; 2020. https://www.who.int/immunization/monitoring_surveillance/data/yem.pdf
35. Bruni LAG, Serrano B, Mena M, Gómez D, Muñoz J, Bosch FX, de Sanjosé. Human papillomavirus and related diseases report YEMEN: summary report. ICO/IARC Information Centre on HPV and Cancer (HPV Information Centre); 2019. www.hpvcentre.net.
36. WHO. An annotated bibliography of scientific studies done on tobacco topic in WHO South-East Asia Region countries: 2003–2014: surveillance, health effects, economics and control efforts. World Health Organization; 2015. Report No.: 9290224940. https://apps.who.int/iris/handle/10665/204785.
37. Abdul Hameed G. Cancer diagnostic pathology centers in Yemen: annual report. National Cancer Control Program. Ministry of Public Health and Population. Aden. Yemen. 2021.
38. WHO. WHO report on cancer: setting priorities, investing wisely and providing care for all. Cairo: World Health Organization; 2020. Report No.: 9240001298. http://www.quotidianosanita.it/allegati/allegato4849716.pdf.
39. Al-Kahiry W, Omer H, Saeed N, Hamid G. Late presentation of breast cancer in Aden, Yemen. Gulf J Oncolog. 2011;9:7–11.
40. Al-Maweri SA, Addas A, Tarakji B, Abbas A, Al-Shamiri HM, Alaizari NA, et al. Public awareness and knowledge of oral cancer in Yemen. Asian Pac J Cancer Prev. 2015;15(24):10861–5.
41. Al-Naggar R, Al-Maktari LAS, H A, J T, B S, SI M. Critical assessment of three decades of breast cancer research in Yemen. Syst Rev Biomed Res Health Adv. 2020;2(1):1008. http://www.medtextpublications.com/biomed-research-and-health-advances-articles-in-press.php
42. Badheeb A, Baamer A. The pattern and distribution of malignancies reported in Hadhramout sector, Yemen-2002-2011. Alandalus For Soc Appl Sci J. 2012;5:7–16.
43. BaSaleem H, Bawazir AA, Moore M, Al-Sakkaf KA. Five years cancer incidence in Aden Cancer Registry, Yemen (2002-2006). Asian Pac J Cancer Prev. 2010;11(2):507.
44. Basaleem HO, Al-Sakkaf KA. Colorectal cancer among Yemeni patients. Characteristics and trends. Saudi Med J. 2004;25(8):1002–5.
45. Bashamakha G, Bin Sumait H, Bashamakha M, Al Serouri A, Khader Y. Risk factors of breast cancer in Hadramout Valley and Desert, Yemen. Int J Prev Med. 2019;10 https://doi.org/10.4103/ijpvm.IJPVM_251_17.
46. Bawazir AA. Deaths, DALY and other related measures of breast cancer in Yemeni women: findings of the global burden of disease study (1990–2010). J Cancer Res Pract. 2017;4(1):14–8.
47. Salim EI, Jazieh AR, Moore MA. Lung cancer incidence in the Arab league countries: risk factors and control. Asian Pac J Cancer Prev. 2011;12(1):17–34.

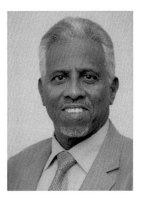

Amen Bawazir, MBBS, Epi DR, PhD, is the Professor and consultant of Epidemiology and Community Medicine at the Faculty of Medicine and Health Sciences, University of Aden, Yemen. He has graduated from Liverpool School of Tropical Medicine, UK. He was a former head of the Aden Cancer Registry and Research Center and the chairman of the Yemeni Society for cancer control/Aden. He has worked as Deputy Dean at the Faculty of Medicine and Health Science, Aden University and consistently contributed to the academic activities for over 35 years in Aden and in KSAU-HS, Saudi Arabia. His publications on cancer were highly cited. Moreover, he has been awarded for his contribution in reviewing articles from many journals.

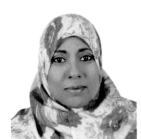

Huda Basaleem is the Professor and consultant in Community Medicine Public Health, Director of Aden Cancer Registry and Research Center, Faculty of Medicine and Health Science and Vice Dean, Faculty of Postgraduate Studies, University of Aden, Yemen. She is a WHO expert for the Eastern Mediterranean Countries on NCDs Surveillance. Dr. Basaleem is the Principal Investigator and consultant for several international organizations like WHO, UNICEF, World Bank, UNHCR, IOM and the Foundation for Future. She is the Editor-In-Chief, Yemeni Journal of Medical and Health Research and editorial member in several journals (regional and international). She was also the winner of the Elsevier Award in Life Sciences for Women Scientists in the Developing World (Arab Region).

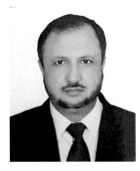

Ahmed Badheeb, MD, is the Professor of Internal Medicine and Medical Oncology. He is the founder and former director of the National Oncology Center-Hadhramout-Yemen. Prof. Ahmed was the former Vice Dean for academic affairs, Hadhramout University, College of Medicine. He has published many papers in the field of Medicine and Oncology. He has a special interest in medical education and the quality of healthcare.

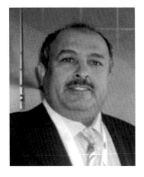

Gamal Abdul Hamid has received his German board in internal medicine and PhD in hematology-oncology from the faculty of medicine, University of Dresden during the period between 1987 and 1993. Currently, he is working as general director of the National Program of Cancer Control, Yemen Republic. Moreover, he is the head of hematology and clinical laboratory in the Faculty of Medicine, University of Aden, general secretary of Yemen Cancer Society and consultant of hematology-oncology in the national oncology center, Aden. He serves as an editorial member of several national and international medical journals. He is a member of ESMO, ASCO, INCTR, Pan Arab Oncology and WAMS.

Chapter 21
General Oncology Care in Qatar, Comoros, and Djibouti

Humaid O. Al-Shamsi ⓘ **and Faryal Iqbal** ⓘ

21.1 Background

The editors of the book contacted authors to write book chapters on cancer care outlook for their respective Arab countries. Every including Arab country in the book has agreed on unanimous effort to bring forward this worthwhile project. However, the editors were unable to find the authors for Qatar, Comoros, and Djibouti. Hence, they decided to compose a short review on oncology care in the aforementioned countries for the book.

H. O. Al-Shamsi (✉)
Department of Oncology, Burjeel Cancer Institute, Burjeel Medical City,
Abu Dhabi, United Arab Emirates

Innovation and Research Center, Burjeel Cancer Institute, Burjeel Medical City,
Abu Dhabi, United Arab Emirates

Emirates Oncology Society, Dubai, United Arab Emirates

University of Sharjah, Sharjah, United Arab Emirates
e-mail: humaid.al-shamsi@medportal.ca

F. Iqbal
Department of Oncology, Innovation and Research Center, Burjeel Cancer Institute,
Burjeel Medical City, Abu Dhabi, United Arab Emirates
e-mail: faryal.iqbal@burjeelmedicalcity.com

© The Author(s) 2022
H. O. Al-Shamsi et al. (eds.), *Cancer in the Arab World*,
https://doi.org/10.1007/978-981-16-7945-2_21

21.2   State of Qatar

21.2.1   Introduction

The Arabian Peninsula encompasses a ministate, the State of Qatar, with a small-scale, comparable young national population. Moreover, it has an extensive ratio of the expatriate population. The country has observed rapid advancement over the last few decades. Subsequently, it has a high per capita Gross Domestic Product (GDP). Cancer has been ranked second among Non-Communicable Diseases (NCDs) in Qatar, first being cardiovascular diseases (CVD). The cancer projection has been estimated to be at threefold elevation between 2010 and 2030, compounded by advanced age and population growth [1].

Qatar has free public health care services, including cancer care for its residents who have paid a minimum health insurance cost. Few charities, including Qatar Cancer Society (QCS) provide accessible ad hoc assistance for cancer treatment on exceptional or humane grounds. The healthcare infrastructure has observed major progress since the launch of the National Cancer Strategy in 2011. Qatar has a formal structural plan and internationally peer-reviewed cancer care services that deliver outcomes proportional to those countries who are ahead in established comprehensive cancer care structures. This has translated into a high assurance level for cancer care services among the population. Hence, substantially increased usage of oncology services can be observed mostly by natives [1].

21.2.2   Oncology Care in the State of Qatar

Qatar has advanced administrative authorities to supervise the strategies, including, a National Cancer Committee that comprises representatives from all sectors to monitor the progress with the established framework (Fig. 21.1) [1].

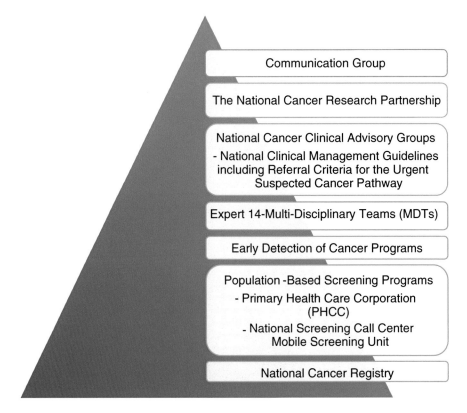

Fig. 21.1 Oncology care strategies framework [1]

21.2.3 Advanced Technology and Breakthroughs in Cancer Care

Qatar's investments in healthcare infrastructure and advanced technologies have improved the clinical practice along with upgraded cancer care facilities across the country. A few top-notch cancer care services available in Qatar are mentioned below [1]:

– *Specialist Palliative Care Unit*: A ten-bedded facility has opened the door for a cancer center. This establishment has been approved to offer an accredited fellowship training program.

- *Radiotherapy*: Qatar's healthcare system comprises many ultra-modern treatment modalities apart from conventional radiotherapy services; subsequently, improved patients' outcomes can be observed. These contemporary technologies, include Cyberknife, MRI guided High Intensity Focused Ultrasound (MRgHIFU), Magnetic Resonance Image Guided Adaptive Brachytherapy (MRIGABT), Radiation Therapy Surface Guided Radiotherapy (SGRT), Total body irradiation (TBI), and Cyclotron.
- *Stem Cell Therapies*: The establishment of the National Stem Cell Transplant Program benefits the adult patients with outstanding outcomes.
- *Gene Chip Development:* The alliance of the Qatar Genome Program (QGP) and local stakeholders catalyzed the gene chip development process. Consequently, a microarray chip content termed as Q-Chip was developed. It is based upon genetic and genomic data of Qatar nationals. Accurate genetic testing for a broad-spectrum of disorders as well as clinical diagnosis of cancer are some significant advantages of Q-Chip.
- *Precision Medicine:* Qatar has introduced a contemporary establishment named "Qatar Precision Medicine Institute (QPMI)." It works closely with local institutional bodies and Healthcare Providers to develop illustrations of precision medicine as an example for patients with predisposition or who have high cancer risk.
- *Cancer Research:* In 2013, the Qatar Cancer Research Partnership (QCRP) was established. The main objective of this system is to supervise the implementation of research programs in addition to academic components of cancer strategies [1].

21.2.4   Cancer Statistics in Qatar

We attained new, sex-specific cancer incidence data along with mortality rates from the International Agency for Research in Cancer (IARC) GLOBOCAN program. A total of 1482 new cancer cases were reported in 2020. Overall, breast cancer (14.7%) was the most commonly occurring cancer in the year 2020, next in order was colorectal (11.7%), followed by prostate (7%) (Fig. 21.2). Breast cancer was at the top among females with 218 cases, while colorectal cancer was highest in males with 112 cases (Table 21.1) [2].

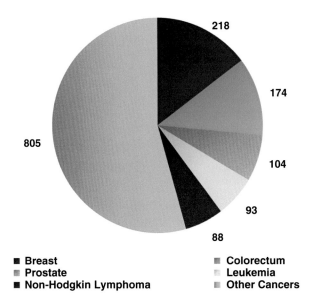

Fig. 21.2 Cancer incident cases in the State of Qatar (2020) [2]. Used with permission from International Agency of Research on Cancer (IARC)/GLOBOCAN

Table 21.1 Sex-specified new cancer cases in the State of Qatar (2020) [2]

Male		Female	
Cancer type	Statistic 2020	Cancer type	Statistic 2020
Colorectum	112 (12.4%)	Breast	218 (37.5%)
Prostate	104 (11.5%)	Colorectum	62 (10.7%)
Leukemia	73 (8.1%)	Thyroid	42 (7.2%)
Lung	71 (7.9%)	Ovary	27 (4.6%)
Non-Hodgkin lymphoma	68 (7.5%)	Cervix uteri	23 (4%)

Source: International Agency of Research on Cancer (IARC)/GLOBOCAN

21.3 Union of the Comoros

21.3.1 Introduction

Union of the Comoros, a group of islands, is an independent state which is located in the Indian Ocean, between Madagascar and the Southeast African mainland. Comoros has witnessed the departure of its educated and skilled workforce to France. Subsequently, a constant decline in Gross Domestic Product (GDP) was observed. The main sources of income in the Comoros are agriculture and farming. Most of its inhabitants live below the subsistence level. The beautiful beaches have always caught the attention of tourists. However, the authorities' struggle to develop a tourism industry which is still in an exploration phase [3].

Each island has its own hospitals. However, the healthcare system has a dearth of medical workforce, state-of-the-art resources, and supplies [3].

21.3.2 Cancer Statistics in Comoros

GLOBOCAN (2020) reported new, sex-specific cancer incidence data in the Comoros. A total of 609 new cancer cases were reported in 2020. Cervix uteri cancer (27.4%) was the most commonly occurring cancer, next in order was prostate (10.7%), followed by breast (10%) cancer (Fig. 21.3). Cervix uteri cancer was at the top among females with 167 cases, while prostate cancer with 65 cases was at the top among males (Table 21.2) [2].

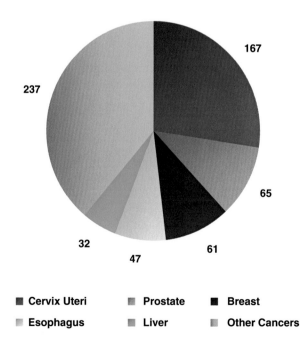

Fig. 21.3 Cancer incident cases in Union of the Comoros (2020) [2]. Used with permission from International Agency of Research on Cancer (IARC)/GLOBOCAN

Table 21.2 Sex-specified new cancer cases in Union of the Comoros (2020) [2]

Male		Female	
Cancer type	Statistic 2020	Cancer type	Statistic 2020
Prostate	65 (28.5%)	Cervix uteri	167 (43.8%)
Esophagus	27 (11.8%)	Breast	61 (16%)
Liver	20 (8.8%)	Esophagus	20 (5.2%)
Bladder	14 (6.1%)	Non-Hodgkin lymphoma	14 (3.7%)
Non-Hodgkin lymphoma	14 (6.1%)	Colorectum	13 (3.4%)

Source: Used with permission from: International Agency of Research on Cancer (IARC)/ GLOBOCAN

The Union of the Comoros is one of the countries that gravitates towards the lowest score on the Human Development Index (HDI). Also, it is included among those countries which have the highest cervical cancer rates. Low HDI countries fail to carry out important systematic affairs including, gender equality, female reproductive health, academic accomplishments, empowerment, and manpower contribution [4].

21.4   Republic of Djibouti

21.4.1   Introduction

The Republic of Djibouti is a small country located on the Northeast coast of the Horn of Africa. Categorically, the 4/5th population is urban, which makes it the top metropolitan country in sub-Saharan Africa. Djibouti has few insufficient natural resources. The restricted capacity of agriculture due to the harsh landscape and industrial activities have affected the socioeconomic situation of the country, resulting in unemployment, a regular shortfall in the budget, and foreign liabilities [5]. Additionally, Djibouti is highly affected by the recurrence of droughts [6]. However, in the recent past, Djibouti has reported development in its economy with 4.5% growth in 2011, 6.5% in 2016, and a 7% expansion in 2017 [7].

A recent study listed the availability of medical devices (including Computed Tomography [CT], Magnetic Resonance Imaging [MRI], Positron Emission Tomography [PET], gamma camera, mammography, radiotherapy equipment) in African countries. Djibouti falls under the category of those countries that have either limited equipment or lack of data [8]. Another study reported countries with demand for radiotherapy (RT) but have no accessibility to them. Djibouti is listed among these countries and had 307 radiotherapy patients, indicating the demand for RT services in 2013 [9].

21.4.2   Cancer Statistics in Djibouti

A total of 765 new cancer cases were reported by GLOBOCAN in 2020. Breast cancer has the highest percentage among new cases (24.7%), followed by cervix uteri and colorectal cancers with 8.2% and 7.6%, respectively (Fig. 21.4). Breast cancer was the leading cancer among females with 189 cases, and prostate cancer was the leading cancer in males with 37 cases (Table 21.3) [2].

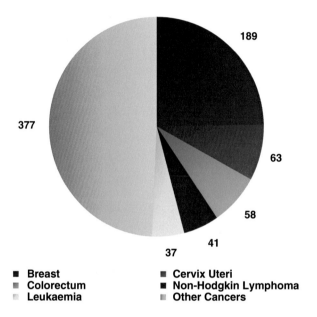

Fig. 21.4 Cancer incident cases in the Republic of Djibouti (2020) [2]. Used with permission from International Agency of Research on Cancer (IARC)/GLOBOCAN

Table 21.3 Sex-specified new cancer cases in the Republic of Djibouti (2020) [2]

Male		Female	
Cancer type	Statistic 2020	Cancer type	Statistic 2020
Prostate	37 (12.9%)	Breast	189 (39.5%)
Colorectum	33 (11.5%)	Cervix uteri	63 (13.2%)
Non-Hodgkin lymphoma	29 (10.1%)	Ovary	27 (5.6%)
Leukemia	21 (7.3%)	Colorectum	25 (5.2%)
Liver	20 (7%)	Thyroid	21 (4.4%)

Source: Used with permission from International Agency of Research on Cancer (IARC)/GLOBOCAN

21.5   Collective Data of Cancer Mortality

The 2020 cancer mortality rates of Qatar, Comoros, and Djibouti are illustrated for the year 2018 (Fig. 21.5) [2, 10–12].

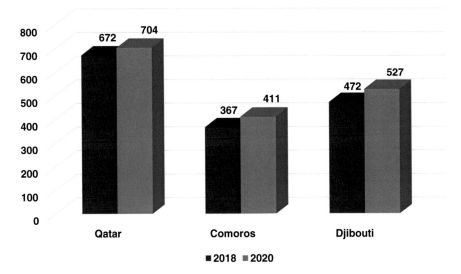

Fig. 21.5 Cancer mortality data of Qatar, Comoros, and Djibouti (2018 & 2020) [2, 10–12]. Used with permission from International Agency of Research on Cancer (IARC)/GLOBOCAN and WHO. (This adaptation is not published by IARC/GLOBOCAN and WHO. Hence, none of them are responsible for the content or accuracy of this adaptation)

21.6 Oncology Care Developmental Systems in Qatar, Comoros, Djibouti

Qatar has one of the highest per capita incomes worldwide. It has been striving to articulate the best strategies that can reform the oncology care infrastructure of the state [1]. Whereas the cancer care data for the Comoros and Djibouti was limited and acquired through the cancer country profiles elucidated by World Health Organization (WHO) (Table 21.4) [10–12].

The data on human resources for Qatar, Comoros, and Djibouti is presented in Fig. 21.6. Few oncology care manpower fields were not available.

Table 21.4 Overview of oncology care profile for Qatar, Comoros, Djibouti [10–12]

Initiatives	Year	Qatar	Comoros	Djibouti
Mapping oncology services				
Integrated NCD plan	2019	N/A	Under development	N/A
NCCP (including cancer types)	2019	Operational	Do not know	Not in effect
No. of treatment services (surgery, radiotherapy, chemotherapy)	2019	3	1	1
Pathology services	2019	Available	Not available	Available
Early detection program/guidelines for 4 cancers (breast, cervix, colon, childhood)	2019	3 cancer(s)	0 cancer(s)	0 cancer(s)
Availability of opioids[a] for pain management	2015–2017	195	4	0
No. of public cancer centers per 10,000 cancer patients	2019	7.9	–	–
Oncology system capacity				
Availability of population-based cancer registry (PBCR)	2019	High quality PBCR	No information	No information
Quality of mortality registration[b]	2007–2016	Low	No coverage	No coverage
No. of external beam radiotherapy[c]	2019	23.8	0.0	0.0
No. of mammographs[c]	2020	111.1	19.6	59.3
No. of CT scanners[c]	2020	246.0	19.6	59.3
No. of MRI scanners[c]	2020	309.5	0.0	14.8
No. of PET or PET/CT scanners[c]	2020	15.9	0.0	0.0

Used with permission from World Health Organization (WHO) (This adaptation is not published by WHO. Hence, WHO is not responsible for the content or accuracy of this adaptation)
[a]Defined daily doses for statistical purposes (S-DDD) per million inhabitants per day
[b]The mortality estimates for this country have a high degree of uncertainty because they are not based on any national NCD mortality data
[c]Per 10,000 cancer patients

State of Qatar

No. of radiation oncologists**	2019	N/A
No. of medical physicists**	2019	158.7
No. of surgeons**	2011	531.7
No. of radiologists**	2019	N/A
No. of nuclear medicine physicians**	2019	39.7
No. of medical & pathology lab scientists**	2006	4000.0

Union of the Comoros

No. of radiation oncologists**	2019	N/A
No. of medical physicists**	2019	0.0
No. of surgeons**	N/A	N/A
No. of radiologists**	2019	N/A
No. of nuclear medicine physicians**	2019	0.0
No. of medical & pathology lab scientists**	2012	N/A

Republic of Djibouti

No. of radiation oncologists**	2019	N/A
No. of medical physicists**	2019	0.0
No. of surgeons**	2013	252.2
No. of radiologists**	2019	N/A
No. of nuclear medicine physicians**	2019	0.0
No. of medical & pathology lab scientists**	2005	44.5

*Per 10,000 cancer patients

Fig. 21.6 Oncology Manpower in Qatar, Comoros, and Djibouti [10–12]. Used with permission from World Health Organization (WHO). (This adaptation is not published by WHO. Hence, WHO is not responsible for the content or accuracy of this adaptation)

21.7 Cancer Care Challenges

Cancer control plans in countries where the health system is still evolving have been aggravated by a lack of skilled professionals, high treatment and diagnostic costs, and the emergence of complicated personalized systematic treatment plans. Moreover, there are many factors, for instance, culture and habits, that contribute to indigent cancer awareness and prevention among the community. The supreme level of public awareness and education in Arab countries is yet to be achieved since Arab women only seek medical check-up when their cancer has developed to locally advanced or metastatic stages. This leads to late presentation, substandard patient outcomes and imprecise epidemiological data. There are a few considerable barriers to improving cancer outcomes in the Arab communities, including hurdles generated by the dissociation of innovative cancer research from service delivery, the fact that public awareness concerning cancer is relatively lower than misconceptions about the disease that are quite high, low uptake of screening programs in the Arab community perhaps owing to health and social beliefs about the disease, family relationships, shame or embarrassment, discomfort, fatalism and social stigma [13]. A few more challenges for optimum cancer care services include reliable diagnostics (in addition to advanced pathology services and staging), fragmented treatment option (chiefly for radiotherapy administration along with complete scope of systematic treatment), establishment and upkeep of cancer data registries for their respective countries, and coordination of multi-disciplinary spheres to broaden outreach programs for the community [13].

There is a lack of cancer data from the Comoros and Djibouti. Moreover, cancer research is nominal in these countries. A patient-centered approach is required to provide excellent care for their patients. Health authorities should implement feasible strategic plans to expand cancer control and prevention measures in the community.

21.8 Conclusion

Qatar has one of the highest per capita incomes across the globe. It has invested in healthcare infrastructure and state-of-the-art technologies, which resulted in upgraded cancer care facilities across the country. The research and other oncology supporting fields are also at an advanced stage. Conversely, oncology care services in the Comoros and Djibouti are still underdeveloped. This chapter highlighted epidemiology and cancer services in the respective countries while indicating unavailable facilities through WHO data.

Conflict of Interest Authors have no conflict of interest to declare.

References

1. Qoronfleh MW. Pathway to excellence in cancer care: learning from Qatar's experience. Precis Med Sci. 2020;9(2):51–61.
2. Ferlay J, Ervik M, Lam F, Colombet M, Mery L, Piñeros M, Znaor A, Soerjomataram I, Bray F. Global cancer observatory: cancer today. Lyon: International Agency for Research on Cancer; 2020. Available from: https://gco.iarc.fr/today. Accessed 21 Aug 2021
3. https://www.britannica.com/place/Comoros. Accessed Aug 2021.
4. Singh GK, Azuine RE, Siahpush M. Global inequalities in cervical cancer incidence and mortality are linked to deprivation, low socioeconomic status, and human development. Int J MCH AIDS. 2012;1(1):17.
5. https://www.britannica.com/place/Djibouti. Accessed Aug 2021.
6. United States Department of State. Bureau of Public Affairs. (1988). Djibouti. Department of State Publication background notes series, p. 1–7.
7. https://www.presidence.dj/sousmenu.php?ID=18. Accessed Aug 2021.
8. Hamdi Y, Abdeljaoued-Tej I, Zatchi AA, Abdelhak S, Boubaker S, Brown JS, Benkahla A. Cancer in Africa: the untold story. Front Oncol. 2021:11.
9. Yap ML, Zubizarreta E, Bray F, Ferlay J, Barton M. Global access to radiotherapy services: have we made progress during the past decade? J Glob Oncol. 2016;2(4):207–15.
10. https://www.who.int/publications/m/item/cancer-qat-2020. Accessed Aug 2021. Used with permission from World Health Organization (WHO) (This adaptation is not published by WHO. Hence, WHO is not responsible for the content or accuracy of this adaptation).
11. https://www.who.int/publications/m/item/cancer-com-2020. Accessed Aug 2021. Used with permission from World Health Organization (WHO) (This adaptation is not published by WHO. Hence, WHO is not responsible for the content or accuracy of this adaptation).
12. https://www.who.int/publications/m/item/cancer-dji-2020. Accessed Aug 2021. Used with permission from World Health Organization (WHO) (This adaptation is not published by WHO. Hence, WHO is not responsible for the content or accuracy of this adaptation).
13. Brown R, Kerr K, Haoudi A, Darzi A. Tackling cancer burden in the Middle East: Qatar as an example. Lancet Oncol. 2012;13(11):e501–8.

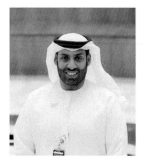

Humaid O. Al-Shamsi is the director of VPS oncology services in the United Arab Emirates, which is the largest cancer care provider network in the UAE. He is also the President of the Emirates Oncology Society and an adjunct professor at the college of medicine—University of Sharjah. Prof. Al-Shamsi holds triple specialty board certifications in medical oncology from the UK, the USA, and Canada. He completed his bachelor of science and bachelor of medicine from Cork University, the national university of Ireland, with honors in 2005. He then completed his internal medicine residency followed by medical oncology fellowship, and he then completed a subspecialty combined fellowship in gastrointestinal and palliative oncology at McMaster University in Canada in 2013. He then joined MD Anderson Cancer Center, The University of Texas, Houston, USA as an assistant professor from 2014 to 2017. Prof. Al-Shamsi is the founder of Burjeel Cancer institute at Burjeel Medical City in Abu Dhabi, UAE, which is the most comprehensive cancer center in the UAE. He has more than 70 peer-reviewed articles and book chapters. His research focus is on precision medicine and health policies related to cancer care in the UAE and the Arab region. He was awarded the researcher of the year in 2020 and 2021 by the Emirates Oncology Society.

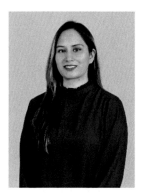

Faryal Iqbal holds an undergraduate degree in Molecular Biology and Biotechnology. Subsequently, she earned a postgraduate qualification in Molecular Genetics from Pakistan, where she worked on finding the association between *XRCC1* gene polymorphism and radiation exposure in healthcare workers. She is currently working with an oncology-specific research group and serving in the domains of scientific writing, data management, supervision of medical internees, and providing editorial assistance. Ms. Iqbal's research interests and publications encompass genetics and oncology. She intends to support research across the oncology key areas, including prevention, diagnosis, and treatment. Her focus is on preparing for future adoption of genomic technology and increased use of genomic information as part of the cancer diagnostic and therapeutic pathways.

Chapter 22
Breast Cancer in the Arab World

Salwa Saadeh and Hikmat Abdel-Razeq

22.1 Introduction

Breast cancer is the most common malignancy diagnosed in females worldwide [1, 2], and despite enormous efforts at early detection and the presence of many new and evolving treatments, it remains the leading cause of cancer-related mortality in females as well [3, 4]. The estimated incidence of new breast cancer cases was around 2.26 million in 2020, with a cumulative of 685,000 breast cancer-related deaths worldwide in that year [2]. Cancer in general, and breast cancer in particular, is a growing health issue in the Arab World.

The Arab world comprises 22 countries with memberships in the Arab League, spanning across the Middle East and North Africa. Unfortunately, many of these countries are troubled with financial and political instabilities, some being active war zones. Although there are significant linguistic and cultural ties and similarities, there are also many significant social and economic differences in addition to some ethnic and genetic variations. According to the World Bank ranking, some Arab countries are ranked as high income (i.e., Gulf countries) while others are ranked as low income (i.e., Syria, Sudan, and Somalia), with many in between [5]. These differences have many implications on education, social perspectives, and health care system development and organization in their respective countries, in addition to direct effects on the policies prioritizing health care resources' allocations.

S. Saadeh
Department of Internal Medicine, King Hussein Cancer Center, Amman, Jordan
e-mail: ss.10559@khcc.jo

H. Abdel-Razeq (✉)
Department of Internal Medicine, King Hussein Cancer Center, Amman, Jordan

School of Medicine, The University of Jordan, Amman, Jordan
e-mail: habdelrazeq@khcc.jo

© The Author(s) 2022
H. O. Al-Shamsi et al. (eds.), *Cancer in the Arab World*,
https://doi.org/10.1007/978-981-16-7945-2_22

353

In the following review, we attempt to discuss the unique features of breast cancer and breast cancer care within Arab Countries. Although the Arab World is viewed as a single region, it is important, as mentioned above, to understand data in the context of the vast variations in political stability and social and economic development variations between the different countries.

22.2   Epidemiology of Breast Cancer in Arab Countries

The exact prevalence and incidence of breast cancer cases in the Arab world are not known due to the lack of well-structured cancer registries in most of these countries. In addition, mortality registries and disease-specific mortality records are lacking and largely unknown. Data on breast cancer in the Arab World mostly stem from literature reviews of published data from individual countries in the forms of retrospective data reports and published individual institution records, many of which are high-quality reports published in peer-reviewed journals.

From available data from the years 2010, 2013, and most recently 2020, breast cancer is thought to be the most common malignancy diagnosed in Arab women, estimating somewhere between 14–42% of all tumors [6, 7] in some reports, and between 17.7–19% of all new cancers in others [8], depending on individual countries and type of reports reviewed. Age-standardized incidence also varies between countries and ranges between 9.5 and 50 cases per 100,000 women per year [7]. Although the incidence of new cases and burden of the disease seem to be lower than that in the more developed Western World and the global averages in general, the incidence has been rising over the past few decades [7, 9, 10], and the rate of increase seems to be similar to the global trend [9]. This increase can be partly attributed to advances in medical care and diagnosis, implementation of limited screening programs leading to better diagnosis of previously unidentified cases, in addition to better reporting. However, this can also be partially attributed to an actual increase in disease burden due to demographic and lifestyle changes. More Arab societies and women are being influenced by Westernized lifestyles such as dietary habits, delayed age at marriage and first pregnancies, lower reproductive rates, in addition to more smoking and more use of oral contraceptives and Hormonal Replacement Therapies (HRTs) [9–11].

The median age at the time of diagnosis of women with breast cancer in the Arab world is almost a decade younger than in industrialized countries such as Europe and the USA. It is estimated in different reports to be around 48–52 years compared to around 63 years, with somewhat between one-half and two-thirds of diagnosed individuals below the age of 50 [7, 10, 12, 13], compared to only about 23% below the age of 50 in the United States [14]. This can largely be attributed however to the young population structure. In addition to the younger median population age, elderly Arab women are also likely to be under-represented and more frequently underdiagnosed in relevant analyses, as they are less likely to obtain a mammogram or seek medical care for breast disease [15, 16].

22.3   Breast Cancer Screening and Early Detection

Unfortunately, most Arab countries lack a structured universal screening program. Several awareness campaigns take place on different occasions, especially in the month of October, Breast Cancer Awareness Month. These kinds of campaigns take place in the form of media interventions, advertisements, public physician interviews, and awareness lectures/speeches. Although some promising screening program initiatives have been recently raised in some countries, most women who undergo screening mammograms are either self-motivated, advised by afflicted family members, or by motivated physicians. These screening procedures are, however, not consistently covered by medical insurances. In addition, there is a lack in the number and distribution of mammography centers, and trained personnel, and the existing units are not universally monitored for quality, results, and reporting by any overseeing agency [10, 17].

Although some researchers and experts have suggested that the younger median age at the time of initial breast cancer diagnosis in the Arab World should trigger a younger age for breast cancer screening advice and target population [7, 10], others have challenged this suggestion since the median age of diagnosis in a population is thought to be less relevant than age-specific incidence when forming policies and recommendations [9, 18, 19].

22.4   Diagnosis and Stage

More women in the Arab World present with more advanced diseases compared to Western countries. More patients are diagnosed with larger tumors, positive lymph nodes, and inflammatory breast cancer, and metastatic diseases [17, 20–24]. Reports assessing tumor size at the time of initial presentation have estimated that as high as 70–80% of tumors were more than 2 cm in diameter [20, 21]. Similarly, lymph node involvement at the time of initial diagnosis has also been reported at high percentages of 50–80% [22–24].

Inflammatory breast cancer, being the most aggressive form of non-metastatic breast cancer, is associated with the highest mortality. It is considered rare and reported in only 1–2% of new breast cancer diagnoses in the United States [25, 26]. In the Arab world, reported rates are as high as 11% of newly diagnosed cases [27, 28]. Unfortunately, the same applies to a higher incidence of de novo metastatic disease with rates as high as 13.4% compared to 6% [17, 29, 30].

There are many proposed reasons for the late diagnosis and advanced initial stage. Although genetic, adverse molecular variations and racial factors have been proposed; delayed presentation and late seeking of medical advice are likely to play a major role, as well. In addition to impaired access to adequate care, several psycho-social aspects also influence women's decisions to delay diagnosis and treatment. This is discussed in an upcoming section.

22.5 Obstacles to High-Quality Standardized Management

One major obstacle to optimal cancer care in general and breast cancer care in particular in the Arab region is the social, financial, and political instability of many countries in this region. Some countries are directly inflicted by wars, leading to the routing of health care resources away from many Non-Communicable Diseases (NCDs) such as cancer. With these wars and conflicted areas, there is a growing refugee crisis, as many people move from politically unstable areas to financially unstable countries. There has been an increasing awareness about this issue in recent years [31]. The repercussions of the Syrian crisis and refugee cancer care status have been comprehensively reviewed in several recent articles, for example [32–35]. Cancer care results in a significant strain on health care systems in hosting countries, both financially and ethically. Although there continue to be international medical relief efforts, both through non-governmental and governmental agencies, the costly nature of cancer care, and the need to prioritize already limited resources, leads in many instances to suboptimal care or even neglect. The need for an increase in funding, in addition to multidisciplinary care teams and evidence-based standard operating procedures in these areas, is highly needed to coordinate and prioritize care and resources, but this is yet to be established [32, 33].

Although the role of multidisciplinary care is well established in cancer care to ensure the best available management approach and treatment outcomes [36], this is seldom available or practiced in the majority of healthcare systems in the Arab region. With few exceptions, many, even though not all, Arab countries lack universal access to comprehensive cancer care centers or patient care by specialized cancer care teams with the adequate advanced oncologic training and expertise needed to provide required complicated treatment plans, leading to suboptimal cancer care. As an example, the rate of modified radical mastectomies in Arab countries is much higher than that in internationally reported literature, reaching up to about two-thirds of cases [10, 20, 37–41], and is as high as 88% in some reports from Syria [42]. Around 21% of patients undergoing modified radical mastectomy will develop clinically significant lymphedema [43], a complication that could potentially be avoided in a subset of patients.

One important reason for a high rate of radical procedures in breast cancer is the advanced stage at the time of disease presentation. However, many of these procedures could otherwise be potentially avoidable, and some reasons for this unexpected high rate have been explored in published reports. Lack of enough radiation therapy centers and accelerator machines in some countries are additional contributing factors [44]. Professional experience in breast-conserving surgery, sentinel lymph node sampling, skin-sparing and nipple-sparing mastectomies is not available in most of the low-income Arab countries and contributes to a higher rate of more radical procedures. Similarly, reconstructive surgeries are not always available, and when they are, not consistently covered by insurance [17].

Cost of cancer treatment in general, and new targeted and immunotherapy in breast cancer, in particular, is a major issue in The Arab World. There has been an approval of several expensive novel agents for breast cancer in recent years. Although these treatments might be readily available in some high-income Arab countries, access to these medications and financial coverage by governmental and non-governmental insurance plans and agencies is limited in many others.

Cost and financial burden also play a role in the limitation of many other aspects of breast cancer care in the Arab world. One major example is genetic testing and counseling. Almost 10–15% of breast cancers worldwide are thought to be inherited [45], and genetic testing for the most prevalent cancer genes such as *BRCA1* and *BRCA2* has become standard in many countries and is recommended by international guidelines [46]. However, this is not widely practiced or standardized in most Arab countries, reports from these areas are limited, and little is known about the role of these and other genetic mutations in Arab patients, although some reports suggest a higher prevalence in Arab women [47]. One report from Jordan, from a single institution's experience, showed that about 14% of screened high-risk breast cancer patients had a deleterious mutation [48]. Two different studies in Tunisia showed contrasting variable results for *BRCA1* testing in selected populations with a reported prevalence of 16% and 38% [49, 50]. Reports from Lebanon, Morocco, Egypt, and a few other countries have also shown variable results [51–57], likely reflecting variations in selection criteria for testing referrals, different testing techniques, and small numbers of patients enrolled [48]. This lack of standardized and universal testing contributes to limitations of proper screening and follow-up in patients and their family members, further leading to late diagnoses and advanced disease stage at presentation. Cost and financial burden are not the only factors contributing to inconsistent genetic testing and counseling in the Arab populations, however, with psycho-social aspects also playing a significant role in patient acceptance of testing, and sharing of results.

22.6   Unique Psycho-Social Aspects of Breast Cancer in the Arab World

Unfortunately, even in this time and age, cancer in general and breast cancer, in particular, is associated with significant social stigmatization in many countries and societies in the Arab world, regardless of socio-economic and educational development in these countries. Women diagnosed with breast cancer often describe a feeling of shame or guilt, and fear of being blamed for having cancer, as at times, it is regarded as a sign of punishment for undisclosed sins [8]. In addition, there is added stress of fearing they can pass their illness to their daughters, or that the females in the family are considered potentially diseased, and thus decreasing their chances of future marriage. This is more pronounced in less urban parts of the Arab world where arranged marriages and consanguinity are still a significant part of these societies. Light has been shed on these issues in several different reports from the area [58–64]. The importance of this particular aspect stems from the fact that this leads many women to conceal their illness, delay seeking medical advice, and delay treatment despite active symptoms and this results in late presentations and more advanced disease stages at the time of diagnosis. In addition, this is an important factor hampering the progress of national efforts for the promotion and implementation of screening programs. Much progress has been made over the past few years in awareness campaigns in many parts of the Arab world, and much more is still needed.

22.7 Conclusion and Future Directions

Breast cancer is the most common cancer diagnosed among women worldwide as well as in Arab countries. More advanced-stage and younger age at presentations are common features in the region. Resources and staff availability are quite variable. Opportunities exist to up-scale the quality of care provided and that should reflect positively on treatment outcomes.

Conflict of Interest Authors have no conflict of interest to declare.

References

1. Ferlay J, Soerjomataram I, Dikshit R, Eser S, Mathers C, Rebelo M, et al. Cancer incidence and mortality worldwide: sources, methods and major patterns in GLOBOCAN 2012. Int J Cancer. 2015;136(5):E359–86.
2. Sung H, Ferlay J, Siegel RL, Laversanne M, Soerjomataram I, Jemal A, et al. Global cancer statistics 2020: GLOBOCAN estimates of incidence and mortality worldwide for 36 cancers in 185 countries. CA Cancer J Clin. 2021b;71(3):209–49. https://doi.org/10.3322/caac.21660.
3. Ferlay J, Shin HR, Bray F, Forman D, Mathers C, Parkin DM. Estimates of worldwide burden of cancer in 2008: GLOBOCAN 2008. Int J Cancer. 2010;127:2893–917.
4. GBD 2015 Eastern Mediterranean Region Cancer Collaborators. Burden of cancer in the Eastern Mediterranean Region, 2005–2015: findings from the global burden of disease 2015 study. Int J Public Health. 2018;63:151–64.
5. The World Bank: Countries Data. https://data.worldbank.org/country
6. El Saghir SN, Abulkhair O. Epidemiology, prevention and management guidelines for breast cancer in Arab countries. Pan Arab J Oncol. 2010;3:12–8.
7. Chouchane L, Boussen H, Sastry K. Breast cancer in Arab populations: molecular characteristics and disease management implications. Lancet Oncol. 2013;14(10):e417–24.
8. Fearon D, Hughes S, Brearly S. Experiences of breast cancer in Arab countries: a thematic synthesis. Qual Life Res. 2020;29(2):313–24.
9. Hashim M, Al-Shamsi F, Al-Marzooqi N, Al-Qasemi S, Mokdad A, Khan G. Burden of breast cancer in the Arab world: findings from global burden of disease, 2016. J Epidemiol Glob Health. 2018;1(1–2):54–8.
10. Al Saghir N, Khalil M, Eid T, et al. Trends in epidemiology and management of breast cancer in developing Arab countries: a literature and registry analysis. Int J Surg. 2007 Aug;5(4):225–33.
11. Ravichandran K, Al-Zahrani AS. Association of reproductive factors with the incidence of breast cancer in Gulf Cooperation Council countries. East Mediterr Health J. 2009;15:612–21.

12. Najjar H, Easson A. Age at diagnosis of breast cancer in Arab nations. Int J Surg. 2010;8:448–52.
13. SEER cancer stat facts: female breast cancer. National Cancer Institute. Bethesda, MD. https://seer.cancer.gov/statfacts/html/breast.html
14. Smigal C, Jemal A, Ward E, Cokkinides V, Smith R, Howe HL, et al. Trends in breast cancer by race and ethnicity: update 2006. CA Cancer J Clin. 2006;56:168–83.
15. Mellon S, Gauthier J, Cichon M, Hammad A, Simon MS. Knowledge, attitude, and beliefs of Arab-American women regarding inherited cancer risk. J Genet Couns. 2013;22:268–76.
16. Brown R, Kerr K, Haoudi A, Darzi A. Tackling cancer burden in the Middle East: Qatar as an example. Lancet Oncol. 2012;13:e501–8.
17. Abdel-Razeq H, Mansour A, Jaddan D. Breast cancer care in Jordan. JCO Glob Oncol. 2020;6:260–8.
18. Corbex M, Harford JB. Perspectives on breast cancer in Arab populations. Lancet Oncol. 2013;14:e582.
19. Harford JB. Breast-cancer early detection in low-income and middle-income countries: do what you can versus one size fits all. Lancet Oncol. 2011;12:306–12.
20. Fakhro AE, Fateha BE, Al-Asheeri N, Al-Ekri SA. Breast cancer: patient characteristics and survival analysis at Salmaniya Medical Complex, Bahrain. East Mediterr Health J. 1999;5:430–9.
21. Missaoui N, Jaidene L, Abdelkrim SB, et al. Breast cancer in Tunisia: clinical and pathological findings. Asian Pac J Cancer Prev. 2011;12:169–72.
22. El-Zaemey S, Nagi N, Fritschi L, Heyworth J. Breast cancer among Yemeni women using the National Oncology Centre Registry 2004–2010. Cancer Epidemiol. 2012;36:249–53.
23. Ezzat AA, Ibrahim EM, Raja MA, Al-Sobhi S, Rostom A, Stuart RK. Locally advanced breast cancer in Saudi Arabia: high frequency of stage III in a young population. Med Oncol. 1999;16:95–103.
24. Zidan J, Sikorsky BW, Sharabi A, Friedman E, Steiner M. Differences in pathological and clinical features of breast cancer in Arab as compared to Jewish women in Northern Israel. Int J Cancer. 2012;131:924–9.
25. Goldner B, Behrendt C, Schollhammer H, Lee B, Chen S. Incidence of inflammatory breast cancer in women, 1992–2009, United States. Ann Surg Oncol. 2014;21(4):1267–70.
26. Anderson WF, Schairer C, Chen BE, Hance KW, Levine PH. Epidemiology of inflammatory breast cancer (IBC). Breast Dis. 2005–2006;22:9–23.
27. Boussen H, Bouzaiene H, Ben Hassouna J, Gamoudi A, Benna F, Rahal K. Infl ammatory breast cancer in Tunisia: reassessment of incidence and clinicopathological features. Semin Oncol. 2008;35:17–24.
28. Soliman AS, Banerjee M, Lo AC, et al. High proportion of inflammatory breast cancer in the population-based cancer registry of Gharbiah, Egypt. Breast J. 2009;15:432–4.
29. National Cancer Institute: Cancer stat facts: Female breast cancer. https://seer.cancer.gov/statfacts/html/breast.html
30. Cancer Research: UK Breast cancer incidence (invasive) statistics. https://www.cancerresearchuk.org/health-professional/cancer-statistics/statistics-by-cancer-type/breast-cancer/incidence-invasive
31. El Saghir NS, Pérez S, de Celis E, Fares JE, Sullivan R. Cancer care for refugees and displaced populations: Middle East conflicts and global natural disasters. Am Soc Clin Oncol Educ Book. 2018;23(38):433–40.
32. Spiegel PB, Cheaib JG, Aziz SA, Abrahim O, Woodman M, Khalifa A, Jang M, Mateen FJ. Cancer in Syrian refugees in Jordan and Lebanon between 2015 and 2017. Lancet Oncol. 2020 May;21(5):e280–91.
33. Spiegel P, Khalifa A, Mateen FJ. Cancer in refugees in Jordan and Syria between 2009 and 2012: challenges and the way forward in humanitarian emergencies. Lancet Oncol. 2014 Jun;15(7):e290–7.
34. Abdul-Khalek RA, Guo P, Sharp F, Gheorghe A, Shamieh O, Kutluk T, Fouad F, Coutts A, Aggarwal A, Mukherji D, Abu-Sittah G, Chalkidou K, Sullivan R, R4HC-MENA

Collaboration. The economic burden of cancer care for Syrian refugees: a population-based modelling study. Lancet Oncol. 2020;21(5):637–44.

35. Akik C, Ghattas H, Mesmar S, Rabkin M, El-Sadr WM, Fouad FM. Host country responses to non-communicable diseases amongst Syrian refugees: a review. Confl Heal. 2019 Mar;22(13):8.

36. Anderson BO, Braun S, Carlson RW, et al. Overview of breast health care guidelines for countries with limited resources. Breast J. 2003;2(Suppl. 9):S42e5035.

37. Elattar I, Zaghloul M, Omar A, Mokhtar N. Breast cancer in Egypt. Cairo: National Cancer Institute of Egypt, NCI Cairo Publications; 2007.

38. Abdel-Fattah M, Lotfy NS, Bassili A, Anwar M, Mari E, Bedwani R, et al. Current treatment modalities of breast cancer patients in Alexandria, Egypt. Breast. 2001;10(6):523e9.

39. Al-Moundhri M, Al-Bahrani B, Pervez I, et al. The outcome of treatment of breast cancer in a developing country-Oman. Breast. 2004;13:139e45.

40. Nissan A, Spira RM, Hamburger T, et al. Clinical profile of breast cancer in Arab and Jewish women in the Jerusalem area. Am J Surg. 2004;188:62e7.

41. Maalej M, Frikha H, Ben Salem S, et al. Breast cancer in Tunisia: clinical and epidemiological study. Bull Cancer. 1999;86:302–6.

42. Mzayek F, Asfar T, Rastam S, Maziak W. Neoplastic diseases in Aleppo, Syria. Eur J Cancer Prev. 2002;11(5):503–7.

43. Morcos BB, Al Ahmad F, Anabtawi I, et al. Lymphedema: a significant health problem for women with breast cancer in Jordan. Saudi Med J. 2013;34:62–6.

44. Semaan S. Breast cancer in Syria. Pan Arab Cancer Congress Proceedings, Damascus, Syria; 2003.

45. Peto J, Collins N, Barfoot R, et al. Prevalence of BRCA1 and BRCA2 gene mutations in patients with early-onset breast cancer. J Natl Cancer Inst. 1999;91:943–9.

46. National Comprehensive Cancer Network: =Clinical practice guidelines in oncology: Genetic/ familial high-risk assessment—Breast, ovarian, and pancreatic. https://www.nccn.org/professionals/physician_gls/pdf/genetics_bop.pdf

47. Rouba A, Kaisi N, Al-Chaty E, Badin R, Pals G, Young C, Worsham MJ. Patterns of allelic loss at the BRCA1 locus in Arabic women with breast cancer. Int J Mol Med. 2000;6(5):565–9.

48. Abdel-Razeq H, Abujamous L, Jadaan D. Patterns and prevalence of germline *BRCA1* and *BRCA2* mutations among high-risk breast cancer patients in Jordan: a study of 500 patients. J Oncol. 2020;2020:8362179.

49. Troudi W, Uhrhammer N, Romdhane KB, Sibille C, Amor MB, Khodjet El Khil H, Jalabert T, Mahfoudh W, Chouchane L, Ayed FB, Bignon YJ, Elgaaied AB. Complete mutation screening and haplotype characterization of BRCA1 gene in Tunisian patients with familial breast cancer. Cancer Biomark. 2008;4(1):11–8.

50. Mahfoudh W, Bouaouina N, Ahmed SB, Gabbouj S, Shan J, Mathew R, Uhrhammer N, Bignon YJ, Troudi W, Elgaaied AB, Hassen E, Chouchane L. Hereditary breast cancer in Middle Eastern and North African (MENA) populations: identification of novel, recurrent and founder BRCA1 mutations in the Tunisian population. Mol Biol Rep. 2012;39(2):1037–46.

51. El Saghir NS, Zgheib NK, Assi HA, Khoury KE, Bidet Y, Jaber SM, et al. BRCA1 and BRCA2 mutations in ethnic Lebanese Arab women with high hereditary risk breast cancer. Oncologist. 2015;20:357–64.

52. Jalkh N, Nassar-Slaba J, Chouery E, Salem N, Uhrchammer N, Golmard L, et al. Prevalance of BRCA1 and BRCA2 mutations in familial breast cancer patients in Lebanon. Hered Cancer Clin Pract. 2012;10:7.

53. Laraqui A, Uhrhammer N, Lahlou-Amine I, Rhaffouli EL, El Baghdadi J, Dehayni M, et al. Mutation screening of the BRCA1 gene in early onset and familial breast/ovarian cancer in Moroccan population. Int J Med Sci. 2013;10:60–7.

54. Ibrahim SS, Hafez EE, Hashishe MM. Presymptomatic breast cancer in Egypt: role of BRCA1 and BRCA2 tumor suppressor genes mutations detection. J Exp Clin Cancer Res. 2010;29:82–91.

55. Awadelkarim KD, Aceto GVS, Elhaj A, Morgano A, Mohamedani AA, et al. BRCA1 and BRCA2 status in a central Sudanese series of breast cancer patients: interactions with genetic, ethnic and reproductive factors. Breast Cancer Res Treat. 2007;102:189–99.
56. Hasan TN, Shafi G, Syed NA, Alsaif MA, Alsaif AA, Alshatwi AA. Lack of association of BRCA1 and BRCA2 variants with breast cancer in an ethnic population of Saudi Arabia, an emerging high-risk area. Asian Pac J Cancer Prev. 2013;14:5671–4.
57. Troudi W, Uhrhammer N, Romdhane KB, Sibille C, Amor MB, El Khil HK, et al. Complete mutation screening and haplotype characterization of BRCA1 gene in Tunisian patients with familial breast cancer. Cancer Biomark. 2008;4:11–8.
58. Al-Azri M, Al-Awisi H, Al-Rasbi S, El-Shafie K, Al-Hinai M, Al-Habsi H, et al. Psychosocial impact of breast cancer diagnosis among Omani women. Oman Med J. 2014;29(6):437–44.
59. Alqaissi NM, Dickerson SS. Exploring common meanings of social support as experienced by Jordanian women with breast cancer. Cancer Nurs. 2010;33(5):353–61.
60. Doumit MA, El Saghir N, Abu-Saad Huijer H, Kelley JH, Nassar N. Living with breast cancer, a Lebanese experience. Eur J Oncol Nurs. 2010;14(1):42–8.
61. Elobaid Y, Aw TC, Lim JNW, Hamid S, Grivna M. Breast cancer presentation delays among Arab and national women in the UAE: a qualitative study. SSM Population Health. 2016;2:155–63.
62. Jassim GA, Whitford DL. Understanding the experiences and quality of life issues of Bahraini women with breast cancer. Soc Sci Med. 2014;107:189–95.
63. McEwan J, Underwood C, Corbex M. "Injustice! That is the cause": a qualitative study of the social, economic, and structural determinants of late diagnosis and treatment of breast cancer in Egypt. Cancer Nurs. 2014;37(6):468–75.
64. Nizamli F, Anoosheh M, Mohammadi E. Experiences of Syrian women with breast cancer regarding chemotherapy: a qualitative study. Nurs Health Sci. 2011;13(4):481–7.

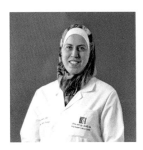

Salwa Saadeh, MBBS, is a Hematologist/Medical oncologist at King Hussein Cancer Center, Amman, Jordan. She obtained her medical degree from Jordan University of Science and Technology, 2008. She completed postgraduate training at King Abdullah University Hospital and King Hussein Cancer Center (Jordan). She completed an advanced fellowship at Mayo Clinic (USA) and received a diploma in Cancer biology and Therapeutics from Harvard University (USA). Dr. Saadeh holds the Jordanian boards in Internal Medicine and Medical Oncology, and MRCP(UK)/Internal Medicine, MRCP(UK)-SCE/Medical Oncology, and European Board of Hematology.

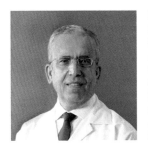

Hikmat Abdel-Razeq, MD, is the chairman of the Department of Internal Medicine, Chief Medical Officer and the Deputy Director General of King Hussein Cancer Center in Amman, Jordan. Additionally, he has been appointed as Professor of Medicine at the School of Medicine, University of Jordan. He obtained his medical degree from the University of Jordan, Amman in 1988 and had his postgraduate training at the Cleveland Clinic Foundation and the New York Medical College. Prof. Abdel-Razeq holds American Board certifications in Internal Medicine, Medical Oncology and Hematology. In addition to breast cancer, Prof. Abdel-Razeq has major interest and research in cancer-related thrombosis.

Chapter 23
Colorectal Cancer in the Arab World

Adhari AlZaabi

23.1 Status of CRC in Arab Countries

23.1.1 Incidence

According to the most recent GLOBOCAN report, Colorectal Cancer (CRC) is considered the third most commonly diagnosed cancer and the second leading cause of cancer-related death worldwide. It accounted for almost 1.8 million new cases, and 860,000 deaths in 2018. It is expected that the global CRC burden will increase by 60% by 2030 [1]. The global incidence and mortality of CRC vary according to the geographical areas and countries, which could be attributed to existing risk factors, ethnicity, comprehensiveness of cancer registries, availability of screening facilities and management protocols [2].

Fortunatly, the CRC incidence and CRC-related death is declining in the western countries [1]. On the other hand, there has been an obvious and rapid rise of CRC incidence and mortality across many developed countries in Asia, Eastern Europe and South America [3]. The Arab population is no exception, although the figures reported for colorectal cancer among Arabs are much lower than that for developed countries, yet the incidence of colorectal cancer in the Arab countries is increasing in the past ten years [4].

The Arab world has a population of >300 million people distributed among 22 countries delimited by Lebanon and Syria to the north, Morocco to the west, Yemen to the south, and Iraq to the east. It includes the 7 Gulf Cooperation Council (GCC) member countries, including Bahrain, Kuwait, Oman, Qatar, Saudi Arabia, United Arab Emirates, and Yemen.

A. AlZaabi (✉)
College of Medicine, Sultan Qaboos University, Muscat, Oman
e-mail: adhari@squ.edu.om

© The Author(s) 2022   363
H. O. Al-Shamsi et al. (eds.), *Cancer in the Arab World*,
https://doi.org/10.1007/978-981-16-7945-2_23

A rapid revolution and modernization have happened in this region at all levels, which cumulatively led to major changes in the disease burden profile where Non-Communicable Diseases exert a huge burden. That is mainly attributed to increased incidence of obesity, physical inactivity, stressful busy life, smoking, and dietary habits, which correlated with a dramatic increase in cancer incidence over the past 10 years [5].

Focusing on Colorectal Cancer (CRC), the incidence and mortality of CRC among Arabs have obviously increased in the last decade. For example, in the GCC countries, CRC is considered the second most common cancer among both genders with reported 2.3 fold and a 2.7 fold increase in newly diagnosed cases of CRC among male and female, respectively [4]. A similar trend has been reported from other Arab countries (Table 23.1).

From table 23.1, Comoros reported the least CRC Age-Standardized Rate (ASR) (4.5/100,000) of both genders among Arab countries, while Gaza Strip reported the maximum ASR (18.6/100,000). It is very noticeable from the GLOBOCAN report that there is a multi-fold increase in the ASR in this region compared to previously reported ASR in the region [4, 6–9].

The National Health Services in the GCC countries and the World Cancer Research Fund Report (WCRF) and the American Institute for Cancer Research (AICR) have linked this increase to the drastic changes in the lifestyle and food consumption patterns such as high daily calorie intake, increased consumption of carbohydrates and sedentary lifestyle plus increased sitting time regardless of physical activity. These factors have synergized with the genetic factors of cancer among Arabs and resulted in a noticeable increase in the incidence of cancer. In fact, studies in food consumption patterns have confirmed the high consumption of this diet that is considered a high-risk dietary profile for cancer in general and CRC specifically [4, 10]. A comprehensive longitudinal study is needed to evaluate the detailed dietary profile and sedentary lifestyle of Arabs and evaluate their correlation with CRC incidence.

23.1.2   Clinicopathological Parameters

23.1.2.1   Age

CRC tends to occur at a younger age among Arabs compared to western population. The median age for CRC among Arabs is found to be 60+/− 15 compared to the average age of 70 years in Westernized countries. The population structure of Arabs might explain this finding as the majority of the Arab population are in this age group [7, 9, 11–16] but more studies are needed to find out if this is a real increase in the incidence in this age group or is it the population structure effect.

Table 23.1 Estimated age-standardized incidence rates of Colorectal Cancer in 2020 across all ages in Arab countries compared to non-Arab countries

Estimated age-standardized incidence rates in 2020, Colorectal Cancer, all ages				
Population	Country	Both gender	Female	Male
Arab Population	Comoros	4.5	5.2	3.7
	South Sudan	5.7	5.1	6.3
	Egypt	6.1	6.2	5.8
	Sudan	6.3	6	6.6
	Djibouti	6.9	5.9	7.8
	Mauritania	7.2	6.1	8.6
	Iraq	8.7	6.9	10.8
	Somalia	9.3	8.6	10.1
	Oman	9.9	7.7	11.2
	Yemen	10.7	9.5	12
	Morocco	11.3	9.9	12.9
	Lebanon	12.2	9.5	15.2
	Kuwait	12.5	11.9	13.1
	Tunisia	12.7	11.7	14
	United Arab Emirates	13.1	17.3	11.5
	Bahrain	13.9	14.6	13.7
	Saudi Arabia	13.9	10.9	16.1
	Algeria	15.3	14.2	16.5
	Libya	15.7	15.1	16.7
	Qatar	15.7	20.6	13.6
	Jordan	17.7	18.4	17.2
	Gaza Strip and West Bank	18.6	16.7	20.7
Non-Arab Population	Democratic Republic of Korea	18.8	15.9	22.8
	Malaysia	19.6	18	21.2
	Turkey	20.6	16.2	26.2
	United States of America	25.6	22.9	28.7
	Germany	25.8	21.8	30.4
	Sweden	27.8	25.2	30.5
	France	30.1	24.9	36.3
	Canada	31.2	27.9	34.7
	Singapore	33	27.4	38.6
	United Kingdom	34.1	29	40
	Japan	38.5	30.5	47.3
	Islamic Republic of Iran	13.9	11.9	15.9

Data Source: Arnold M, Rutherford M, Lam F, Bray F, Ervik M, Soerjomataram I (2019). ICBP SURVMARK-2 online tool: International Cancer Survival Benchmarking. Lyon, France: International Agency for Research on Cancer. Available from: http://gco.iarc.fr/survival/survmark, accessed [05/Feb/2021]

23.1.2.2 Stage

Most CRC clinicopathological studies in the region reported an advanced stage (stage III and IV) cancer at diagnosis. Majority of CRC patients are diagnosed late when the tumor has already grown into a clinically detectable size causing alarming symptoms and signs [7, 9, 11–16]. It has been attributed mainly to lack of screening, poor awareness of the disease early symptoms and disconnected healthcare system. These patients either have ignored their symptoms since they are non-specific, or the primary care providers do not have high suspicion for cancer for such symptoms.

23.1.2.3 Lateralization

There are no consistent findings on the lateralization of CRC among the Arab population. Majority of studies of CRC in Arab countries found that the most affected site is the rectum, followed by sigmoid and distal colon. This is similar to reports from western and regional countries [7, 9, 11–17]. In fact, there is a noticeable shift toward proximal colon cancer in western countries which has been explained by the high success rate of CRC screening for detection of rectal and distal colon tumors, leaving the proximal colon cancer undetected till late in the disease [1, 18, 19].

23.1.3 Survival and Mortality

The CRC survival rate is lower in Arab countries compared to western countries. This is mainly because the majority of patients are detected late in an advanced stage due to lack of screening and poor awareness of signs and symptoms [9, 20]. The Age-standardized mortality rate in the Arab population compared to non-Arab countries is listed in Table 23.2 (constructed from Globocan 2018 report).

Egypt has the least estimated age-standardized mortality among Arab population (3.4) and Gaza strip has the highest among all Arab countries (11.2).

Prognosis of CRC that is diagnosed at a late stage is unfavorable with very limited treatment options available. The 5-years survival of CRC is highly dependent on the stage of the disease, being 95% for stage I CRC and decreasing to 70% for stage IV CRC [21]. This explains the relatively low survival rate of CRC among Arabs compared to western countries [16, 20, 22].

Table 23.2 Estimated age-standardized mortality rates of colorectal cancer in 2020 across all ages in Arab countries compared to non-Arab countries

Estimated age-standardized mortality rates in 2020, Colorectal Cancer, all ages				
Population	Country	Both gender	Female	Male
Arab Population	Egypt	3.4	3.4	3.3
	Sudan	3.9	3.6	4.2
	South Sudan	4.5	4	5.1
	Djibouti	5.3	4.6	6.1
	Iraq	5.4	4.4	6.8
	Mauritania	5.4	4.6	6.5
	Oman	5.7	4.5	6.2
	Morocco	6.2	5.4	7.2
	Tunisia	6.4	5.6	7.3
	Kuwait	6.6	6.1	7
	Lebanon	6.7	5	8.8
	United Arab Emirates	6.9	8.7	6.2
	Bahrain	7.1	7.5	6.8
	Saudi Arabia	7.3	5.6	8.7
	Somalia	7.7	7.1	8.4
	Yemen	7.7	6.9	8.6
	Syrian Arab Republic	8.2	7.2	9.4
	Algeria	8.3	7.7	9
	Qatar	9	10.9	8
	Jordan	9.6	9.6	9.7
	Libya	10.2	9.8	11
	Gaza Strip and West Bank	11.2	9.9	12.7
Non-Arab Population	Canada	9.9	8	12
	United States of America	8	6.7	9.4
	Germany	9.9	7.3	12.9
	Turkey	10.1	7.8	13
	Malaysia	10.2	9.4	11
	France	10.4	8.1	13.3
	Sweden	10.8	9.7	12.1
	Democratic Republic of Korea	10.9	8.7	13.5
	United Kingdom	11.4	9.6	13.5
	Japan	11.6	8.9	14.7
	Singapore	16.2	12.8	19.8
	Islamic Republic of Iran	7.3	6.3	8.3

Data Source: Arnold M, Rutherford M, Lam F, Bray F, Ervik M, Soerjomataram I (2019). ICBP SURVMARK-2 online tool: International Cancer Survival Benchmarking. Lyon, France: International Agency for Research on Cancer. Available from: http://gco.iarc.fr/survival/survmark, accessed [05/Feb/2021]

23.2   CRC Screening in the Arab Region

23.2.1   Status of CRC Screening in the Arab Region and Barriers to Its Implementation

Screening is known to be the most powerful intervention to reduce the incidence and mortality of cancer [23]. In fact, the nationwide screening programs implemented in the western courtiers have resulted in a noticeable reduction in both incidence and mortality rate of the screened cancers [1].

Unfortunately, there is no established CRC screening program in most of the Arab countries, and even in those countries that have established such a program as a trial at a smaller scale, for instance, in the UAE, the uptake is very low [24]. The barriers were studied and collectively listed as system based and patients' based barriers. The system based barriers include lack of resources, disintegrated medical systems and lack of test recommendation to patient by the treating physicians. Patients based barriers include unawareness of symptoms and risk factors of CRC, lack of knowledge of screening tests and their significance, embarrassment from doing the test and stigma about being diagnosed with cancer [4, 24–30]. A study from UAE reported that almost 95% of participants were not advised to do the CRC screening by their physicians [31]. This necessitates significant efforts to be directed toward increasing the awareness of both patients and healthcare providers, primary healthcare providers specifically, about the suspicious symptoms and the significance of early detection and screening. Furthermore, primary healthcare providers should be involved in the CRC screening program construction as they are the ones who can reach people and advocate for such campaigns.

In parallel to these findings, Arab Americans were found to have low adherence to CRC screening in the USA compared to Americans from other ethnic groups as well. The same local cultural, religious, and familiarity barriers do exist in the Arab American population despite being in a non-Arab country with well-established screening programs. Poor communication with the healthcare providers was highlighted as a major factor either due to language and culture barriers or distrust of the western recommendation. Other significant factors are costs and inaccurate understanding of risk factors [29, 32]. Such sociocultural barriers necessitate innovative awareness campaigns for Arabs to correct misconceptions and stress on the cost-effectiveness of screening programs. Furthermore, statistics of CRC status in the country and symptoms of the disease should be clearly communicated with people to influence their uptake of the screening program.

23.2.2   How to Improve CRC Screening in Arab Region

Every country has its own cancer burden that necessitates the construction of a cancer control plan with goals and objectives tailored to the available infrastructures and resources. In general, cancer screening programs are constructed either to target the whole population or high-risk group specifically. There are so many determinants for such a decision. Since the number of CRC among Arabs is relatively low compared to western nations, a screening program targeting high-risk groups would be a suitable starting step. Large-scale nationwide screening is expensive and needs a well-built infrastructure which is not the case in most of the Arab countries.

The reported insufficient screening uptake and poor awareness of CRCs among Arabs reflect the need for the involvement of all stakeholders; primary healthcare providers, ministry of health, media sector, schools, Non-Governmental Organizations, etc. Primary healthcare providers should be aware of the gap in knowledge in the population and work hard to ensure proper understanding of issues related to the risk of CRC and the usefulness of the screening programs [33]. Non-governmental and governmental organizations should be involved to spread awareness and correct misconceptions and negative attitudes related to the disease and the screening program. Media is a very powerful platform to spread awareness where it should be extensively used to stress on the significance of screening, increase awareness of the risk factors, CRC signs and symptoms. In fact, a study conducted in UAE showed that 66% of participants claimed that their main source of cancer information is media channels [31]. The other significant hallmark of succcessful screening program is the preparation of a strong and connected healthcare infrastructure in order to handle suspicious and confirmed cases systematicly and offer the needed management plans promptly.

23.3   CRC in Arab: Hereditary, Familial, or Sporadic?

The mode of presentation of CRC follows one of three patterns: sporadic, inherited, and familial.

- Sporadic CRC is the most common and accounts for approximately 70–75% of all diagnosed CRCs. It is characterized by an absence of family history. Early onset CRC cases in Arabs are thought to be sporadic, which necessitates further research to decipher the main molecular, environmental, and behavioral mechanisms.
- Inherited CRC represents only 10% of all diagnosed CRCs. Patients usually are diagnosed with inherited syndromes that predispose them to develop CRC. The inherited syndromes are divided into two categories, polyp associated syndromes such as Familial Adenomatous Polyposis (FAP), MUTYH-Associated Polyposis (MAP) and hamartomatous polyposis syndromes and non-polyp associated syndromes such as Lynch syndrome (HNPCC). Having a family member with CRC due to any of these syndromes necessitates early screening and sometimes prophylactic procedures for all people in the family who are at risk to reduce their chance of developing CRC.

- The third and least well-understood pattern is known as "familial" CRC, which accounts for up to 25% of cases. In this category, the CRC patients have a family history of CRC, but there is no clear pattern that is consistent with any of the known inherited syndromes. If a family member developed a familial CRC, it increases the risk of other members to develop CRC up to 1.7-fold, especially if the affected person is below the age of 55.

Unfortunately, data about the pattern of CRC and the molecular characteristics from Arab countries is scarce. That could be explained by the retrospective nature of the majority of the available studies where molecular markers and detailed family history are not routinely available. Furthermore, until recently, suspicious hereditary CRC cases are identified through the application of specific clinical criteria listed in the Amsterdam and Bethesda guidelines without the use of a laboratory-based screening test [34]. Therefore, there is not enough molecular or genetic data to determine the pattern and molecular signatures of CRC among Arabs, which is a fertile area for future research.

23.3.1 Biological Markers

The development of colorectal cancer is an accumulative process that necessitates a sequence of genetic mutations and epigenetic events at different sites that transforms the cells into cancerous cells [35]. There are several mutations that have been investigated and found to play a role in the initiation of CRC. Some of them have reached the clinic as biological markers for personalized medicine and prognosis prediction, such as mutations in KRAS, BRAF, and MMR, which are critical genes that are involved in cell proliferation, angiogenesis, cell motility and apoptosis. In fact, clinical evaluation and consideration of these genetic markers along with other clinicopathological parameters have revolutionized CRC management and improved patient outcome and prognosis. For example, KRAS-wild CRC showed 40–60% good response to anti-EGFR agents such as cetuximab. While KRAS mutant CRC and extended RAS family mutant tumors do not respond to anti-EGFR agents. Understanding the status of these biological markers in the Arab population is crucial to compare with other non-Arab populations and support international guidelines.

23.3.1.1 KRAS

It is the Kirsten Rat Sarcoma (KRAS) gene, one of the commonly mutated oncogenes that has been linked to CRC. The KRAS protein is involved in signaling pathways that play a major role in cell proliferation, differentiation, and apoptosis. KRAS testing is now considered as part of the standard of care of metastatic CRC being recommended by international guidelines. The frequency of KRAS in the

Arab population has been found to range from 30% to 50%, which is similar to reported data from western population. Majority of KRAS mutations occur in codon 12, which is found to be the same among Arab, Middle Eastern and Western populations [36–43]. KRAS mutant tumors are claimed to be associated with a more advanced stage CRC. Studies from the Arab world in patients at different stages of CRC did not find such association [43]. Therefore, the prognostic value of KRAS mutation was conflicting among studies. It has been associated with poor prognosis and outcome regardless of the stage of the tumor in a study done in Saudi Arabia [43], but it did not show that association in other studies. This could be explained by the variation in study design, especially study parameters that are related to sample size, ethnic group, modality of testing the KRAS mutation and timing of the reported tumor stage, whether the reported stage was at the time of diagnosis or at the time of data collection.

23.3.1.2 BRAF

BRAF is another attributed genetic marker for the initiation of CRC. The BRAF gene encodes a protein that is part of the Ras-Raf-MEK-ERK [44]. The frequency of BRAF mutation among Arabs with CRC was found to range from 2.4% to 4%, which is similar to nearby Asian and Middle Eastern countries, 4.9%, 4.6%, respectively, but lower than that reported from western countries (9.2%) [38, 39, 45].

The BRAF and KRAS mutations were not significantly associated with any clinicopathological parameters, tumor lateralization, gender, age, compared to western countries, which were significantly associated with right-side tumor, female gender and metastatic tumor. This could be explained by the small sample size again from Arab studies and the method used to test these molecular markers [37, 38].

23.3.1.3 PIK3CA

This gene plays a role in the cell survival signaling pathway. Mutations in this gene have been found to be similar in Arabs and Western countries, which is about 12–13% [36, 38, 46].

23.3.1.4 APC

The tumor suppressor gene APC plays an important role in CRC development. The absence of the APC protein leads to the accumulation of beta-catenin in the cytoplasm, resulting in constitutive transcriptional activation of TCF-responsive genes, which enhances tumor progression [47]. The frequency from the pooled results in Middle Eastern countries is (33%), which is consistent with the frequency rate in

Asian countries (32.4%), but it is lower than the frequency rate in Western countries (44.8%) [38, 48].

23.3.1.5 Mismatch Repair (MMR) Genes

A mutation in Mismatch Repair (MMR) genes (MLH1, MSH2, MSH6, and PMS2) is linked to the most common hereditary autosomal dominant CRC syndrome "Lynch syndrome (LS). The presence of Microsatellite Instability (MSI) is the hallmark of this syndrome. Several studies from the Middle East reported LS families, and the clinical features of these families appear to be similar to those seen in Western families. About 0.9% of newly diagnosed CRC in Saudi Arabia has LS, which is similar to other countries [49–51]. Siraj et al. reported 11.2% of CRC in Saudi Arabia patients to have MSI high that was related to LS [51], compared to 9.4% found in the CRC population from UAE [52] and 11.6% from Israeli Arabs [53]. It is worth mentioning that MSI high is not only correlated to LS but also has been found in 10% of sporadic CRC. The presence of a hotspot mutation in the BRAF oncogene with the MSI indicates a sporadic tumor because the BRAF mutation is never detected in LS [52]. MSI in sporadic CRC was associated with more proximal, poorly differentiated tumors and young male predominance [52, 54]. More studies are needed among Arabs in the genetic predisposition of CRC as early identification of individuals at high risk would allow earlier screening, intervention and subsequently improve outcomes.

23.3.1.6 Consensus Molecular Subtypes of CRC

Recent studies have evaluated the Consensus Molecular Subtypes (CMS) of CRC tumors and if there are any differences in these signatures related to the age of onset, the anatomical location or the prognosis. Interestingly, a CMS classification system has been constructed, which divided the CRC into four distinct subtypes, CMS1 (Microsatellite Instability Immune), CMS2 (Canonical), CMS3 (Metabolic), and CMS4 (Mesenchymal) [55]. These subtypes differ in their clinical, genetic and biological signatures and subsequently treatment response. Since the construction of this CMS classification in 2015, it has been implemented largely in basic and clinical cancer research but not yet integrated into clinical practice [56, 57]. More intensive research projects with multidisciplinary collaboration are required in order to decipher the correlation between these classifications and other clinicopathological parameters before integrating them into routine clinical practice. There are no studies conducted on the prevalence of CMS subtypes among Arabs yet. In fact, Korphaisarn. et al. analyzed them among different populations and concluded that there is a substantial variation by geographic region [58]. Further studies are needed in global populations to understand the pattern and validate their findings which ultimately might add a new transcriptomic dimension for CRC management strategy.

23.4 Early Onset Colorectal Cancer (EOCRC) in Arabs

Early Onset Colorectal Cancer (EOCRC) is defined as a colorectal cancer that is diagnosed before the screening age, i.e., < 50 years of age. As stated earlier, there was a noticeable decrease in incidence of adult-onset CRC (> 50 years) by 2% per year in the western countries compared to an annual increase of 1.5% per year among patients 20 to 49 years old. In fact, there is a prediction that by 2030 in the USA, 10% of all colon and 22% of all rectal cancers are expected to be diagnosed in patients <50 years old [4]. Almost all reports on CRC in the Arab region reported predominant young age at diagnosis, even younger than western population at diagnosis. 17–38% of CRC patients diagnosed in Arab were younger than 40 years old [6, 7, 20, 54, 59–62]. This increase in EOCRC incidence has not been fully understood till now. A key question in understanding the factors responsible for increasing incidence of EOCRC is whether EO- and LO-CRC are the same disease, or if EOCRC is caused by unique underlying biological pathways that synergize with different risk factors. It was strongly believed that EOCRC is highly linked to genetic factors and hereditary familial syndrome. Surprisingly, recent evidence do not support this belief. Genetic risk assessment of a cohort of young CRC patients revealed that only 1 in 5 of these patients do carry a germline genetic mutation and about 25% of them had a first-degree relative with CRC. The remaining majority of patients are sporadic [63, 64].

Retrospective studies to understand sporadic EOCRC revealed distinctive histologic features in terms of the anatomical location of the tumor and stage at diagnosis compared to late-onset CRC and inherited EOCRC. Sporadic young-onset CRC has been found to present at advanced stages and often in the distal colon and the rectum. Several studies have shown that sporadic EOCRC exhibit mucinous and signet ring features or poorly differentiated histology. Furthermore, they usually present with metastasis at diagnosis and are shown to have early disease recurrence and subsequently lower survival [63–65]. At the molecular level, investigation is going on to decipher its molecular profile. The most recent findings showed that sporadic EOCRC is associated with a higher percentage of synchronous and metachronous tumors [66]. The genetic profile of this cancer entity is different as well, where most of these tumors are microsatellite and chromosomal stable (MACS), lack DNA repair mechanism abnormalities and have significantly fewer *BRAF* and *APC* mutations than late-onset CRC [38, 66, 67]. More studies are needed to understand the molecular and clinicopathological signatures of EOCRC among Arabs in order to construct the best preventive and intervention measures.

23.5 Cancer Genetic Counseling in Arabs

As discussed earlier, hereditary cancer occurs in high frequency in several Arab populations due to high rates of consanguinity; 25–60% of consanguineous marriages among Arabs [33]. In fact, a comprehensive genetic study conducted in Saudi

Arabia on children with cancer found that 4 in 10 children with cancer have hereditary cancer syndrome. They reported 38% consanguinity among the studied group. Unfortunately, there are a smaller number of studies on familial and hereditary cancer among the Arab population. Several initiatives have been initiated from many Arab countries, such as the Saudi Human Genome Project (SGHP) and similar programs in Qatar, Egypt, and the United Arab Emirates aiming to understand the genetic profile and distribution of cancer among their population.

At the same time, healthcare planners envisioned the huge demand for familial cancer genetic counseling in the Arab world and worldwide in general [33]. The definition of Genetic counseling is a "process of helping people understand and adapt to the medical, psychological and familial implications of genetic contributions to disease" [68]. These facilities provide screening, monitoring and offer prophylactic interventions to reduce the risk of cancer development.

It is true that these facilities have been found to positively reduce the cost of care and improve the cancer awareness and care satisfaction among patients and their relatives, but they have raised few other negative issues related to the psychological distress of doing the genetic test, misinterpretation of genetic results and sometimes unnecessary interventions [33, 69]. Therefore, professionally trained personnel are needed to run these clinics in order to overcome these challenges. Genetic counselors must successfully communicate risk perception to their patients and to provide significant levels of long-term psychosocial support to patients and their families.

Such clinics were established in several Arab countries such as in Saudi Arabia [33], Oman [70] and others. They have constructed guidelines and recommendations for different types of cancer [33]. These clinics receive referrals for patients who are genetically high-risk in order to do the needed genetic or clinical screening and proper counseling and interventions. Such genetic counseling and prophylactic intervention coupled with increase in public awareness of risk factors, signs, and symptoms will collectively help in reducing the impact of CRC in the societies.

23.6 Conclusion

The burden of CRC is increasing worldwide. There is an unmet need for primary and secondary prevention measures in Arab countries. Cancer prevention programs should be implemented within an organized program with all infrastructure and resources tailored to ensure offering a comprehensive cancer care through all steps of the cancer continuum. Cost-effectiveness studies of either high-risk population or nationwide screening options are needed by every country to tackle their own cancer burden.

Conflict of Interest Authors have no conflict of interest to declare.

Acknowledgment The author wishes to acknowledge Dr. Humaid Al-Adawi, consultant colorectal surgeon from Sultan Qaboos University Hospital for proofreading the chapter and adding his expert opinion.

References

1. Siegel RL, Miller KD, Goding Sauer A, Fedewa SA, Butterly LF, Anderson JC, et al. Colorectal cancer statistics, 2020. CA Cancer J Clin. 2020;70(3):145–64.
2. Rawla P, Sunkara T, Barsouk A. Epidemiology of colorectal cancer: Incidence, mortality, survival, and risk factors. Prz Gastroenterol. 2019;14(2):89–103.
3. Arnold M, Sierra MS, Laversanne M, Soerjomataram I, Jemal A, Bray F. Global patterns and trends in colorectal cancer incidence and mortality. Gut. 2017;66(4):683–91.
4. Arafa MA, Farhat K. Colorectal cancer in the Arab world - screening practices and future prospects. Asian Pacific J Cancer Prev. 2015;16(17):7425–30. [Internet].Available from http://koreascience.or.kr/journal/view.jsp?kj=POCPA9&py=2015&vnc=v16n17&sp=7425
5. Al-Zalabani AH. Cancer incidence attributable to tobacco smoking in GCC countries in 2018. 2020 [cited 2021 Jan 15]; Available from https://doi.org/10.18332/tid/118722.
6. Veruttipong D, Soliman AS, Gilbert SF, Blachley TS, Hablas A, Ramadan M, et al. Age distribution, polyps and rectal cancer in the Egyptian population-based cancer registry. World J Gastroenterol. 2012;18(30):3997–4003.
7. Khachfe HH, Salhab HA, Fares MY, Khachfe HM. Probing the colorectal cancer incidence in Lebanon: an 11-year epidemiological study. Springer [Internet]. 2029 [cited 2021 Jan 18]; Available from https://doi.org/10.1007/s12029-019-00284-z.
8. Missaoui N, Jaidaine L, Ben AA, Trabelsi A, Mokni M, Hmissa S. Colorectal cancer in Central Tunisia: Increasing incidence trends over a 15-year period. Asian Pacific. J Cancer Prev. 2011;12(4):1073–6.
9. Awad H, Abu-Shanab A, Hammad N, Atallah A, Abdulattif M. Demographic features of patients with colorectal carcinoma based on 14 years of experience at Jordan University Hospital. Ann Saudi Med. 2018;38(6):427–32. [Internet] Available from http://www.annsaudimed.net/doi/10.5144/0256-4947.2018.427
10. Al-Jawaldeh A, Taktouk M, Nasreddine L. Food consumption patterns and nutrient intakes of children and adolescents in the eastern mediterranean region: A call for policy action. Nutrients. 2020;12(11):1–28.
11. Al-Shamsi SR, Bener A, Al-Sharhan M, Al-Mansoor TM, Azab IA, Rashed A, et al. Clinicopathological pattern of colorectal cancer in the United Arab Emirates. Saudi Med J. 2003;24(5):518–22.
12. El-Bolkainy TN, Sakr MA, Nouh AA, El-Din NHA. A comparative study of rectal and colonic carcinoma: demographic, pathologic and TNM staging analysis. J Egypt Natl Canc Inst. 2006;18(3):258–63.
13. Aljebreen AM. Clinico-pathological patterns of colorectal cancer in Saudi Arabia: Younger with an advanced stage presentation. Saudi J Gastroenterol. 2007;13(2):84–7.
14. Kumar S, Burney IA, Zahid KF, Souza PCD, Al Belushi M, Mufti TD, et al. Colorectal cancer patient characteristics, treatment and survival in Oman - A single center study. Asian Pacific J Cancer Prev. 2015;16(12):4853–8. [Internet; cited 2020 Dec 6]. Available from https://pubmed.ncbi.nlm.nih.gov/26163603/
15. Smirnov M, Lazarev I, Perry ZH, Ariad S, Kirshtein B. Colorectal cancer in southern Israel: comparison between Bedouin Arab and Jewish patients. Int J Surg. 2016 Sep;1(33):109–16.

16. Alsanea N, Abduljabbar AS, Alhomoud S, Ashari LH, Hibbert D, Bazarbashi S. Colorectal cancer in Saudi Arabia: Incidence, survival, demographics and implications for national policies. Ann Saudi Med. 2015;35(3):196–202.
17. Amin TT, Suleman W, Al Taissan AA, Al Joher AL, Al Mulhim O, Al Yousef AH. Patients' profile, clinical presentations and histopathological features of colorectal cancer in Al Hassa region, Saudi Arabia. Asian Pacific J Cancer Prev. 2012;13(1):211–6.
18. de Leon MP, Marino M, Benatti P, Rossi G, Menigatti M, Pedroni M, et al. Trend of incidence, subsite distribution and staging of colorectal neoplasms in the 15-year experience of a specialised cancer registry. Ann Oncol. 2004;15(6):940–6.
19. Phipps AI, Scoggins J, Rossing MA, Li CI, Newcomb PA. Temporal trends in incidence and mortality rates for colorectal cancer by tumor location: 1975-2007. Am J Public Health. 2012;102(9):1791–7.
20. Al-Ahwal MS, Shafik YH, Al-Ahwal HM. First national survival data for colorectal cancer among Saudis between 1994 and 2004: What's next? BMC Public Health. 2013;13(1):1–6.
21. Jemal A, Clegg LX, Ward E, Ries LAG, Wu X, Jamison PM, et al. Annual report to the nation on the status of cancer, 1975-2001, with a special feature regarding survival. Cancer. 2004;101(1):3–27.
22. Panato C, Abusamaan K, Bidoli E, Hamdi-Cherif M, Pierannunzio D, Ferretti S, et al. Survival after the diagnosis of breast or colorectal cancer in the GAZA Strip from 2005 to 2014. BMC Cancer. 2018;18(1):632. [Internet]. Available from http://www.ncbi.nlm.nih.gov/pubmed/29866055
23. Lawton C. Colorectal-cancer incidence and mortality with screening flexible sigmoidoscopy. Yearb Med. 2013;2013:139–40.
24. Al Abdouli L, Dalmook H, Abdo MA, Carrick FR, Rahman MA. Colorectal cancer risk awareness and screening uptake among adults in the United Arab Emirates. Asian Pacific J Cancer Prev. 2018;19(8):2343–9.
25. Qumseya BJ, Tayem YI, Dasa OY, Nahhal KW, Abu-Limon IM, Hmidat AM, et al. Barriers to colorectal cancer screening in Palestine: A national study in a medically underserved population. Clin Gastroenterol Hepatol. 2014;12(3):463–9.
26. Al-Dahshan A, Chehab M, Bala M, Omer M, AlMohamed O, Al-Kubaisi N, et al. Colorectal cancer awareness and its predictors among adults aged 50–74 years attending primary healthcare in the State of Qatar: a cross-sectional study. BMJ Open. 2020;10(7):e035651. [Internet]. Available from https://bmjopen.bmj.com/lookup/doi/10.1136/bmjopen-2019-035651
27. Al-Sharbatti S, Muttappallymyalil J, Sreedharan J, Almosawy Y. Predictors of colorectal cancer knowledge among adults in the United Arab Emirates. Asian Pacific J Cancer Prev. 2017;18(9):2355–9.
28. Al-Azri M, Al-Kindi J, Al-Harthi T, Al-Dahri M, Panchatcharam SM, Al-Maniri A. Awareness of stomach and colorectal cancer risk factors, symptoms and time taken to seek medical help among public attending primary care Setting in Muscat Governorate, Oman. J Cancer Educ. 2019;34(3):423–34.
29. Saad F, Ayyash M, Ayyash M, Elhage N, Ali I, Makki M, et al. Assessing knowledge, physician interactions and patient-reported barriers to colorectal cancer screening among Arab Americans in Dearborn, Michigan. J Community Health. 2020;45(5):900–9.
30. Tfaily M, Naamani D, Kassir A. SS-A of global, 2019 undefined. Awareness of colorectal cancer and attitudes towards its screening guidelines in Lebanon. ncbi.nlm.nih.gov [Internet]. [cited 2021 Jan 18]; Available from https://www.ncbi.nlm.nih.gov/pmc/articles/PMC6634322/
31. Al Abdouli L, Dalmook H, Akram Abdo M, Carrick FR, Abdul RM. Colorectal cancer risk Awareness and screening uptake among adults in the United Arab Emirates. Asian Pac J Cancer Prev. 2018;19(8):2343–9. [Internet]. Available from http://www.ncbi.nlm.nih.gov/pubmed/30141313
32. Alsayid M, Tlimat NM, Spigner C, Dimaano C. Perceptions of colorectal cancer screening in the Arab American community: a pilot study. Prim Health Care Res Dev. 2019;20:e90.
33. AlHarthi FS, Qari A, Edress A, Abedalthagafi M. Familial/inherited cancer syndrome: a focus on the highly consanguineous Arab population. NPJ Genomic Med. 2020;5(1):3. [Internet]. Available from http://www.nature.com/articles/s41525-019-0110-y

34. Umar A, Boland CR, Terdiman JP, Syngal S, de la Chapelle A, Rüschoff J, et al. Revised Bethesda guidelines for hereditary nonpolyposis colorectal cancer (Lynch syndrome) and microsatellite instability. J Natl Cancer Inst. 2004;96(4):261–8.

35. Abdel-Malak C, Darwish H, Elsaid A, El-Tarapely F, Elshazli R. Association of APC I1307K and E1317Q polymorphisms with colorectal cancer among Egyptian subjects. Familial Cancer. 2016;15(1):49–56. [Internet]. Available from: https://link.springer.com/article/10.100 7%2Fs10689-015-9834-8

36. Ibrahim T, Saer-Ghorra C, Trak-Smayra V, Nadiri S, Yazbeck C, Baz M, et al. Molecular characteristics of colorectal cancer in a Middle Eastern population in a single institution. Ann Saudi Med. 2018;38(4):251–9.

37. Zahrani A, Kandil M, Badar T, Abdelsalam M, Al-Faiar A, Ismail A. Clinico-pathological study of K-ras mutations in colorectal tumors in Saudi Arabia. Tumori. 2014;100(1):75–9.

38. Al-Shamsi HO, Jones J, Fahmawi Y, Dahbour I, Tabash A, Abdel-Wahab R, et al. Molecular spectrum of KRAS, NRAS, BRAF, PIK3CA, TP53, and APC somatic gene mutations in Arab patients with colorectal cancer: determination of frequency and distribution pattern. J Gastrointest Oncol. 2016;7(6):882–902. [Internet]. Available from http://jgo.amegroups.com/article/view/10606/9407

39. Beg S, Siraj AK, Prabhakaran S, Bu R, Al-Rasheed M, Sultana M, et al. Molecular markers and pathway analysis of colorectal carcinoma in the Middle East. Cancer. 2015;121(21):3799–808.

40. Zhang J, Zheng J, Yang Y, Lu J, Gao J, Lu T, et al. Molecular spectrum of KRAS, NRAS, BRAF and PIK3CA mutations in Chinese colorectal cancer patients: Analysis of 1, 110 cases. Sci Rep. 2015;5:1–8.

41. Soliman AS, Bondy ML, El-Badawy SA, Mokhtar N, Eissa S, Bayoumy S, et al. Contrasting molecular pathology of colorectal carcinoma in Egyptian and Western patients. Br J Cancer. 2001;85(7):1037–46.

42. Mao C, Yang ZY, Hu XF, Chen Q, Tang JL. PIK3CA exon 20 mutations as a potential biomarker for resistance to anti-EGFR monoclonal antibodies in KRAS wild-type metastatic colorectal cancer: A systematic review and meta-analysis. Ann Oncol. 2012;23(6):1518–25.

43. Zekri J, Al-Shehri A, Mahrous M, Al-Rehaily S, Darwish T, Bassi S, et al. Mutations in codons 12 and 13 of K-ras exon 2 in colorectal tumors of Saudi Arabian patients: frequency, clincopathological associations, and clinical outcomes. Genet Mol Res. 2017;16(1):1–6. [Internet]. Available from http://www.funpecrp.com.br/gmr/year2017/vol16-1/pdf/gmr-16-01-gmr.16019369.pdf

44. Dhomen N, Marais R. New insight into BRAF mutations in cancer. Curr Opin Genet Dev. 2007;17(1):31–9.

45. Tran B, Kopetz S, Tie J, Gibbs P, Jiang ZQ, Lieu CH, et al. Impact of BRAF mutation and microsatellite instability on the pattern of metastatic spread and prognosis in metastatic colorectal cancer. Cancer. 2011;117(20):4623–32.

46. Abubaker J, Bavi P, Al-Harbi S, Ibrahim M, Siraj AK, Al-Sanea N, et al. Clinicopathological analysis of colorectal cancers with PIK3CA mutations in Middle Eastern population. Oncogene. 2008;27(25):3539–45.

47. Béroud C, Soussi T. APC gene: database of germline and somatic mutations in human tumors and cell lines. Nucleic Acids Res. 1996;24(1):119–20.

48. Abdel-Malak C, Darwish H, Afaf E, El-Tarapely F, Elshazli R. Association of APC I1307K and E1317Q polymorphisms with colorectal cancer among Egyptian subjects. Familial Cancer. 2016;15(1):49–56.

49. Schofield L, Grieu F, Amanuel B, Carrello A, Spagnolo D, Kiraly C, et al. Population-based screening for Lynch syndrome in Western Australia. Int J Cancer. 2014;135(5):1085–91.

50. Abu Freha N, Leibovici Weissman Y, Fich A, Barnes Kedar I, Halpern M, Sztarkier I, et al. Constitutional mismatch repair deficiency and Lynch syndrome among consecutive Arab Bedouins with colorectal cancer in Israel. Familial Cancer. 2018;17(1):79–86.

51. Siraj AK, Prabhakaran S, Bavi P, Bu R, Beg S, Hazmi MAL, et al. Prevalence of Lynch syndrome in a Middle Eastern population with colorectal cancer. Cancer. 2015;121(11):1762–71.

52. Kamat N, Khidhir MA, Alashari MM, Rannug U. Microsatellite instability and loss of hetero-zygosity detected in middle-aged patients with sporadic colon cancer: A retrospective study. Oncol Lett. 2013;6(5):1413–20.
53. Vilkin A, Niv Y, Nagasaka T, Morgenstern S, Levi Z, Fireman Z, et al. Microsatellite instabil-ity, MLH1 promoter methylation, and BRAF mutation analysis in sporadic colorectal cancers of different ethnic groups in Israel. Cancer. 2009;115(4):760–9.
54. Ashktorab H, Brim H, Al-Riyami M, Date A, Al-Mawaly K, Kashoub M, et al. Sporadic colon cancer: Mismatch repair immunohistochemistry and microsatellite instability in Omani sub-jects. Dig Dis Sci. 2008;53(10):2723–31.
55. Guinney J, Dienstmann R, Wang X, De Reyniès A, Schlicker A, Soneson C, Marisa L, Roepman P, Nyamundanda G, Angelino P, Bot B. The consensus molecular subtypes of colorectal can-cer. Nat Med. 2015;21(11):1350–6.
56. Sawayama H, Miyamoto Y, Ogawa K, Yoshida N, Baba H. Investigation of colorectal can-cer in accordance with consensus molecular subtype classification. Ann Gastroenterol Surg. 2020;4(5):528–39.
57. Álvaro E, Cano JM, García JL, Brandáriz L, Olmedillas-López S, Arriba M, et al. Clinical and molecular comparative study of colorectal cancer based on age-of-onset and tumor location: Two main criteria for subclassifying colorectal cancer. Int J Mol Sci. 2019;20(4):968.
58. Korphaisarn K, Lam M, Loree JM, Ruiz E, Aguiar S, Kopetz S. Consensus molecular subtypes in colorectal cancer differ by geographic region. J Clin Oncol. 2020;38(15_suppl):4061.
59. Guraya SY, Eltinay OE. Higher prevalence in young population and rightward shift of colorec-tal carcinoma. Saudi Med J. 2006;27(9):1391–3.
60. Abdalla AA, Musa MT, Khair R. Presentation of Colorectal Cancer in Khartoum Teaching Hospital. Sudan. J Med Sci. 2008;2(4):263–5.
61. Fireman Z, Sandler E, Kopelman Y, Segal A, Sternberg A. Ethnic differences in colorectal cancer among Arab and Jewish neighbors in Israel. Am J Gastroenterol. 2001;96(1):204–7.
62. Al-Shamsi O, H, Abdullah Alzaabi A, Hassan A, Abu-Gheida I, Alrawi S. Early onset colorectal cancer in the United Arab Emirates, where do we stand? Acta Sci Cancer Biol. 2020;4(11):24–7.
63. Stoffel EM, Koeppe E, Everett J, Ulintz P, Kiel M, Osborne J, et al. Germline genetic features of young individuals with colorectal cancer. Gastroenterology. 2018;154(4):897.e1–905.e1.
64. Cavestro GM, Mannucci A, Zuppardo RA, Di Leo M, Stoffel E, Tonon G. Early onset sporadic colorectal cancer: worrisome trends and oncogenic features. Dig Liver Dis. 2018;50:521–32. Elsevier B.V.
65. Refaat G. Early onset colorectal cancer: a major health problem. Int J Cell Sci Mol Biol. 2017;3(2):1–3.
66. Siegel RL, Jemal A, Ward EM. Increase in incidence of colorectal cancer among young men and women in the United States. Cancer Epidemiol Biomark Prev. 2009;18(6):1695–8.
67. Ballester V, Rashtak S, Boardman L. Clinical and molecular features of young-onset colorectal cancer. World J Gastroenterol. 2016;22(5):1736–44. [Internet; cited 2020 Dec 16] Available from /pmc/articles/PMC4724605/?report=abstract
68. Jenkins S, Kirwan C. Principles and practice of genetic counselling for inherited cardiac condi-tions. Cardiovasc Genet Genomics Princ Clin Pract. 2018;2018:71–95.
69. Donnai D, Kerzin-Storrar L, Craufurd D, Evans G, Clayton-Smith J, Kingston H. Tensions in implementing the new genetics. Genetic counsellors could be based in genetic centres but be formally linked to general practice. BMJ. 2000;321(7255):241.
70. Rajab A, Al Rashdi I, Al SQ. Genetic services and testing in the Sultanate of Oman. Sultanate of Oman steps into modern genetics. J Community Genet. 2013;4(3):391–7.

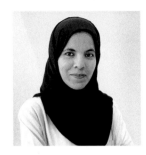

Adhari AlZaabi (MD/PhD) is an assisstant professor at the college of Medicine and Health Sciences at Sultan Qaboos University. She got her Medical degree with honor from Sultan Qabos University. She was aworded a full PhD scholership to the USA. She completed her doctorate studies in serum biomarkers for early detection of cancer metastasis from Brigham Young University, USA. She was a fellow in the cancer control and prevention summer program at National cancer Institute in the United State in 2018. Her research interests is in early-onset colorectal cancer, omics predictive models and artificial intelligence applications in medicine. Adhari was nominated for the award committee membership of Human proteomic organization (HUPO) in 2020. She has received multiple awards for her scientific and community contribution in raising awarness about cancer and healthy lifestyle at the national and international levels. She received IBRO Global Engagement Seed Grant Award in 2020. Adhari is the founder of the National Cancer Awareness Program Siyaj (twitter and instegram: "@Siyaj_CAP") in Oman that has national reputations." Adhari and her team have published different books and articles in Arabic to raise awareness and reduce stigma about cancer among the Arabs.

Chapter 24
Palliative Care in the Arab World

Hibah Osman and Rana Yamout

24.1 Role of Palliative Medicine in Cancer Care

Palliative Care is the active holistic care of patients with serious or life-threatening illnesses. It aims to improve the quality of life of patients and families by managing symptoms such as pain and preventing and relieving suffering [1, 2]. Patients diagnosed with advanced cancer tend to experience an enormous symptom burden, aggressive medical care, as well as emotional and spiritual distress, all of which can result in poor quality of life throughout the course of the disease [3, 4]. Palliative care aims to support cancer patients by managing sources of distress throughout the course of treatment. This includes early detection and management of pain and other symptoms, providing psychosocial support to help patients and their families cope with cancer and its treatment, and supporting them as they make decisions about their treatment goals [4].

There is a common misconception that palliative care should only be offered towards the end of life and only after options for disease-directed therapies are exhausted. However, in recent years research has demonstrated that involvement of palliative care providers early in the cancer trajectory has advantages to patients, their families, and the healthcare system [4–7]. Patients receiving early palliative

H. Osman (✉)
Dana-Farber Cancer Institute, Boston, MA, USA

Harvard Medical School, Boston, MA, USA

Balsam – Lebanese Center for Palliative Care, Beirut, Lebanon
e-mail: hibah_osman@dfci.harvard.edu

R. Yamout
Balsam – Lebanese Center for Palliative Care, Beirut, Lebanon

American University of Beirut Medical Center, Beirut, Lebanon
e-mail: Ry30@aub.edu.lb

© The Author(s) 2022
H. O. Al-Shamsi et al. (eds.), *Cancer in the Arab World*,
https://doi.org/10.1007/978-981-16-7945-2_24

care have a better quality of life, less depression, and longer survival while receiving less aggressive care compared to patients receiving standard oncological care [4]. Research evidence has led the American Society of Clinical Oncology (ASCO) to recommend that patients with advanced cancer begin receiving palliative care early in the course of their illness and in parallel to active cancer treatment [8].

Palliative care is in the early stages of development in the Arab world. It was first introduced in Jordan and Saudi Arabia in the early 1990s [9]. Several other countries followed over the next 30 years, but many countries still have no palliative care activity [1, 9, 10].

Cancer is among the leading causes of death in Arab countries, and cancer incidence is projected to continue to increase. Patients diagnosed with cancer in the region tend to present at later stages of illness and therefore have high palliative care needs [11, 12]. Unfortunately, few of the patients who could benefit from palliative care receive it. The number of palliative care providers in the region are not enough to meet the needs of the population, and services tend to be concentrated in urban areas and less accessible to people living in more remote rural communities [12].

24.2   Cost-Effectiveness of Palliative Care

Health expenditure among patients with cancer and patients near the end of life tends to be high. Research has shown that palliative care significantly reduces the cost of cancer care [10, 13]. Patients who receive palliative care have fewer visits to physicians and emergency departments primarily because pain and other symptoms are adequately managed. The role of palliative care in promoting open conversations about prognosis and clarifying goals of care also plays an important role in mitigating health care costs by reducing medical interventions that are unlikely to be of benefit and may in fact increase suffering. Palliative care has been associated with reduced hospital admissions, decreased hospital length of stay, and decreased ICU admissions [10].

In addition to reducing the direct costs to the healthcare system, the early introduction of palliative care during the course of the cancer trajectory decreases unnecessary and burdensome personal and societal costs [4]. Palliative care can have a significant impact on the cost of informal caregivers and productivity loss which can be responsible for almost half of the total cost of illness [14].

24.3   Palliative Care Needs in Arab Countries

There are several approaches to estimating the palliative care needs of a country. Population-based methods estimate palliative care needs using mortality statistics, cause of death, hospital data on symptom prevalence, and data on opioid consumption [2, 15]. It is estimated that less than 1% of the 23,569 people who needed palliative care in 2017 in the Eastern Mediterranean Regional Office (EMRO) in the Eastern Mediterranean received it [10].

In 2017, the Lancet Commission on Global Access to Palliative Care and Pain Relief (GAPCPR) introduced an approach to estimating Serious Health-related Suffering (SHS) as a proxy for the unmet palliative care needs of populations [16]. The Lancet Commission report was the culmination of a broader project that estimated the palliative care needs of countries across the globe. Table 24.1 is a summary of the data on SHS for Arab countries based on the work for the GAPCPR [17].

There are no published estimates of the projected increase in SHS in Arab countries specifically. However, an analysis by the World Health Organization (WHO) region projects the highest proportional increase of the burden of SHS (170%) to be in the EMRO in between 2016 and 2060. Cancer is predicted to be among the five health conditions that will contribute to the largest increase in SHS and contribute to the largest number of deaths [18].

Table 24.1 People experiencing serious health suffering (SHS) for cancer, leukemia, and other diseases who could have benefited from palliative care in 2015 in Arab countries [17]

Country	Cancer (#)	Cancer (Per 1000 pop)	Leukemia (#)	Leukemia (Rate per 1000)	People with SHS (#)	Rate of people with SHS (Per 1000 pop)
Algeria	40,000	1.016	1140	0.0288	157,000	3.96
Bahrain	1000	0.444	20	0.0131	2000	1.64
Comoros	1000	0.863	10	0.0068	4000	5.02
Djibouti	1000	0.880	30	0.0352	13,000	14.73
Egypt	127,000	1.385	3620	0.0408	428,000	4.67
Iraq	31,000	0.855	1560	0.0429	143,000	3.93
Jordan	7000	0.921	240	0.0320	24,000	3.16
Kuwait	1000	0.381	70	0.0174	7000	1.82
Lebanon	9000	1.617	230	0.0401	31,000	5.29
Libya	6000	1.034	190	0.0301	26,000	4.17
Mauritania	3000	0.637	20	0.0059	32,000	7.80
Morocco	42,000	1.234	760	0.0221	163,000	4.75
Oman	2000	0.399	100	0.0219	9000	2.02
Palestine	No data	No data	No data	No data	No data	No data
Qatar	1000	0.411	40	0.0189	3000	1.27
Saudi Arabia	18,000	0.559	650	0.0207	83,000	2.65
Somalia	10,000	0.901	280	0.0258	98,000	9.11
Sudan	28,000	0.688	970	0.0242	229,000	5.68
Syria	23,000	1.243	800	0.0434	123,000	6.64
Tunisia	13,000	1.198	310	0.0277	62,000	5.51
UAE	3000	0.291	100	0.0105	11,000	1.15
Yemen	15,000	0.547	1030	0.0386	105,000	3.91

24.4 Palliative Care Policies

National health policies are an important indicator of healthcare priorities. They outline strategies and define resource allocation, which are both essential for the development of programs and services. The inclusion of palliative care in national health plans and legislation are essential steps towards the integration of palliative care into healthcare systems [19]. National policies, funding for palliative care services, and the presence of a dedicated palliative care unit within the ministry of health are all considered important indicators of palliative care development [20].

The data on these indicators is limited in most Arab countries. Palliative care is only recognized as a specialty in Lebanon and Saudi Arabia [21]. More recently, other countries such as the UAE have moved towards the recognition of palliative care as a specialty. Tunisia is the only country with a stand-alone national palliative care strategy. Several Arab countries have a palliative care strategy included in their national cancer control plan or their non-communicable disease (NCD) action plan. In general, palliative care services are covered in countries with publicly funded healthcare, but patients must pay for palliative care in countries with private healthcare systems such as Lebanon and Jordan.

24.5 Palliative Care Services

There are several models for palliative care service delivery. Services can be delivered at home, in the ambulatory setting, in the hospital, in nursing homes or in dedicated hospices. Most palliative care programs in the region are hospital-based, either in the form of hospital-based consultation services or dedicated inpatient units. Saudi Arabia, Jordan, and Egypt have the highest number of palliative care programs. No palliative care service providers have been identified in Syria, Libya, Yemen, Djibouti, or Somalia [11, 20, 21]. Figure 24.1 shows the number of palliative care programs in the Eastern Mediterranean Region (EMR) [21].

Even in countries with the most developed palliative care services, the services remain at the early stages of development and are not yet integrated into the national health system [10, 11]. Palliative care remains restricted to patients who have a limited prognosis and are no longer candidates for disease-directed therapies [22]. Most palliative care service providers in the region are located in large urban cities and primarily in tertiary care centers resulting in limited access to people living in rural areas [12].

Oncology patients can receive palliative care through their primary care providers, by their oncologist, or by a palliative care specialist. Regardless of who is providing the care, they should be able to address different sources of distress associated with illness which include the physical, the psychosocial and the existential. This usually requires the involvement of a multidisciplinary team that includes physicians, nurses, social workers, psychologists, and a spiritual care provider. With few exceptions, palliative care programs in Arab countries are physician-led with limited involvement of other disciplines and treatment is largely focused on physical symptoms with limited attention to psychosocial or spiritual needs [22].

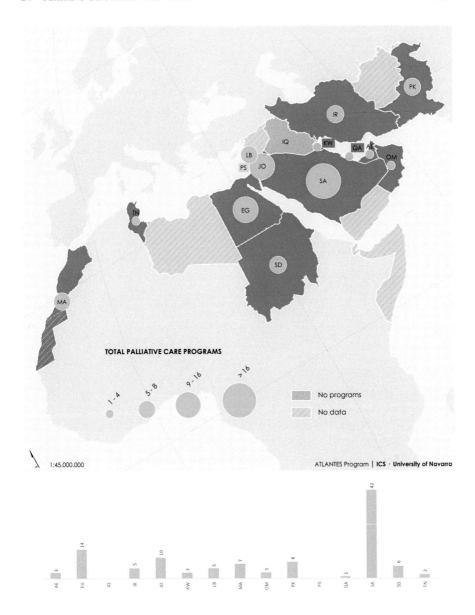

Fig. 24.1 Number of palliative care programs in countries of the Eastern Mediterranean. Reproduced with authorization from the IAHPC [21]

The Worldwide Hospice Palliative Care Alliance (WHPCA) assessed and categorized countries according to the level of development of their palliative care system into four categories. Group 1 includes countries with no known hospice or palliative care activity; group 2 includes countries with capacity building activity; group 3 consists of countries with isolated or generalized palliative care services; and finally, group 4 comprises countries with hospice or palliative care services integrated into mainstream service provision (Table 24.2) [10].

Table 24.2 Arab countries by level of palliative care development according to World Palliative Care Alliance (WPCA) [10]

Level of palliative care development	Countries
Level 1—No known palliative care activity	Comoros, South Sudan, Djibouti, Iraq, Somalia, Somaliland, Syria, Yemen
Level 2—Capacity building palliative care activity	UAE
Level 3 a—Isolate palliative care provision	Algeria, Mauritania, Bahrain, Egypt, Kuwait, Lebanon, Libya, Morocco, Palestine, Sudan, Tunisia
Level 3 b—Generalized palliative care provision	Jordan, Oman, Qatar, Saudi Arabia
Level 4 a—Palliative care services at preliminary stage of integration	None
Level 4 b—Palliative care at advanced stage of integration	None

24.6 Medication Availability

Access to opioids is regulated by governments to minimize diversion. Governments have employed different approaches to balance having safe access to opioid analgesia for the treatment of pain while minimizing diversion. Both prescribing and dispensing are closely regulated and require special forms and documentation. There is major variability in prescribing regulations among Arab countries. They include restricting prescribing by medical speciality, by diagnosis, by location or level of care, by dose or by number of days supplied.

Pain control is an essential component of palliative care, and opioid consumption is widely utilized as an indicator of pain control and palliative care development. The ability to switch patients from one opioid to another (opioid rotation), when they develop side effects or there are contraindications to using one of the opioid analgesics, is essential to proper pain management. Therefore, access to different formulations is important for proper pain management. Opioid consumption is usually reported in oral morphine equivalents (OME).

Overall, morphine consumption in Arab countries is relatively low compared to the global average and very low compared to opioid consumption in Europe and North America. The mean opioid consumption in the Eastern Mediterranean Region (EMR) in 2014 was 0.384 mg/person, which is 16 times less than the average global consumption [11]. Table 24.3 includes a list of the opioids available in Arab countries and the opioid consumption in 2017 according to data from the International Narcotics Control Board (INCB). The average consumption in Arab countries was 3.23 OME per person in 2017 compared to the average global consumption of 75.98 OME per person in the same year [23]. Misconceptions about the use of opioid analgesics, limited training of physicians and nurses in pain management, and prescribing restrictions all contribute to low consumption of opioid analgesics and inadequate pain control in the region.

Table 24.3 Opioid consumption in Arab countries in oral morphine equivalence (OME) (mg/person) [10]

| Country | Opioid use in Morphine equivalence (mg/person) | | | | | | | | Total opioid consumption in Morphine equivalence (mg/person) |
	Morphine	Codeine	Fentanyl	Oxycodone	Hydro-morphone	Pethidine	Methadone		
Algeria	0.2	0	0.8	0	0	0	0		1
Bahrain	3.1	0	2.2	0.8	0	0.4	0		6.5
Comoros	0.19	0	0.03	0	0	0	0		0.22
Djibouti	N/A	N/A	N/A	N/A	N/A	N/A	N/A		N/A
Egypt	0.2	0	2.1	0.016	0.014	0	0		2.33
Iraq	N/A	N/A	N/A	N/A	N/A	N/A	N/A		N/A
Jordan	1.3	0	2.2	0.25	0	0.3	0.23		4.28
Kuwait	0.4	0.1	4.4	0.8	0	0.4	0.2		6.3
Lebanon	1.1	0	3.05	0.2	0	0.2	0		4.55
Libya	0.012	0.01	0.5	0	0	0.05	0		0.572
Mauritania	N/A	N/A	N/A	N/A	N/A	N/A	N/A		N/A
Morocco	0.8	0	0.6	0	0	0	5.6		7
Oman	0	0	1.1	0	0	0	0		1.1
Palestine	N/A	N/A	N/A	N/A	N/A	N/A	N/A		N/A
Qatar	1.08	0	3.3	0.05	0	0.04	0.3		4.77
Saudi Arabia	0.8	1.2	4.6	0.3	0	0.2	0.3		7.4
Somalia	N/A	N/A	N/A	N/A	N/A	N/A	N/A		N/A
Sudan	0.116	0	0.064	0	0	0.031	0		0.211
Syria	0.05	0	0.7	0	0	0.1	0		0.85
Tunisia	2.9	0	1.2	0	0	0	0		4.1
UAE	0.4	0	3	0	0.	0	0.3		3.7
Yemen	N/A	N/A	N/A	N/A	N/A	N/A	N/A		N/A
Global	4.93	0.18	15.03	10.84	2.21	0.062	42.73		75.982

24.7   Education and Research

Palliative care has not yet been universally integrated into medical and nursing school curricula across the region. Some medical schools in Jordan, Lebanon, Oman are teaching palliative care as a separate module. Other countries like Egypt and Kuwait have integrated palliative care teaching in their undergraduate curriculum as part of modules in oncology or pulmonary medicine [21]. However, most medical schools have yet to include palliative care as part of their standard undergraduate curriculum. Few nursing schools in Jordan, Lebanon, and Tunisia have integrated palliative care principles into their nursing curricula or offer dedicated courses in palliative care [9, 21].

When palliative care first came to the Arab world, there were no specialist training programs in palliative care in the region and most experts practicing in Arab countries were trained internationally. The first palliative care fellowship program was established at the King Faisal Specialist Hospital and Research Center (KFSHRC) in Saudi Arabia in 2000. The program was later accredited in 2013. Many of its graduates have gone on to practice, build programs, teach, and mentor young clinicians in other Arab countries. However, the specialty has yet to be listed under the Arab Board of Medical Specialties, and Arab Board certification in Palliative Medicine is not yet an option for medical graduates.

Over the past 20–30 years, workshops, short courses, and certificate programs have been offered through cancer centers, universities, and organizations across the region. Many of these have been developed and delivered in collaboration with international partners such as the American Society of Clinical Oncology (ASCO), Hospice Africa Uganda, San Diego Hospice, OhioHealth, and Yale University.

Research funding and output in palliative care in the region remain limited. A scoping review of publications on palliative care from the EMR region between 2005–2016 identified 73 unique articles [21].

24.8   Professional Associations

Medical societies are commonly seen as sources of information sharing and educational opportunities. However, they can also play a critical role in setting professional standards, encouraging and supporting research initiatives, advocating for change in the health system, and advancing a medical specialty.

Since palliative care was introduced to the region relatively recently, the activity of palliative care societies in the region remains limited. National palliative care societies have been established in Jordan, Kuwait, Morocco, Saudi Arabia, and Tunisia with varying degrees of activity. However, attempts at establishing a regional palliative care organization have not been successful to date.

24.9 Pediatric Palliative Care

There is a paucity of healthcare experts in pediatric oncology in most Arab countries [24]. The few clinicians trained in pediatric palliative care in the region mostly practice without the support of a multidisciplinary team, program, or department. A manual search of organizations dedicated to pediatric palliative care listed on the website of the International Children's Palliative Care Network (ICPCN) revealed only two organizations in Kuwait: the Kuwait Association for the Care of Children in Hospital (KACCH) and Bayt Abdullah Children's Hospice (BACCH) Sheikh Khalifa Medical City.

Approximately 14,000 children younger than 15 years are diagnosed with cancer each year in Arab countries [25]. Cancer is a primary cause of illness-related mortality among children. However, even in countries with more advanced palliative care systems like Egypt, Lebanon, and Jordan, there are no policies or guidelines dedicated to pediatric palliative care. In some countries, like Morocco, opioid regulations are more restrictive for pediatric patients [26]. The absence of national guidelines, limited knowledge, inadequate training, restricted access to opioids, and limited resources are all barriers to the advancement of pediatric palliative care in the region [27].

24.10 Arab Culture and Palliative Care

Culture and social norms are central to the way people cope with pain, cancer, treatment choices as well as death and dying. The role of the family, social values, religion, and health beliefs all have an important impact on how treatment options are communicated, how decisions are made, and what treatments are received when a patient is sick.

As in many other countries, misconceptions and stigma associated with the use of opioid analgesics create barriers to pain management. Fear of addiction and the belief that opioids should be reserved for the final days of life are prevalent in Arab countries.

The family unit plays a very central role in Arab culture. When someone has a serious illness, the extended family generally contributes to caregiving and providing support to a patient. Decision-making usually rests with the family or a family spokesperson rather than the individual [22]. Family members often withhold information as disclosure of a terminal illness or a cancer diagnosis can be perceived as harmful to the patient [12, 22].

Choosing costly medical interventions and hospital-based care can be one way for the family to express how much their loved one is valued. Families are less likely to choose to keep a patient at home and minimize aggressive interventions towards the end of life. There can be significant social pressure to demand more aggressive care [22]. Misconceptions about palliative care, pain management, and opioids can be important barriers to patients receiving the care that they need.

Religion also plays a central role in the lives of most patients and frequently influences the choices they make about their care. Families may reach out to a religious resource for guidance in medical decision-making. Religious interpretations vary, and there can be a lack of clarity around legal issues related to medical care at the end of life [22]. These include inconsistent interpretation of the position of Islam on medical interventions that may be considered futile and even pain management. Policies allowing choice around aggressive medical interventions towards the end of life are variable across countries and institutions based on the interpretation of Islamic law.

24.11 Future of Palliative Care

Given the overwhelming evidence regarding the benefit of palliative care to oncology patients, Arab countries should strive to make palliative care a standard component of cancer care and accessible to patients who need it. Current efforts to build palliative care in the region include many innovative programs and successful initiatives led by forward-thinking pioneers with great skills and commitment. However, more often than not, leaders work in isolation from the broader palliative care community. Collaborations and coordination of efforts across borders have been limited. This is indicated by the absence of a functional Arab palliative care association after 30 years of regional activity.

Coordination of regional efforts can encourage the development of policies, guidelines, standards, and regulations. Collaborative efforts can expand training programs and advocate successfully for registration of palliative care as a specialty with the Arab Board of Medical Specializations and eventual board certification. Regional efforts can be helpful in coordinating access to opioid analgesics at the regional level, increasing awareness, engaging communities, and mobilizing resources for education, research, and service delivery.

An example of such an effort is the Palliative Care Regional Expert Network which was launched by the WHO Eastern Mediterranean Regional Office (EMRO) in September 2019. The network was the outcome of a regional meeting held in Beirut with the aim of setting priorities, drafting a roadmap for the development of palliative care in the region, and providing input and technical guidance to support governments as they implement national palliative care priorities, structures, and activities in line with regional and global commitments. The group has brought together leaders in palliative care from 9 countries to think together, share information, and collaborate on projects.

24.12 Conclusion

Serious health-related suffering due to cancer is high in Arab countries and projected to increase through the first half of the twenty-first century. There is great variability in the level of palliative care development across the region, but even in the most advanced countries, services do not meet the needs of the population in the setting of high incidence of cancer at advanced stages. The lack of national policies and funding; limited training opportunities, human resources, and service providers; restricted access to medications; poor public awareness; and the lack of coordination and collaboration among palliative care professionals have hindered the integration of palliative care into health systems in the region. Political instability and regional conflicts have forced many governments to focus on crisis management leaving limited resources to invest in health infrastructure. Regional planning must address all these dimensions to allow healthcare systems to meet the palliative care needs of cancer patients across the Arab world.

Conflict of Interest Authors have no conflict of interest to declare.

References

1. Radbruch L, De Lima L, Knaul F, Wenk R, Zippporah A, Bhatnaghar S, et al. Redefining palliative care - a new consensus-based definition. J Pain Symptom Manag. 2020;60(4):754–64.
2. WHO Palliative care. 2020. Retrieved from https://www.who.int/news-room/fact-sheets/detail/palliative-care.
3. Bauman J, Temel J. The Integration of early palliative care with oncology care: the time has come for a new tradition. J Natl Compr Cancer Netw. 2014;12(12):1763–71.
4. Temel J, Greer J, Muzikansky A, Gallagher E, Admane S, Jackson V. Early palliative care for patients with metastatic non-small-cell lung cancer. N Engl J Med. 2010;363(8):733–42.
5. Davis MP, Temel JS, Balboni T, Glare P. A review of the trials which examine early integration of outpatient and home palliative care for patients with serious illnesses. Ann Palliat Med. 2015;4(3):99–121. https://doi.org/10.3978/j.issn.2224-5820.2015.04.04.
6. Dionne-Odom, J. N., Azuero, A., Lyons, K. D., Hull, J. G., Tosteson, T., Li, Z., . . . Bakitas, M. A. (2015). Benefits of early versus delayed palliative care to informal family caregivers of patients with advanced cancer: outcomes from the ENABLE III randomized controlled trial. J Clin Oncol, 33(13), 1446–1452. doi:https://doi.org/10.1200/JCO.2014.58.7824.
7. Hannon B, Swami N, Rodin G, Pope A, Zimmermann C. Experiences of patients and caregivers with early palliative care: a qualitative study. Palliat Med. 2017;31(1):72–81. https://doi.org/10.1177/0269216316649126.
8. Ferrell, B. R., Temel, J. S., Temin, S., Alesi, E. R., Balboni, T. A., Basch, E. M., . . . Smith, T. J. (2017). Integration of palliative care into standard oncology care: American Society of Clinical Oncology clinical practice guideline update. J Clin Oncol, 35(1), 96–112. doi:https://doi.org/10.1200/JCO.2016.70.1474.
9. Zeinah GFA, Al-Kindi SG, Hassan AA. Middle East experience in palliative care. Am J Hosp Palliat Care. 2013;30(1):94–9.

10. Connor SR, editor. Global atlas of palliative care. 2nd ed. London: World Hospice and Palliative Care Alliance; 2020.
11. Fadhil I, Lyons G, Payne S. Barriers to, and opportunities for, palliative care development in the Eastern Mediterranean Region. Lancet Oncol. 2017;18(3):e176–84.
12. Shamieh O, Jazieh A-R. Modification and Implementation of NCCN Guidelines™ on Palliative Care in the Middle East and North Africa Region. J Natl Compr Cancer Netw. 2010;8(Suppl_3):S-41–7.
13. May, P., Garrido, M. M., Cassel, J. B., Kelley, A. S., Meier, D. E., Normand, C., . . . Morrison, R. S. (2016). Palliative care teams' cost-saving effect is larger for cancer patients with higher numbers of comorbidities. Health Aff (Millwood), 35(1), 44–53. doi:https://doi.org/10.1377/hlthaff.2015.0752.
14. Haltia, O., Farkkila, N., Roine, R. P., Sintonen, H., Taari, K., Hanninen, J., . . . Saarto, T. (2018). The indirect costs of palliative care in end-stage cancer: a real-life longitudinal register- and questionnaire-based study. Palliat Med, 32(2), 493–499. doi:https://doi.org/10.1177/0269216317729789.
15. Murtagh FE, Bausewein C, Verne J, Groeneveld EI, Kaloki YE, Higginson IJ. How many people need palliative care? A study developing and comparing methods for population-based estimates. Palliat Med. 2014;28(1):49–58.
16. Knaul FM, Farmer PE, Krakauer EL, et al. Alleviating the access abyss in palliative care and pain relief-an imperative of universal health coverage: The Lancet Commission report. Lancet. 2018;391(10128):1391–454. http://www.thelancet.com/commissions/palliative-care.
17. IAHPC. Global data platform to calculate HS and palliative care need: International Association for Hospice and Palliative Care. 2020. Retrieved from https://hospicecare.com/what-we-do/resources/global-data-platform-to-calculate-shs-and-palliative-care-need/.
18. Sleeman, K. E., de Brito, M., Etkind, S., Nkhoma, K., Guo, P., Higginson, I. J., . . . Harding, R. (2019). The escalating global burden of serious health-related suffering: projections to 2060 by world regions, age groups, and health conditions. Lancet Glob Health, 7(7), e883-e892. doi:https://doi.org/10.1016/s2214-109x(19)30172-x.
19. Stjernswärd J, Foley KM, Ferris FD. The public health strategy for palliative care. J Pain Symptom Manag. 2007;33(5):486–93.
20. Rhee JY, Luyirika E, Namisango E, Powell RA, Garralda E, Pons-Izquierdo JJ, et al. APCA atlas of palliative care in Africa. Houston: IAHPC Press; 2017.
21. Osman H, Rihan A, Garralda E, Rhee JY, Pons-Izquierdo JJ, Lima L, et al. Atlas of palliative care in the eastern Mediterranean region. Houston: IAHPC Press; 2017.
22. Al-Awamer A, Downar J. Developing a palliative care service model for Muslim Middle Eastern countries. Support Care Cancer. 2014;22(12):3253–62.
23. WaltherCenter. Global essential medicines consumption: Walther Center in global palliative care & supportive oncology. 2017. Retrieved from https://walthercenter.iu.edu/essential-medicines/global-data.html.
24. Silbermann, M., Arnaout, M., Daher, M., Nestoros, S., Pitsillides, B., Charalambous, H., . . . Khleif, A. (2012). Palliative cancer care in Middle Eastern countries: accomplishments and challenges. Ann Oncol, 23(suppl_3), 15–28.
25. Sultan I. Pediatric oncology in the Arab World. In: Laher I, editor. Handbook of healthcare in the Arab World. Cham: Springer International Publishing; 2020. p. 1–25.
26. Hessissen L, Madani A. Pediatric oncology in Morocco: achievements and challenges. J Pediatr Hematol Oncol. 2012;34:S21–2.
27. Mojen LK, Rassouli M, Eshghi P, Sari AA, Karimooi MH. Palliative care for children with cancer in the Middle East: A comparative study. Indian J Palliat Care. 2017;23(4):379.

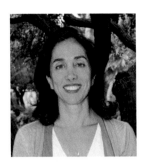

Hibah Osman is the founder of Balsam—the Lebanese Center for Palliative Care and founding director of the Palliative and Supportive Care Program at the American University of Beirut Medical Center. She is currently a palliative care physician at Dana-Farber Cancer Institute where she is also Associate Medical Director for oncology at the International Patient Center. Dr. Osman is committed to developing palliative care in the MENA region and globally. She is a member of the Board of the International Association for Hospice and Palliative Care and a member of the WHO EMRO Palliative Care Expert Network.

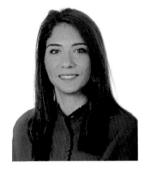

Rana Yamout, MD, has been playing an active role in integrating palliative care into the Lebanese healthcare system. After completing her Master of Research in Palliative Care Medicine at Paris Descartes and medical training in France, she led the establishment of the palliative care mobile unit at the Clemenceau Medical Center. She was also a founding member of the palliative care unit at Hospital Hotel-Dieu de France. Dr. Yamout is currently the Director of the Palliative and Supportive Care Program at the American University of Beirut Medical Center and a member of the palliative care team at Balsam- Lebanese Center for Palliative Care.

Chapter 25
Cancer Research in the Arab World

Randah R. Hamadeh ⓘ, Haitham Jahrami ⓘ, and Khaled Nazzal ⓘ

25.1 Introduction

Health research productivity in the Arab countries is lagging than other non-Arab countries in the Middle East and the world [1–3]. It is below the world average except for four countries (Qatar, Tunisia, Lebanon, and Kuwait) [2]. However, there has been an increase in scientific productivity since the start of the 1990s [4]. A study on the toxicology research output among Middle Eastern Arab countries has also shown that Arab countries are falling behind in the number of publications and noted a rise in the research activity [5].

The Arab world was delayed in the number of publications in top journals and the number of citations [2]. International collaborations have contributed to the recent increase in citations and publishing in top quartile journals [2]. It has been reported that common metrics that assess health research are missing from some Arab countries [6]. Research in the Arab region has been criticized for several issues, including the underinvestment in research and development, production, and use of research [4, 7, 8]. Arab countries have low Gross domestic Expenditure on Research and Development (GERD) as a percentage of Gross Domestic Product (GDP), with Libya (0.86) and Morocco (0.73) having the highest GERD/GDP ratios [9]. It is worth noting that most Arab countries suffer from brain drain except for the

R. R. Hamadeh (✉)
College of Medicine and Medical Sciences, Arabian Gulf University, Manama, Bahrain
e-mail: randah@agu.edu.bh

H. Jahrami
College of Medicine and Medical Sciences, Arabian Gulf University, Manama, Bahrain

Ministry of Health, Manama, Bahrain
e-mail: hjahrami@health.gov.bh

K. Nazzal
Ibn Al Nafees Hospital, Manama, Bahrain

© The Author(s) 2022
H. O. Al-Shamsi et al. (eds.), *Cancer in the Arab World*,
https://doi.org/10.1007/978-981-16-7945-2_25

Gulf Cooperation Council (GCC) countries who, on the contrary, attract professionals, including academicians and researchers from the Arab world and elsewhere [10]. Conflict, political turmoil, and difficulty in publishing in journals with high impact factors are among the other reasons given to the Arab countries' delay in comparison to the world [1, 11]. Further, few faculty members and graduate students in the Arab world publish, and those who do mostly published in journals that are not indexed in Scopus or Web of Science. Moreover, not all Arab universities require publications for academic promotions. For the 11 Arab countries that have available data, the number of researchers per million inhabitants ranges from 19 in Sudan to 1394 in Tunisia [9]. Another challenge that some Arab countries, GCC countries, in particular, face in conducting research is the heterogeneity of the non-national population and their transient nature with implications such as sampling, the need for translating questionnaires into several languages if used as a tool and conducting longitudinal studies [12].

25.2   Cancer Research Output in the Arab World

There is a rise in cancer incidence rates in the Eastern Mediterranean Region (EMR) countries that include 19 Arab countries in addition to Afghanistan, Iran, and Pakistan. This rate is expected to increase twofold from 2012 to 2030. The top five cancers among males are lung, prostate, colorectal, liver, and urinary bladder [13]. The corresponding cancers for females are breast, cervical, colorectal, ovarian, and stomach cancers. Despite this burden, cancer research output in the Arab countries is low, which is a disadvantage to the academic community [13]. Further, none of the institutions in the Arab world were listed among the 2020 top 200 institutions in cancer research based on the Nature Index [14]. Globally, cancer research has been increasing, with the United States and China taking the lead [14, 15].

Of all the research performed worldwide, 4% was on cancer research in 2014 [15]. A study comparing the health research output and burden of disease in Palestine indicated that cancer is seldom addressed in the country's publications relative to its burden [16]. On the other hand, a scoping review of Non-Communicable Diseases (NCDs) from seven Arab countries reported that there was a relative surplus of cancer publications compared to cardiovascular diseases [17]. Only one study assessed the cancer research output of Arab countries, however, it was limited to seven countries out of the twenty-two [18]. Another study examined breast cancer research in all Arab countries [19]. Two studies assessed cancer publications output in Qatar [20] and Egypt [21]. The Qatari study reported that cancer publications represented 17% out of total publications from 2000–2012, below the world average (24%) with the number of cancer publications per 1000 population increasing from nil in 2000 to 0.02% in 2012 [20]. The Egyptian study concluded that the Egyptian cancer and biomedical publications comprised 0.13% of the world's cancer publications between 1991 and 2010 [21].

The review of cancer research productivity in seven Arab countries that covered 14 years starting 2000, ending 2013, indicated that the productivity in Arab countries is lower than Europe, Japan, and the United States, which was attributed to the lower number of researchers, lack of financing, research support, networking, and difficulties in accessing reliable and valid data. Furthermore, the review highlighted the role of political unrest in hindering research output [18]. In a publication on global cancer research, none of the Arab countries were listed as contributors of at least 1% of the global cancer publications, although few low development index countries were included [22].

As far as the last cancer research publications review of Arab countries is concerned, only seven Arab countries were included that covered a 14-year period which ended in 2012. Thus, we identified cancer publications for the last decade starting 2010 and ending 2019 to include all Arab countries. We searched using Scopus, PubMed/Medline, and Google Scholar using the keywords "Arab" and "cancer" and repeated the search for each of the 22 Arab countries and "cancer."

The review that we conducted included 4541 publications confirmed that the publications almost doubled in 2019 compared to 2010, with a steady increase since 2017 (Fig. 25.1). Among the seven Arab countries included in the review by Hamadeh et al., [18] Morocco had the highest proportion of publications (40.8%),

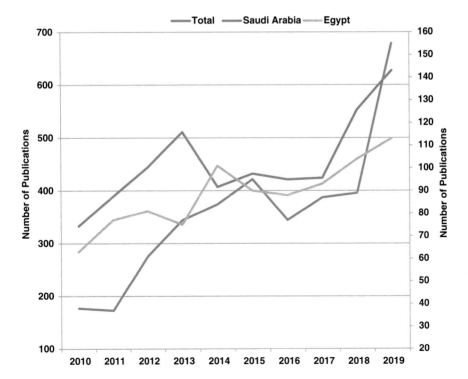

Fig. 25.1 Annual number of cancer publications in the Arab world, Egypt, and Saudi Arabia, 2010–2019

followed by Lebanon (25.3%), Kuwait (19%), Iraq (5.8%), Sudan (5.4%), Bahrain (2.1%), and Palestine (1.6%). In our review, there was a large variation between the countries where some contributed to most of the output and some hardly had any publications. Few studies included several Arab countries or were regional like those conducted in the GCC countries, Maghreb countries and the North African countries. The top five countries that had major contribution to the cancer research productivity were Egypt (19.5%), Saudi Arabia (17.6%), Morocco (11.8%), Tunisia (8.5%), and Jordan (8.2%), accounting for almost two-thirds of the cancer publications in this period excluding their contribution to regional or global studies. Egypt and Saudi Arabia had a steady rise in the number of publications in recent years in line with the increase in total publications (Fig. 25.1). However, there was a dearth in cancer publications from the Arab Sub-Saharan African countries (Comoros Islands, Djibouti, Mauritania, and Somalia). The majority (92.2%) of the publications were in English and the remaining in French (mostly from the Maghreb countries) except for one in Italian, and the other in Spanish.

25.3 Arab Cancer Regional Studies

There were several articles that included Arab or EMR countries or were regional, focusing on all cancers or specific cancers with various themes. Among those is the one by (Hamadeh et al. 2017) that examined cancer research [18], one examining mutations in hereditary breast and ovarian cancers [23], prostate cancer [24], liver cancer [25], cervical cancer [26] and colorectal cancer [27]. As for the regional, from the Maghreb, and GCC countries, among the most recent publications that included all cancers were those by Ben Abdelaziz et al. 2019, and Al-Zalabani 2020 [28, 29]. Others investigated specific cancers like cervical and breast cancers [30, 31].

25.4 Cancer Research in Arab Countries Based on Cancer Registries

Most Arab countries have Population-Based Cancer Registries (PBCR), yet they are not fully utilized for research. There is a deficiency in population-based studies that can provide incidence, prevalence, mortality, survival, and other data [13]. A recent survey by the International Agency for Research on Cancer (IARC) and the World Health Organization (WHO) Eastern Mediterranean Regional Office on PBCR in 12 Arab and one non-Arab country in the EMR showed that such data has limited availability, including mortality data [32]. During the past 10 years, most Arab countries did not utilize the PBCR to their full potential. Breast cancer was the most PBCR based researched cancer, followed by lung cancer. In contrast, Saudi Arabia had several publications based on PBCR that included all cancers and a landscape of specific cancers [33–37]. There were several PBCR based studies from other countries during 2019 and 2020 [38–42].

25.5 Most Researched Cancers

Out of the 4541 publications, 712 articles included all cancers or were nonspecific. Of the remaining, the ten commonest cancers that were researched in the last decade were breast cancer, colorectal cancer, liver cancer, leukemia, childhood cancers, lung cancer, cervical cancer, bladder cancer, prostate cancer, and Non-Hodgkin's Lymphoma (NHL), with variable contributions (Fig. 25.2). It is gratifying to know that cancer publications in the Arab world focused on most of the commonest five cancers among males and females [13] with the exception of stomach and ovarian cancers.

It has been previously reported that breast cancer research output was low in the 1970s and 1980s and started to increase in the mid-1990s. However, it was lower than that of non-Arab countries in the region. Further, Egypt and Saudi Arabia were the major contributors to breast cancer research, and there was a sharp increase in the two countries in the decade preceding 2012 [19].

In our review, almost a quarter of the Arab cancer publications in the last decade focused on breast cancer. The top five Arab countries that contributed the most in breast cancer research during the last decade were Saudi Arabia (17.5%), Egypt (16.2%), Morocco (11.1%), Tunisia (9.6%) while Iraq and Jordan equally contributed to 7.8%. There was a variation between the countries with respect to the proportion of the country's cancer research focusing on breast cancer. Of all the cancer

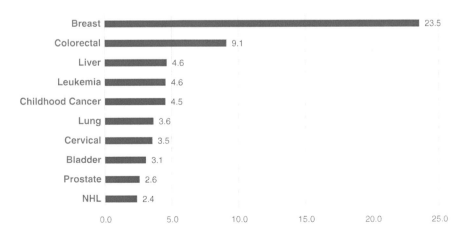

Fig. 25.2 The top ten cancers that were researched in the Arab publications, 2010–2019

research that was conducted in the country, the proportion of breast cancer articles ranged from 14.3% in Mauritania to 44.2% in Bahrain (Fig. 25.3).

The proportion of publications focusing on lung cancer was 3.6% of all the publications. Over two-thirds of the lung cancer publications were from five countries: Morocco, Tunisia, Egypt, Lebanon, and Saudi Arabia. There was a large variation between the countries by the proportion of colorectal cancer research. Saudi Arabia was the leading contributor to almost one-third (32.5%) of the research on colorectal cancer in the Arab world, followed by Egypt (14.4%), Tunisia (14%), Morocco (8.4%) and Jordan (6.5%). Out of all the prostate cancer publications in the last ten years, Saudi Arabia contributed 17.9%, Egypt, 15.4%, Jordan, 12%, Tunisia, 10%, and Algeria, 8.5%. As for liver cancer, the major contributor among the Arab states was Egypt, which provided almost three-quarters of the publications, with Saudi Arabia being next contributing 10.9%. Egypt contributed the most (44.8%) of the bladder cancer publications, followed by Tunisia (13.4%) and Morocco (9.7%). Egypt (26.1%), Lebanon (14%), Morocco (14%) and Saudi Arabia (13.5%) contributed significantly to the cancer research on leukemia. About a quarter of the articles on cervical cancer were from Saudi Arabia. Morocco (19.9%), Tunisia (14%) and Egypt (9.9%) also made high contributions. Over one-third (34.5%) of the publications on childhood cancers were from Egypt. The rest were mainly from Jordan (13.1%), Lebanon (10.2%) and Saudi Arabia (10.2%). Around half of the NHL cancer publications were from Morocco and Egypt, almost equally distributed. Tunisia and Saudi Arabia contributed 20%.

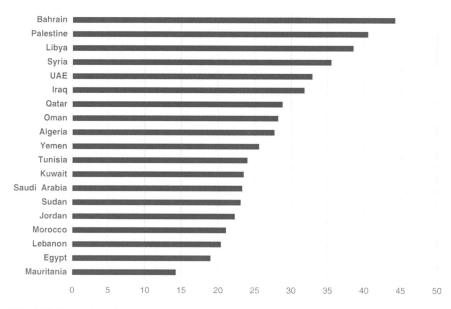

Fig. 25.3 Proportion of cancer publications allocated to breast cancer by Arab country, 2010–2019

25.6 Journals

Table 25.1 shows the top 5 ranked journals for the total cancer publications and the countries that contributed the most to the cancer research output in the Arab world during the last ten years. The Asian Pacific Journal of Cancer Prevention and the Pan African Medical Journal were the only non-Arab journals among the top 5 most popular journals for cancer publications from Arab countries. The former was also among the top 5 ranked journals in Egypt, Saudi Arabia, Morocco, Tunisia, and Jordan. It accounted with the Saudi Medical Journal for 20% of all the Saudi publications. In Morocco, 20% of the articles were published in the Pan African Medical Journal. It is worth noting that all the countries except for Morocco had a local journal amongst its top selected journal for cancer publications. The Saudi Medical Journal was reported to be the most popular journal for breast cancer research in Arab countries [19] and one of the top five in our review, contributing to 2.8% of the total breast cancer publications. In our review, the Saudi Medical Journal was second (2.5%) after The Asian Pacific Journal of Cancer Prevention (9.5%) for the breast cancer publications. The third, fourth, and fifth journals were Pan African Medical Journal (2.3%), BMC Cancer (2.1%) and PLoS ONE (1.7%), respectively.

The top 20 journals where Arab cancer research publications in the last decade were published are presented by quartile and Scimago Journal Rank (SJR) in Table 25.2. Their SJRs ranged from 0.11 to 1.627, with an average of 0.487. These top 20 journals had published 28.1% of the research manuscripts in the region in the last ten years, 40% of which were Q4 journals. There were few publications in the Q1 journals with high SJR like The Lancet, Lancet Oncology, Cancer Discovery, and Cancer Cell International, but their contribution was 0.7% only.

25.7 First Authors

Usually, the country of the first author is where the study is conducted. However, in the Arab region, there are several publications whereby first authors have affiliations from other Arab countries or even from non-Arab countries. Some of these publications as well do not have a co-author from the concerned country. There are several possible explanations for this phenomenon. In assigning the affiliation of the first author, we usually consider the first affiliation written as the primary affiliation if the author holds more than one. Moreover, on some occasions, the first author writes one of his affiliations that might not be corresponding to that of the country where the study was undertaken. In addition, there are some cases where an Arab individual is studying or working abroad and is affiliated to a university or a non-academic institution elsewhere but conducting the research in his country of residence.

Table 25.1 Percentage contribution of the top five journals of total Arab cancer publications and top five contributing countries, 2010–2019

	Total	Egypt	Saudi Arabia	Morocco	Tunisia	Jordan
1	Asian Pacific Journal of Cancer Prevention (7.5%)	Asian Pacific Journal of Cancer Prevention (6.8%)	Saudi Medical Journal (10.6%)	Pan African Medical Journal (19.9%)	Tunisie Medicale (13.3%)	Asian Pacific Journal of Cancer Prevention (11%)
2	Pan African Medical Journal (2.8%)	Journal of the Egyptian National Cancer Institute (5.2%)	Asian Pacific Journal of Cancer Prevention (9.4%)	Journal African du Cancer (3.9%)	Asian Pacific Journal of Cancer Prevention (5.5%)	Jordan Medical Journal (5.4%)
3	Saudi Medical Journal (2.5%)	Journal of Pediatric Hematology/Oncology (1.5%)	Annals of Saudi Medicine (3.9%)	Asian Pacific Journal of Cancer Prevention (3.7%)	Bulletin du Cancer (4.3%)	Journal of Cancer Education (3.8%)
4	Tunisie Medicale (1.4%)	Egyptian Journal of Radiology and Nuclear Medicine (1.1%)	PLoS One (2.2%) Saudi Journal of Gastroenterology (2.2%)	BMC Research Notes (3.2%)	Tumor Biology (4%)	Eastern Mediterranean Health Journal (1.9%) Saudi Medical Journal (1.9%)
5	Gulf Journal of Oncology (1.2%) Journal of the Egyptian National Cancer Institute (1.2%)	Applied Immunohistochemistry and Molecular Morphology (1%) Chinese-German Journal of Clinical Oncology (1%) Medical Oncology (1%)	Journal of Cancer Education (2.1%)	BMC Cancer (1.9%) World Journal of Surgical Oncology (1.9%)	Pan African Medical Journal (3.1%)	Cancer Nursing (1.6%)

Table 25.2 The quartiles, and Scimago Journal Ranks of the 20 top journals of cancer publications of Arab countries, 2010–2019

S. No	Name of Journal	Quartile	Scimago Journal Rank
1	Asian Pacific Journal of Cancer Prevention	Q2	0.813
2	Pan African Medical Journal	Q3	0.203
3	Saudi Medical Journal	Q3	0.276
4	Gulf Journal of Oncology	Q3	0.143
5	Journal of the Egyptian National Cancer Institute	Q3	0.424
6	Tunisie Medicale	Q3	0.149
7	PLoS One	Q1	1.395
8	Journal African du Cancer	Q4	0.188
9	Journal of Cancer Education	Q2	0.525
10	BMC Cancer	Q1	1.627
11	Eastern Mediterranean Health Journal	Q2	0.328
12	Annals of Saudi Medicine	Q3	0.24
13	Kuwait Medical Journal	Q4	0.11
14	Indian Journal of Public Health Research and Development	Q4	0.105
15	Bahrain Medical Bulletin	Q3	0.135
16	Pediatric Blood and Cancer	Q1	1.505
17	Oman Medical Journal	Q2	0.309
18	Medical Oncology	Q2	0.837
19	Journal of Pediatric Hematology/Oncology	Q2	0.452
20	Bulletin du Cancer	Q3	0.297

Scimago Journal List Ranking–2019. https://www.scimagojr.com/journalrank.php

Further, there are instances where non-Arab faculty members leave the region and publish papers on the country they had worked in but with their new affiliations.

25.8 COVID 19 Pandemic and Cancer Research

Several researchers from the Arab world were active and published on cancer and COVID-19 (Coronavirus disease 2019). Since many Arab patients, including cancer patients, seek treatment abroad, a review examined the challenges that cancer patients and their families faced during the pandemic [43]. Arab researchers also studied the impact of the pandemic on the management of cancer patients [44]. Oncologists from the Gulf and Arab countries examined managing cancer patients virtually, the challenges they encountered and had a collaborative international study on a novel approach to manage cancer patients [45, 46]. Another study provided treatment guidelines for cancer patients during the pandemic [47], and one looked into screening for COVID-19 in hospitals among asymptomatic patients with cancer [48]. A study from Jordan examined the "do not resuscitate" policy during the pandemic in the largest cancer center in Jordan [49]. Researchers from Gaza, a city with several challenges, studied the additional ones faced by cancer patients in Gaza due to COVID-19 [50].

25.9 Conclusion

The Arab countries are mostly low to middle-income countries with few considered high income. Several countries are in conflict and political turmoil that makes research funding not a priority. Further, the research enabling environment in such a situation is not optimal, and some countries face brain drain of researchers. This partly explains why Arab countries fall behind in cancer research productivity. Nevertheless, there has been a steady increase in the cancer research yield with variable contributions between countries. Breast cancer, the commonest cancer among females in the region, is given priority over other leading cancers with respect to research output. The PBCR are not used as expected to generate cancer studies. The main journals targeted by researchers in the Arab world are international journals with low ranking and local journals. There is an urgent need to examine the challenges and barriers facing researchers in Arab countries, allocate funds for cancer research and collaborate with researchers in notable institutions regionally and globally to improve the quantity and quality of cancer research. Concerted efforts should be made to narrow the knowledge gaps with respect to the less researched cancers and generate evidence. PBCR data should be made more accessible to researchers to assist in generating knowledge that contributes to cancer control and prevention.

Conflict of Interest Authors have no conflict of interest to declare.

References

1. Benamer HT, Bakoush O. Arab nations lagging behind other Middle Eastern countries in biomedical research: a comparative study. BMC Med Res Methodol. 2009;9:26. https://doi.org/10.1186/1471-2288-9-26.
2. El Rassi R, Meho LI, Nahlawi A, Salameh JS, Bazarbachi A, Akl EA. Medical research productivity in the Arab countries: 2007-2016 bibliometric analysis. J Glob Health. 2018;8(2):020411. https://doi.org/10.7189/jogh.08.020411.
3. Al-Khader AA. Enhancing research productivity in the Arab world. Saudi Med J. 2004;25(10):1323–7.
4. Ismail SA, McDonald A, Dubois E, Aljohani FG, Coutts AP, Majeed A, et al. Assessing the state of health research in the Eastern Mediterranean Region. J R Soc Med. 2013;106(6):224–33. https://doi.org/10.1258/jrsm.2012.120240.
5. Zyoud SH, Al-Jabi SW, Sweileh WM, Awang R. A bibliometric analysis of toxicology research productivity in Middle Eastern Arab countries during a 10-year period (2003-2012). Health Res Policy Syst. 2014;12:4. https://doi.org/10.1186/1478-4505-12-4.
6. Blair I, Grivna M, Sharif AA. The "Arab world" is not a useful concept when addressing challenges to public health, public health education, and research in the Middle East. Front Public Health. 2014;2:30. https://doi.org/10.3389/fpubh.2014.00030.

7. Kennedy A, TAM K, Abou-Zeid AH, Ghannem H, Ijsselmuiden C, Group W-ECGNC. National health research system mapping in 10 Eastern Mediterranean countries. East Mediterr Health J. 2008;14(3):502–17.
8. Elsayed AMA, Sabtan YMN. Reality of scientific research in the Arab world and suggestions for development. Int J Adv Soc Sci Humanit. 2019;7(1):31–5.
9. Zou'bi MR, Mohamed-Nour S, El-Kharraz J, Hassan N. Chapter 17. The Arab States. UNESCO science report: towards 2030. Paris: UNESCO Publishing; 2015.
10. El Saghir NS. Modern cancer management and research in the Middle East. Lancet Oncol. 2012;13(11):1076–8. https://doi.org/10.1016/S1470-2045(12)70479-5.
11. Maziak W. Geography of biomedical publications. Lancet. 2004;363(9407):490. https://doi.org/10.1016/S0140-6736(04)15500-1.
12. Aw TC, Zoubeidi T, Al-Maskari F, Blair I. Challenges and strategies for quantitative and qualitative field research in the United Arab Emirates. Asian Pac J Cancer Prev. 2011;12(6):1641–5.
13. Arafa MA, Rabah DM, Farhat KH. Rising cancer rates in the Arab world: now is the time for action. East Mediterr Health J. 2020;26(6):638–40. https://doi.org/10.26719/emhj.20.073.
14. Nature S: Nature Index 2020 Cancer. https://www.nature.com/collections/hfgbcehage/tables. 2020. Accessed 2 Dec 2020.
15. Elsevier: cancer research: current trends & future directions. https://www.elsevier.com/?a=230374. 2016. Accessed 1 Dec 2020.
16. Albarqouni L, Elessi K, Abu-Rmeileh NME. A comparison between health research output and burden of disease in Arab countries: evidence from Palestine. Health Res Policy Syst. 2018;16(1):25. https://doi.org/10.1186/s12961-018-0302-4.
17. Sibai AM, Singh NV, Jabbour S, Saleh S, Abdulrahim S, Naja F, et al. Does published research on non-communicable disease (NCD) in Arab countries reflect NCD disease burden? PLoS One. 2017;12(6):e0178401. https://doi.org/10.1371/journal.pone.0178401.
18. Hamadeh RR, Borgan SM, Sibai AM. Cancer research in the Arab world: a review of publications from seven countries between 2000-2013. Sultan Qaboos Univ Med J. 2017;17(2):e147–e54. https://doi.org/10.18295/squmj.2016.17.02.003.
19. Sweileh WM, Zyoud SH, Al-Jabi SW, Sawalha AF. Contribution of Arab countries to breast cancer research: comparison with non-Arab Middle Eastern countries. BMC Womens Health. 2015;15:25. https://doi.org/10.1186/s12905-015-0184-3.
20. Zeeneldin AA, Taha FM. Qatar biomedical and cancer publications in PubMed between 2000 and 2012. Qatar Med J. 2014;5:31–7.
21. Zeeneldin AA, Taha FM, Moneer M. Past and future trends in cancer and biomedical research: a comparison between Egypt and the world using PubMed-indexed publications. BMC Res Notes. 2012;5:349. https://doi.org/10.1186/1756-0500-5-349.
22. Cabral BP, da Graca Derengowski Fonseca M, Mota FB. The recent landscape of cancer research worldwide: a bibliometric and network analysis. Oncotarget. 2018;9(55):30474–84. https://doi.org/10.18632/oncotarget.25730.
23. Abdulrashid K, AlHussaini N, Ahmed W, Thalib L. Prevalence of BRCA mutations among hereditary breast and/or ovarian cancer patients in Arab countries: systematic review and meta-analysis. BMC Cancer. 2019;19(1):256. https://doi.org/10.1186/s12885-019-5463-1.
24. Al-Abdin OZ, Al-Beeshi IZ. Prostate cancer in the Arab population. An overview. Saudi Med J. 2018;39(5):453–8. https://doi.org/10.15537/smj.2018.5.21986.
25. Alavian SM, Haghbin H. Relative importance of hepatitis B and C viruses in hepatocellular carcinoma in EMRO countries and the Middle East: a systematic review. Hepat Mon. 2016;16(3):e35106. https://doi.org/10.5812/hepatmon.35106.
26. Ali S, Skirton H, Clark MT, Donaldson C. Integrative review of cervical cancer screening in Western Asian and Middle Eastern Arab countries. Nurs Health Sci. 2017;19(4):414–26. https://doi.org/10.1111/nhs.12374.
27. Arafa MA, Farhat K. Colorectal cancer in the Arab world--screening practices and future prospects. Asian Pac J Cancer Prev. 2015;16(17):7425–30. https://doi.org/10.7314/apjcp.2015.16.17.7425.

28. Ben Abdelaziz A, Melki S, Nouira S, Ben Abdelaziz A, Khelil M, Azzaza M, et al. Cancers in the Central Maghreb: epidemiology from 1990 to 2017 and trends in 2040. Tunis Med. 2019;97(6):739–70.
29. Al-Zalabani AH. Cancer incidence attributable to tobacco smoking in GCC countries in 2018. Tob Induc Dis. 2020;18:18. https://doi.org/10.18332/tid/118722.
30. Albeshan SM, Mackey MG, Hossain SZ, Alfuraih AA, Brennan PC. Breast cancer epidemiology in Gulf Cooperation Council countries: a regional and international comparison. Clin Breast Cancer. 2018;18(3):e381–e92. https://doi.org/10.1016/j.clbc.2017.07.006.
31. Alkhalawi E, Al-Madouj A, Al-Zahrani A. Cervical cancer incidence and trends among nationals of the Gulf Cooperation Council states, 1998-2012. Gulf J Oncolog. 2019;1(31):7–13.
32. Znaor A, Fouad H, Majnoni d'Intignano F, Hammerich A, Slama S, Pourghazian N, et al. Use of cancer data for cancer control in the Eastern Mediterranean Region: results of a survey among population-based cancer registries. Int J Cancer. 2020;148(3):593–600. https://doi.org/10.1002/ijc.33223.
33. Jazieh AR, Da'ar OB, Alkaiyat M, Zaatreh YA, Saad AA, Bustami R, et al. Cancer incidence trends from 1999 to 2015 and contributions of various cancer types to the overall burden: projections to 2030 and extrapolation of economic burden in Saudi Arabia. Cancer Manag Res. 2019;11:9665–74. https://doi.org/10.2147/CMAR.S222667.
34. Alghamdi IG, Alghamdi MS. The incidence rate of liver cancer in Saudi Arabia: an observational descriptive epidemiological analysis of data from the Saudi Cancer Registry (2004-2014). Cancer Manag Res. 2020;12:1101–11. https://doi.org/10.2147/CMAR.S232600.
35. Alshehri BM. Trends in the incidence of oral cancer in Saudi Arabia from 1994 to 2015. World J Surg Oncol. 2020;18(1):217. https://doi.org/10.1186/s12957-020-01989-3.
36. Belgaumi AF, Pathan GQ, Siddiqui K, Ali AA, Al-Fawaz I, Al-Sweedan S, et al. Incidence, clinical distribution, and patient characteristics of childhood cancer in Saudi Arabia: a population-based analysis. Pediatr Blood Cancer. 2019;66(6):e27684. https://doi.org/10.1002/pbc.27684.
37. Da'ar OB, Zaatreh YA, Saad AA, Alkaiyat M, Pasha T, Ahmed AE, et al. The burden, future trends, and economic impact of lung cancer in Saudi Arabia. Clinicoecon Outcomes Res. 2019;11:703–12. https://doi.org/10.2147/CEOR.S224444.
38. Alawadhi E, Al-Awadi A, Elbasmi A, Coleman MP, Allemani C. Cancer survival trends in Kuwait, 2000-2013: a population-based study. Gulf J Oncolog. 2019;1(29):39–52.
39. Al-Lawati NA, Shenoy SM, Al-Bahrani BJ, Al-Lawati JA. Increasing thyroid cancer incidence in Oman: a joinpoint trend analysis. Oman Med J. 2020;35(1):e98. https://doi.org/10.5001/omj.2020.16.
40. Cherif A, Dhaouadi S, Osman M, Hsairi M. Lung cancer burden of disease in the northern Tunisia. Eur J Pub Health. 2019;29(Supplement 4):ckz186.234. https://doi.org/10.1093/eurpub/ckz186.234.
41. Al-Lawati JA, Al-Bahrani BJ, Al-Lawati NA, Al-Zakwani I. Epidemiology of lung cancer in Oman: 20-year trends and tumor characteristics. Oman Med J. 2019;34(5):397–403. https://doi.org/10.5001/omj.2019.74.
42. Baum C, Soliman AS, Brown HE, Seifeldin IA, Ramadan M, Lott B, et al. Regional variation of pancreatic cancer incidence in the Nile Delta region of Egypt over a twelve-year period. J Cancer Epidemiol. 2020;2020:6031708. https://doi.org/10.1155/2020/6031708.
43. Al-Shamsi HO, Abu-Gheida I, Rana SK, Nijhawan N, Abdulsamad AS, Alrawi S, et al. Challenges for cancer patients returning home during SARS-COV-19 pandemic after medical tourism - a consensus report by the emirates oncology task force. BMC Cancer. 2020;20(1):641. https://doi.org/10.1186/s12885-020-07115-6.
44. Kattan C, Badreddine H, Rassy E, Kourie HR, Kattan J. The impact of the coronavirus pandemic on the management of cancer patients in Lebanon: a single institutional experience. Future Oncol. 2020;16(17):1157–60. https://doi.org/10.2217/fon-2020-0313.
45. Tashkandi E, Zeeneldin A, AlAbdulwahab A, Elemam O, Elsamany S, Jastaniah W, et al. Virtual management of patients with cancer during the COVID-19 pandemic: web-based questionnaire study. J Med Internet Res. 2020;22(6):e19691. https://doi.org/10.2196/19691.

46. Al-Shamsi HO, Alhazzani W, Alhuraiji A, Coomes EA, Chemaly RF, Almuhanna M, et al. A practical approach to the management of cancer patients during the novel coronavirus disease 2019 (COVID-19) pandemic: an international collaborative group. Oncologist. 2020;25(6):e936–e45. https://doi.org/10.1634/theoncologist.2020-0213.
47. Bitar N, Kattan J, Kourie H, Mukherji D, N ES. The Lebanese Society of Medical Oncology (LSMO) statement on the care of patients with cancer during the COVID-19 pandemic. Future Oncol. 2020;16(11):615–7.
48. Al-Shamsi HO, Coomes EA, Alrawi S. Screening for COVID-19 in asymptomatic patients with cancer in a hospital in the United Arab Emirates. JAMA Oncol. 2020;6(10):1627–8. https://doi.org/10.1001/jamaoncol.2020.2548.
49. Shamieh O, Richardson K, Abdel-Razeq H, Harding R, Sullivan R, Mansour A. COVID-19-impact on DNR orders in the largest cancer center in Jordan. J Pain Symptom Manag. 2020;60(2):e87–e9. https://doi.org/10.1016/j.jpainsymman.2020.04.023.
50. AlWaheidi S, Sullivan R, Davies EA. Additional challenges faced by cancer patients in Gaza due to COVID-19. Ecancermedicalscience. 2020;14:ed100. https://doi.org/10.3332/ecancer.2020.ed100.

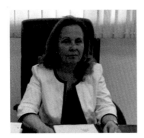

Randah R. Hamadeh is a professor of community medicine and is currently working as a consultant to the Dean, College of Medicine and Medical Sciences (CMMS), Arabian Gulf University (AGU), Bahrain. She served as the Vice Dean for Graduate Studies and Research from 2010–2020 at CMMS, AGU and chaired the Department of Family and Community Medicine from 2005–2010 and was an acting chair during 2016-2017. She attained both her BSc in Environmental Health and MSc in Epidemiology from the American University of Beirut and her DPhil in Community Medicine from the University of Oxford.

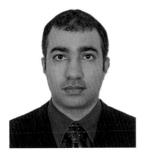

Haitham Jahrami is the Chief, Rehabilitation Services at Governmental Hospitals, Ministry of Health, Kingdom of Bahrain. He is also an Associate Professor, Department of Psychiatry, College of Medicine and Medical Sciences, Arabian Gulf University, Kingdom of Bahrain. Research active staff with approximately 200 papers. Dr. Jahrami attained his PhD from the University of Ulster, UK in 2006 and research training at Harvard Medical School in 2015.

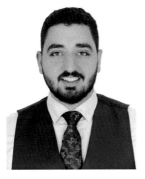

Khaled Nazzal is a graduate of the College of Medicine and Medical Sciences, Arabian Gulf University, Bahrain. He is currently a surgical resident. He is interested in the medical and humanitarian aspects of cancer. His goal is to be a surgeon to manage each patient with care and professionalism.

Chapter 26
Pediatric Oncology in the Arab World

Dua'a Zandaki and Iyad Sultan

26.1   Introduction

Childhood cancer represents a unique challenge in medical care. No other disease receives such emotional sympathy from the public. Yet, it remains to be challenging to allocate resources to offer proper therapy. Nowadays, survival rates for the most common childhood cancers surpass 80% in developed countries, while the average survival approximates 20% in resource-limited settings [1].

The Arab League has 22 member countries that have a population of over 420 million, with one-third of them below the age of 15 (140 million, 33%). There is a great heterogeneity in the region of the world. The Gross Domestic Product (GDP) per capita ranges from 631 to 63,281 USD per capita. This is reflected on all other parameters, including infant mortality rate, for example, which ranges from 6 to 74 per 1000 live births (Table 26.1).

The disparities in the level of care exist even within individual countries. Access to care can be readily available for patients who live close to medical centers, while this can be difficult to reach for those living in less privileged areas. The immigrants and non-nationals who reside in some Arab countries may not be able to afford the expensive care of childhood cancer, and a considerable gap continues to exist.

On the other hand, language and cultural background represent a common background that makes collaboration more feasible. The work of Non-Governmental Organizations (NGOs) may use this as a background for fundraising and health

D. Zandaki
Department of Pediatrics Oncology, King Hussein Cancer Center, Amman, Jordan

I. Sultan (✉)
Department of Pediatrics Oncology, Cancer Care Informatics Program, King Hussein Cancer Center, Amman, Jordan

Department of Pediatrics, University of Jordan, Amman, Jordan
e-mail: isultan@khcc.jo

© The Author(s) 2022
H. O. Al-Shamsi et al. (eds.), *Cancer in the Arab World*,
https://doi.org/10.1007/978-981-16-7945-2_26

Table 26.1 Selected World Bank indicators of Arab countries [2]

Country	GDP	Anemia (%)	Death by NCD (%)	Hospital beds	Health expenditure (%)	Health exp. per capita	Birth rate	Infant mortality	Children (%)	Population
Algeria	4700	30	79	2	6	256	24	20	31	43,053,054
Bahrain	20,913	30	86	2	4	994	14	6	19	1,641,172
Comoros	1399	48	45	2	5	65	31	48	39	850,886
Djibouti	1343	42	52	1	2	71	21	48	29	973,560
Egypt	3010	32	86	1	5	126	26	17	34	100,388,073
Iraq	5589	24	67	1	4	239	29	22	38	39,309,783
Jordan	3326	31	80	1	8	330	21	13	34	10,101,694
Kuwait	32,702	25	79	2	5	1711	13	7	22	4,207,083
Lebanon	5792	25	89	3	8	686	17	6	26	6,855,713
Libya	8122	29	75	3	6	310	18	10	28	6,777,452
Mauritania	1756	68	37	0	5	54	33	50	40	4,525,696
Morocco	3396	34	84	1	5	175	18	18	27	36,471,769
Oman	15,082	38	80	1	4	678	19	10	22	4,974,986
Qatar	63,282	26	77	1	2	1716	9	6	14	2,832,067
Saudi Arabia	20,542	38	73	2	6	1485	17	6	25	34,268,528
Somalia	N/A	56	30	1	N/A	N/A	42	74	46	15,442,905
Sudan	1724	57	54	1	5	60	32	41	40	42,813,238
Syria	N/A	35	75	1	4	70	23	18	31	17,070,135
Tunisia	4405	29	86	2	7	252	17	14	24	11,694,719
UAE	41,420	27	77	1	4	1817	10	6	15	9,770,529
Palestine	2939	26	N/A	1	N/A	N/A	29	17	39	4,685,306
Yemen	631	84	50	1	5	73	30	44	39	29,161,922

World Bank Data (2); values were provided for the most recent available data entry since 2016, and decimals were rounded to the nearest number. Indicator names were abbreviated to construct the table: GDP, GDP per capita (constant 2010 US$); Anemia, Prevalence of anemia among children (% of children under 5); Death by NCD, Cause of death by non-communicable diseases (% of total); Hospital beds, Hospital beds (per 1000 people); Health expenditure, Current health expenditure (% of GDP); Health exp. per capita, Current health expenditure per capita (current US$); Birth rate, Birth rate, crude (per 1000 people); Infant mortality, Mortality rate, infant (per 1000 live births); Children, Population ages 0–14 (% of the total population); N/A, data not available initiatives that may help countries with fewer resources. The collaboration and sharing expertise are also feasible and can easily extend to successful twinning.

According to GLOBOCAN, it is estimated that 18,114 children were diagnosed with cancer during the year 2020, and 6910 died (Mortality: incidence ratio of 0.38). The annual incidence of childhood cancer in Arab countries ranges from 7.5 per 100,000 children (Djibouti) to 12.8 (Morocco), and variations may be attributed to registration accuracy (Fig. 26.1) [3]. The top five childhood cancers in the Arab World in 2020 are similar to those reported in the rest of the world (Fig. 26.2) [3].

It is noted that major gaps in our knowledge regarding the true burden of pediatric cancer in the Arab world exists. In a scoping review by Gheorghe et al., where all literature from three Arab countries and Turkey were reviewed, it was revealed that much needs to be done to appreciate the impact of this problem [4]. One particular area of concern was the lack of reliable data regarding the outcome of

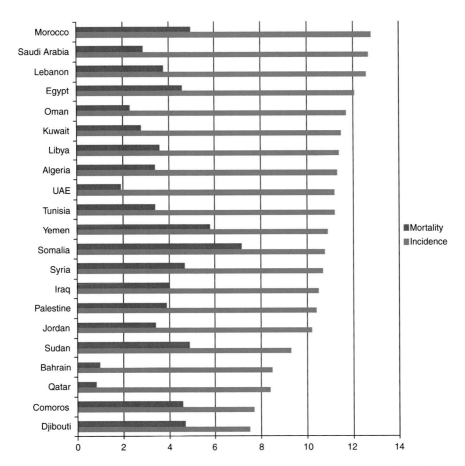

Fig. 26.1 Incidence and mortality rates (per 100,000 children <15 years old) in Arab Countries as estimated by Globocan for the year 2020 [3]

pediatric cancer on national levels. This reflects the need to improve cancer registration and integrate survival data.

Ward et al. developed a microsimulation model to estimate childhood cancer survival across all countries. Their initial estimates were based on CONCORD-2 and CONCORD-3 studies, which were based on data obtained from national cancer registries when it was available [5, 6]. These estimates were then modeled using a computational approach to simulate the effect of different interventions on the outcome of children with cancer. The study estimated that the global 5-year net childhood cancer survival was 37.4% (34.7–39.8%). They found that seven interventions provided small gains in survival, while a comprehensive approach of all policy interventions could raise the global survival of childhood cancer to 80.8%, if fully implemented. The estimates of 5-year net survival in North Africa and West Asia were 30.3% and 56.7%, respectively, which might be increased to 79.2% and 81.4% if all policies adopted [7]. While the estimates for North Africa seem to be alarming, this study was based on data provided by cancer registries, which may overestimate cancer mortality, if diagnosis is not linked properly to survival data. We used the estimates provided in this analysis to draw a map of survival estimates of Acute Lymphoblastic Leukemia (ALL), the most common pediatric malignancy. Figure 26.3 shows the 5- year net survival of ALL estimates using Ward et al. data [7].

Fig. 26.2 A pie chart representing the proportions of the pediatric cancers in the Arab World as provided by Globocan using 2020 estimates [3]

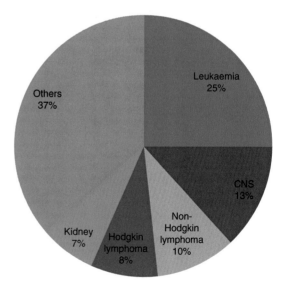

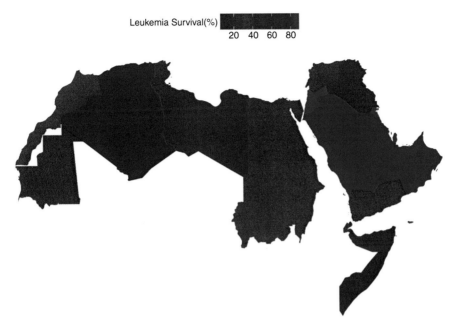

Fig. 26.3 Five-year net survival of Acute Lymphoblastic Leukemia estimates [8]

26.2 Diagnosis Delay and Abandonment

The timely diagnosis of cancer requires the cooperation of parents and pediatricians; parents must seek medical care early on, typically within a month of onset of new persistent symptoms that may initially mimic common childhood illnesses; pediatricians and other practitioners need to be aware of the manifestations of childhood cancer, some can be subtle and require careful history taking and physical examination. This is followed by essential investigations and timely referral to a pediatric oncology unit.

It was suggested that physicians contributed to more delay than parents, and this is consistent with our observations [9]. The delay in diagnosis leads to disease progression, which makes treatment challenging. According to Soliman et al., the rate of delayed diagnosis of retinoblastoma in Alexandria, Egypt was 62%, and it was significantly associated with advanced stage at presentation; 25% of delayed diagnosis was due to misdiagnosis by the first physician, and 21% was due to misjudgment of parents [10].

A study conducted in Egypt to investigate the cancer diagnosis delay in children found that while patient-related causes led to a median delay of 8 days, physician-related causes led to a median of 28 days delay, with a misdiagnosis rate of 40% [11]. As most general physicians are not educated enough about early signs of cancer, especially in the pediatric age, many families get reassured at their first physician's visit. Even after a physician suspects a serious diagnosis like cancer, confirmation can be challenging, as it requires advanced imaging and biopsy modalities, which are very limited in number and access in many Arab countries. For example, delayed diagnosis in Sudanese children with brain tumors was referred to the fact that there was only one Computed Tomography (CT) machine in the governmental hospital and one Magnetic Resonance Imaging (MRI) machine in the private practice [12, 13].

The initiation and continuation of cancer care are challenging, mainly on the parents' side. Accommodating safe and fast transportation is not always feasible. Many poor families can barely adjust the cost of monthly visits to and from the hospital. Needless to say, this burden has doubled in the COVID-19 era, as many countries imposed curfew hours that limit public transportation. Additionally, the number of hospital visits has increased in number due to the testing for COVID-19 before admissions.

Continuing medical care for children with cancer, which can take as long as 3 years, also requires dedicated human power to accompany the child. Many families find this challenging, as it can lead to job abandonment for parents, and it can lead to negligence towards the child's siblings, especially that the average family size in the Arab world is around 5 in most countries.

One study in Morocco showed that one-third of the children with rhabdomyosarcoma abandoned therapy [14]. A report from Iraq showed that 29 patients with high-grade B- Non-Hodgkin Lymphoma (11% out of 261) abandoned therapy, and that was a major cause for lower outcomes among these patients [15]. The abandonment among patients with Hodgkin Lymphoma in Morocco was also reported to be at 12.5% [16]. A report from Morocco showed that almost 1 out of 5 patients with Wilms tumor abandoned therapy, leading to suboptimal event free survival [17]. A recent report from Jordan showed that 2.5% of families of children with CNS tumors (Total = 473) abandoned therapy while 3% refused a part of treatment [18].

The "My Child Matters" project is a multi-institutional, multi-national initiative. Howard et al. reported their results as 55 institutions were mentored to decrease treatment abandonment, diagnosis delays and toxic death. A median improvement in 5-year survival of 5.1% was noticed. The key elements of successful interventions to overcome these hurdles include strong and sustained local leadership, community engagement, international engagement, capacity building and governmental support [19].

26.3 Pediatric Cancer Treatment

26.3.1 Chemotherapy

Most pediatric malignancies are systemic diseases with a risk of distant spread. Chemotherapy is the sole treatment for most cases of leukemia and lymphoma. Even for solid tumors, chemotherapy is typically essential to reduce volume, facilitate surgery, and prevent local and distant metastasis. Examples include Wilms tumor, germ cell tumors, bone, and soft tissue sarcomas. Autologous and allogeneic transplantation are essential interventions to cure many patients, particularly those with relapsed leukemia and lymphoma as well as children with neuroblastoma and infants with brain tumors.

Balancing benefits and risks are essential to achieve the best results. Using aggressive protocols that require intensive care may be feasible if needed resources and infrastructure are available. In most cases, adopting regiments designed for High Income Countries (HIC) in Low and Middle Income Countries (LMIC) is not wise, and modifications should be applied to address the unequal health capacity [20].

Each version of the WHO List of Essential Medicines (updated every 2 years) is found to expand the section of antineoplastic drugs. The latest version issued in 2019 contains 21 antineoplastic drugs, and 5 targeted therapies. In our experience, the two essential drugs that suffer from frequent shortages in the Arab World are actinomycin D (essential for rhabdomyosarcoma and Wilms tumor) and L-asparaginase (essential for the treatment of ALL). Concerns regarding the efficacy of generic formulations of these essential drugs deserve careful attention [21]. Data concerning the shortage of essential chemotherapy in the Arab world is sparse. In one report from Iraq, more than half of patients with ALL between 2000 and 2002 received less than 50% of their prescribed chemotherapy. These patients had significantly worse outcomes [22].

In 2001, World Trade Organization (WTO) Members adopted a special Ministerial Declaration at the WTO Ministerial Conference in Doha, termed the Doha declaration, to clarify some terms on Trade-Related Aspects of Intellectual Property Rights (TRIPS). Some of these items included compulsory licensing and parallel importation. These guarantee that LMIC will get access to essential medicines without being subjected to patent-holders [23].

Administering chemotherapy still comes at a significant cost, including the cost of drugs, drug administration, and accommodations needed for inpatient chemotherapy, as well as the cost of treating side effects. For example, Elshahoubi et al. found that Head Start protocol for children with Central Nervous System (CNS) tumors costs approximately 100,000 USD per patient with chemotherapy constituting 40% of the total treatment cost that includes investigations, surgical intervention, radiotherapy, and accommodation. They also found that lower-cost protocols could be used if reliable risk-stratification systems were available, an option that in itself carries an economical burden, due to the need of molecular testing [24].

There are some applicable solutions to cut on treatment costs. For example, treating Ewing sarcoma patients with an outpatient-based interval compression approach was found to save about 21% of the cost in Jordan [25]. Another area of concern is the hesitancy in applying cost-effective evidence-based approaches. For example, despite the well-established fact that cisplatin monotherapy has similar efficacy to the more toxic combination chemotherapy, many institutions continue to use the latter regimen [26].

26.3.2 Radiotherapy

Radiotherapy is an essential part of treating cancer, especially in LMIC, given the higher prevalence of advanced stages at presentation due to delayed diagnosis. The investment in radiotherapy is a continuous one; as it only starts with providing radiotherapy machines and continues with the need for continuous medical expertise, technical support, and machine maintenance.

According to the Directory for Radiotherapy Centers, the Arab world, whose population averages 420 million, hosts a total of 353 megavoltage machines, 3 kilovoltage machines, and 71 brachytherapy machines. This compares to the USA, of about 75% the Arab population (328 million) that hosts a total of 3727 megavoltage machines, 6 kilovoltage machines, 768 brachytherapy machines, in addition to 37 light ion therapy machines [27].

This scarcity of radiotherapy machines is a major challenge to treating cancer in the Arab world. A report by the commission of Lancet Oncology in 2015 showed that an adequate number of radiotherapy machines was noted in Arab Gulf countries, Jordan and Lebanon [28], while severe shortages were noted in Syria, Iraq, and Yemen. It must be noted that economic challenges are not the only obstacle for establishing this service, as shown by Mousa et al. In their analysis, the number of physicians per 1000 capita was the strongest predictor for the number of machines per capita in the Arab world [29].

The demand for radiation is expected to grow with the increasing incidence of cancer as most Arab populations are undergoing transformation with increased survival. This means that competition for radiation with children may be even worse in the future. A report from Iraq mentions that radiotherapy waiting lists can reach up to 6 months for pediatric patients [30]. This issue deserves immediate attention to improve cancer care for both children and adults.

26.3.3   Surgery

Surgical management is essential in treating childhood solid tumors. Surgical expertise is needed to manage complications of therapy as well, e.g., fungal infections, abscesses, typhlitis, and fasciitis. Surgeons aid in getting biopsies for diagnosis and inserting central lines, which requires special expertise in children. Some surgical interventions also require advanced equipment; a good example is neurosurgical procedures, which are currently witnessing huge improvements in HIC with brain labs and robotic surgery. The complexity of postoperative care is perhaps best represented by orthopedic management of limb sarcomas [31].

One under-studied subject here is the competition of the private sector for surgical expertise. In most cases, pediatric oncology units reside in academic institutions or public hospitals where surgeons are paid less and have difficulty getting tools and equipment. This makes retaining expert surgeons challenging. One example is retinoblastoma, where recruiting and retaining qualified ophthalmologists seems to be extremely challenging. One solution would be cooperation with the private sector and special attention to retention plans that attempt to close the financial gap for highly qualified medical staff.

26.3.4 New Targeted Therapy

The previously mentioned World Health Organization (WHO) list of essential medicines has been updated in the latest versions to include five targeted therapies: All-trans retinoic acid, dasatinib, imatinib, nilotinib, and rituximab. Although highly effective, targeted therapy comes at considerable financial cost; monthly averages of $5000 to $10,000 and annual totals over $100,000 are common [32]. An example of the financial load would be children with cancers related to Constitutional Mismatch Repair Deficiency (CMMRD), a condition that is more prevalent in the region due to high rates of consanguinity [33, 34]. These patients are now successfully treated with long-term targeted therapy. However, the financial capacity to maintain them for the long run is challenging.

26.3.5 Multidisciplinary Care

Coordinating the use of different treatment modalities and the integration of ancillary services, including psychologists, dieticians, social workers, physical therapists and others, is essential in improving outcomes [35, 36]. In our opinion, exchanging medical reports can never be sufficient to treat children with cancer. Direct interactions and discussions with careful coordination, planning, and adjustment of therapy is needed to reach a good outcome. Implementing a successful model of multidisciplinary care can be challenging. Twinning programs can facilitate this and help programs efficiently assemble their teams and initiate their own meetings. Multiple successful examples in the Arab world published their experiences [30, 37, 38].

26.4 Challenges

26.4.1 Research/Collaboration

One of the major heralds to cancer research in the Arab world is the lack of meticulous cancer registries. There are few population-based cancer registries, with only 2% to 5% of populations reporting high-quality incidence data [39, 40]. Like other parts of the world, cancer registration needs to deal with issues related to the accuracy of diagnosis, duplication of entries due to patient referral, abandonment of treatment, and accurate registration of death certificates.

Areas of research that deserve special consideration include cost-effectiveness of pediatric cancer care and outcome studies [4]. Cutting-edge research is available in multiple centers in the Arab world, and many centers are already involved in collaborative international trials.

Another major obstacle for research in the Arab world is financial support. According to the United Nations Education, Scientific, and Cultural Organization (UNESCO), total regional gross expenditure on research and development in all Arab countries collectively for 2019 was 19.5 million US dollars compared to 581.5 million dollars in the US alone [41]. Needless to say, political instability may prevent researchers from conducting research as it becomes very challenging to provide resources and secure follow-up [42].

The International Society of Pediatric Oncology- Pediatric Oncology in Developing Countries (SIOP-PODC) is an initiative that the SIOP established in 1990. It has constructed many committees over the years to support SIOP's vision "no child should die of cancer" in LMIC. It now holds an integral part of SIOP's annual meetings, and it has developed many adapted guidelines to approach pediatric cancer in LMIC settings [43]. The SIOP protocols are more welcoming to countries outside Europe, and many Arab countries participate in their trials.

26.4.2 Political Instability

The Arab region has witnessed major political turmoil, especially in the past decade. This was most notable in Syria and Yemen, where local medical data are not available to measure the effect, however, the health crisis is evident in refugees in neighboring countries. Charity is the major source of funding treatment for refugee children with cancer; however, it cannot always be granted, which impairs care in this subset of patients, especially those with advanced disease at presentation.

Turkish investigators conducted a study to compare the survival of Turkish and Syrian refugee children with cancer and found that Syrian refugees had significantly lower survival, independent of cancer type or stage, even though cancer care is financially covered for Syrian refugees in Turkey. The authors attributed this to economic and bureaucratic measures needed to establish the care and seek the first physician, which leads to advanced stages of presentation in this subset [44].

Saab et al. nicely reported the experience of the Childhood Cancer Center of Lebanon (CCCL) in managing Syrian refugees between 2011 and 2017. During this period, 575 Syrian children with cancer presented to their center. Less than one-fifth (N = 107) received full coverage for their treatment, while 264 (46%) received consultation only. This highlights the importance of charity and fundraising to cover refugees [45].

Mansour et al. reviewed the burden of cancer among Syrian refugees in Jordan. Around 900 cases of cancer are diagnosed annually among this population (adults and pediatrics). The cost of their treatment using average estimates is more than 22 million USD. This represents an extra challenge on the King Hussein Cancer Foundation (KHCF), which provides financial coverage in most cases [46].

26.4.3 Human Resources

Few guidelines have been issued regarding the human resources required for childhood cancer care in LMIC, including Arab countries. Human resources are often unfortunately neglected while planning for cancer care facilities. Human resources for each country should be planned in accordance with total population and cancer incidence. Unfortunately, resources are allocated to buildings and facilities rather than personnel, which leads to major challenges, including chronically understaffed facilities, and low staff morale, with subsequent poor patient handling.

The National Cancer Institute Division of Cancer Treatment and Diagnosis has issued some guidelines regarding appropriate staff numbers for each LMIC based on population and GLOBOCAN data. They are available on their website [47].

26.4.4 Limited Resources

One would make the uneducated guess that all cancer treatment needs are the direct treatment methods: chemotherapeutic drugs, surgical capacity, inpatient wards, and radiotherapy units, all of which are barely available in most Arab countries. However, cancer treatment is in fact a long and branching process. Pediatric ICU care is a mainstay of cancer treatment, isolation units, nutrition team support, and patient support groups. This is in addition to resources needed for survivors, including continuous medical follow-up, medications like hormone supplement, equipment such as artificial limbs, and management of late chemotherapy effects.

26.4.5 COVID-19

COVID-19 has affected Pediatric Oncology in many ways. A survey was conducted among the heads of pediatric departments in the Pediatric Oncology East and Mediterranean (POEM) group in April 2020. The survey covered multiple hospitals and patient-related aspects that affected overall patient care. It was shown that patient visits were restricted for off-therapy patients in 91% and to the absolute essential on-therapy patients in 50%. LMIC witnessed a delay in administering chemotherapy and doing surgery or radiation by 31% and 46%, respectively. 31% of centers also reported a delay in accepting new cases. Outpatient visits witnessed cancelations in 65% of centers and were challenged due to travel restrictions in 18%. Up to 70% of centers witnessed a decreased staff number, and 29% reported that medical care was affected due to it. As for resource availability, medication and drug supply were in shortage in 50% and 70% of centers, respectively. Bed availability was compromised in 18% of centers due to bed reallocation, and 32% of centers reported a delay in financial approval for cases [48].

26.5   The Global Initiative for Childhood Cancer (GICC)

GICC is an initiative launched by the WHO with the intent of improving survival for childhood cancer. It was launched in 2018 with an aim to make childhood cancer survival reach 60% by 2030, aiming at saving one million more lives. These goals come in line with the 2030 United Nations (UN) Agenda for Sustainable Development, and Non-Communicable Diseases (NCDs) agenda.

By first prioritizing awareness of childhood cancer, and second, supporting countries to offer better cancer care in terms of diagnosis and treatment medicines and technologies, GICC hopes to alleviate the survival gap between upper and lower middle income countries [49].

With the help of host partners, including International Society of Pediatric Oncology (SIOP) and the St. Jude Children's Research Hospital in the USA, GICC is set to accomplish its aims on a national, regional, and global level. Since its establishment in 2018, ten countries have been in the GICC pilot focus group, Morocco being the only Arab country.

The initiative defined its pillars in the term: CURE ALL, to stand for: Center for excellences, Universal health coverage for essential quality services, Regimens and roadmaps for diagnosis and treatment, Evaluation and monitoring, Advocacy, Leveraged financing, and Linked governance. It has also developed many tools to help implement and undertake its pillars, including:

1. Tools to support priority setting, budgeting, and health system planning.
2. Tools to facilitate national dialog in health workforce planning.
3. WHO management guidelines or guidance for six index childhood cancers and supportive care.
4. Access to cancer medicines program.
5. Defined global research priorities.
6. Dataset for cancer registries and monitoring of programs.

All these pillars are being addressed in focused countries through many steps (Table 26.2)

As GICC set its goals in line with 2030 United Nations (UN) Agenda for Sustainable Development, it also is served by the UN sustainable development goals (Table 26.3).

GICC has chosen six main childhood cancers to address, based on their large prevalence all around the world (constitute 50–60% of all childhood cancers), and on their high cure rate with implementation of good treatment practices. These cancers are Acute Lymphoblastic Leukemia, Burkitt lymphoma, Hodgkin lymphoma, Retinoblastoma, Wilms tumor, and low-grade glioma.

Table 26.2 Steps of implementing GICC pillars in focus countries [49]

CURE ALL core projects	Phases of country action			
	Assess	Plan, cost, & finance	Implement	Monitor and modify
Analysis of cancer health system	x			
National Cancer Control strategy development/implementation		X	X	X
Implementation of cancer workforce training packages			X	
National network and referral pathway strengthening			X	
Defining national standards and guidelines for index cancers	x		X	
Essential medicines and technologies strengthening, including via UN	x	X	X	X
Economic analysis and benefit packages review of cancer	x	X		
Strengthening and linking cancer registries (population- and hospital-based)	x	X	X	X
Country dashboard for childhood cancer monitoring	x			X
Local/regional advocacy portfolios: case studies, awareness campaigns			X	X

Table 26.3 GICC goals are in line with 2030 United Nations (UN) agenda for sustainable development goals [49]

UN SDG No. 1	Financial protection from catastrophic illness like cancer reduces poverty
UN SDG No. 2	Reducing hunger and malnutrition improves childhood cancer outcomes
UN SDG No. 3	Investing in childhood cancer supports the attainment of multiple health-related targets
UN SDG No. 4	Educational services needed for children with cancer requiring prolonged hospitalization
UN SDG No. 5	Promote access to care that is not discriminatory against girls and enables mothers and families
UN SDG No. 6	Universal access to clean water and sanitation can reduce rates of infection-related complications
UN SDG No. 8	Investing in diverse occupation required for care stimulates local economic growth and employment
UN SDG No. 10	Promote access to care for all communities to reduce catastrophic health expenditure and inequalities
UN SDG No. 16	Investing in child health promotes social stability and reduces exploitation and discrimination
UN SDG No. 17	Multi-sectoral collaboration and international cooperation improve childhood cancer outcomes

26.6 Conclusion

Pediatric oncology faces many challenges in many Arab countries, including diagnosis delay and treatment abandonment, limited research activities, political instability, recruitment and training of human resources, and limited financial support, which all affect the way children with cancer receive their treatment; be it chemotherapy, radiotherapy, surgery, or targeted therapy. The COVID-19 pandemic added more weight to these challenges collectively. Acknowledging and addressing all these challenges is a responsibility that rests upon policy makers and health care workers trying to care for these children. Some suggested solutions are addressing shortages of essential drugs, improving the infrastructure in health care facilities and tailoring evidence-based approaches to develop tolerable and cost-effective treatment regimens personalized to the area. There is a need to establish more twinning programs with advanced centers to quickly improve this discipline. Similar language and cultural backgrounds provide a unique opportunity to collaborate and help in decreasing gaps among countries in the region. We mention the Global Initiative for Childhood Cancer as one of the remarkable global efforts that aim to improve the global outcome of childhood cancer and alleviate the survival gap between high and low middle income countries.

Conflict of Interest Authors have no conflict of interest to declare.

References

1. Gupta S, Howard S, Hunger S, Antillon F, Metzger M, et al. Treating childhood cancers in low- and middle-income countries. In: Gelband H, Jha P, Sankaranarayanan R, Horton S, editors. Disease control priorities, Cancer, vol. 3. 3rd ed. Washington, DC: World Bank. [Internet]. [cited 2020 Nov 23]. Available from: http://dcp-3.org/chapter/900/treating-childhood-cancers-low-and-middle-income-countries.
2. World development indicators and other world bank data: WDI-R package (v 2.7.4) https://cran.r-project.org/web/packages/WDI/index.html. Accessed 10 May 2021.
3. Globocan 12. International Agency for Research on Cancer Global Cancer Observatory: estimated number of new cases in 2018 ac, both sexes, ages 0–14. https://gco.iarc.fr/today/home. Accessed on 1 May 2021
4. Gheorghe A, Chalkidou K, Shamieh O, Kutluk T, Fouad F, Sultan I, et al. Economics of pediatric cancer in Four Eastern Mediterranean countries: a comparative assessment. JCO Glob Oncol. 2020;6:1155–70. Epub 2020/07/23
5. Allemani C, Matsuda T, Di Carlo V, Harewood R, Matz M, Niksic M, et al. Global surveillance of trends in cancer survival 2000-14 (CONCORD-3): analysis of individual records for 37 513 025 patients diagnosed with one of 18 cancers from 322 population-based registries in 71 countries. Lancet. 2018;391(10125):1023–75. Epub 2018/02/06
6. Allemani C, Weir HK, Carreira H, Harewood R, Spika D, Wang XS, et al. Global surveillance of cancer survival 1995-2009: analysis of individual data for 25,676,887 patients from 279 population-based registries in 67 countries (CONCORD-2). Lancet. 2015;385(9972):977–1010. Epub 2014/12/04
7. Ward ZJ, Yeh JM, Bhakta N, Frazier AL, Girardi F, Atun R. Global childhood cancer survival estimates and priority-setting: a simulation-based analysis. Lancet Oncol. 2019;20(7):972–83. Epub 2019/05/28

8. Ward Z, Yeh J, Bhakta N, Frazier AL, Girardi F, Atun R. Simulation results: global childhood cancer survival. V1 ed. Harvard Dataverse; 2019.

9. Haimi M, Peretz Nahum M, Ben Arush MW. Delay in diagnosis of children with cancer: a retrospective study of 315 children. Pediatr Hematol Oncol. 2004;21(1):37–48. Epub 2003/12/09

10. Soliman SE, Eldomiaty W, Goweida MB, Dowidar A. Clinical presentation of retinoblastoma in Alexandria: A step toward earlier diagnosis. Saudi J Ophthalmol. 2017;31(2):80–5. Epub 2017/06/01

11. Abdelkhalek E, Sherief L, Kamal N, Soliman R. Factors associated with delayed cancer diagnosis in egyptian children. Clin Med Insights Pediatr. 2014;8:39–44. Epub 2014/09/19

12. Elhassan MMA, Osman HHM, Parkes J. Posterior cranial fossa tumours in children at National Cancer Institute, Sudan: a single institution experience. Child's Nerv Syst. 2017;33(8):1303–8. Epub 2017/04/23

13. Parkes J, Hess C, Burger H, Anacak Y, Ahern V, Howard SC, et al. Recommendations for the treatment of children with radiotherapy in low- and middle-income countries (LMIC): A position paper from the Pediatric Radiation Oncology Society (PROS-LMIC) and Pediatric Oncology in Developing Countries (PODC) working groups of the International Society of Pediatric Oncology (SIOP). Pediatr Blood Cancer. 2017;64(Suppl 5) Epub 2018/01/04

14. Hessissen L, Kanouni L, Kili A, Nachef MN, El Khorassani M, Benjaafar N, et al. Pediatric rhabdomyosarcoma in Morocco. Pediatr Blood Cancer. 2010;54(1):25–8. Epub 2009/09/12

15. Moleti ML, Al-Hadad SA, Al-Jadiry MF, Al-Darraji AF, Al-Saeed RM, De Vellis A, et al. Treatment of children with B-cell non-Hodgkin lymphoma in a low-income country. Pediatr Blood Cancer. 2011;56(4):560–7. Epub 2011/02/08

16. Hessissen L, Khtar R, Madani A, El Kababri M, Kili A, Harif M, et al. Improving the prognosis of pediatric Hodgkin lymphoma in developing countries: a Moroccan Society of Pediatric Hematology and Oncology study. Pediatr Blood Cancer. 2013;60(9):1464–9. Epub 2013/04/23

17. Madani A, Zafad S, Harif M, Yaakoubi M, Zamiati S, Sahraoui S, et al. Treatment of Wilms tumor according to SIOP 9 protocol in Casablanca, Morocco. Pediatr Blood Cancer. 2006;46(4):472–5. Epub 2005/07/22

18. Amayiri N, Bouffet E. Treatment abandonment and refusal among children with central nervous system tumors in Jordan. Pediatr Blood Cancer. 2021;68(8):e29054. Epub 2021/05/23

19. Howard SC, Zaidi A, Cao X, Weil O, Bey P, Patte C, et al. The My Child Matters programme: effect of public-private partnerships on paediatric cancer care in low-income and middle-income countries. Lancet Oncol. 2018;19(5):e252–e66. Epub 2018/05/05

20. Rodriguez-Galindo C, Friedrich P, Alcasabas P, Antillon F, Banavali S, Castillo L, et al. Toward the cure of all children with cancer through collaborative efforts: pediatric oncology as a global challenge. J Clin Oncol Off J Am Soc Clin Oncol. 2015;33(27):3065–73. Epub 2015/08/26

21. Sankaran H, Sengupta S, Purohit V, Kotagere A, Moulik NR, Prasad M, et al. A comparison of asparaginase activity in generic formulations of E.coli derived L- asparaginase: In-vitro study and retrospective analysis of asparaginase monitoring in pediatric patients with leukemia. Br J Clin Pharmacol. 2020;86(6):1081–8. Epub 2020/01/12

22. Frangoul H, Al-Jadiry MF, Shyr Y, Ye F, Shakhtour B, Al-Hadad SA. Shortage of chemotherapeutic agents in Iraq and outcome of childhood acute lymphocytic leukemia, 1990-2002. N Engl J Med. 2008;359(4):435–7. Epub 2008/07/25

23. The Doha declaration on the trips agreement and public health. https://www.who.int/medicines/areas/policy/doha_declaration/en/. Accessed on 1 May 2021

24. Elshahoubi A, Khattab E, Halalsheh H, Khaleifeh K, Bouffet E, Amayiri N. Feasibility of high-dose chemotherapy protocols to treat infants with malignant central nervous system tumors: Experience from a middle-income country. Pediatr Blood Cancer. 2019;66(1):e27464. Epub 2018/09/27

25. Elshahoubi A, Alnassan A, Sultan I. Safety and cost-effectiveness of outpatient administration of high-dose chemotherapy in children with Ewing Sarcoma. J Pediatr Hematol Oncol. 2019;41(3):e152–e4. Epub 2019/01/05

26. Perilongo G, Maibach R, Shafford E, Brugieres L, Brock P, Morland B, et al. Cisplatin versus cisplatin plus doxorubicin for standard-risk hepatoblastoma. N Engl J Med. 2009;361(17):1662–70. Epub 2009/10/23

27. Directory of radiotherapy centers webpage https://dirac.iaea.org/Home/Equipment. Accessed on 1 May 2021

28. Atun R, Jaffray DA, Barton MB, Bray F, Baumann M, Vikram B, et al. Expanding global access to radiotherapy. Lancet Oncol. 2015;16(10):1153–86. Epub 2015/10/01

29. Mousa AG, Bishr MK, Mula-Hussain L, Zaghloul MS. Is economic status the main determinant of radiation therapy availability? The Arab world as an example of developing countries. Radiother Oncol. 2019;140:182–9. Epub 2019/07/20

30. Al-Hadad SA, Al-Jadiry MF, Al-Darraji AF, Al-Saeed RM, Al-Badr SF, Ghali HH. Reality of pediatric cancer in Iraq. J Pediatr Hematol Oncol. 2011;33(Suppl 2):S154–6. Epub 2011/10/05

31. Shehadeh A, El Dahleh M, Salem A, Sarhan Y, Sultan I, Henshaw RM, et al. Standardization of rehabilitation after limb salvage surgery for sarcomas improves patients' outcome. Hematol Oncol Stem Cell Ther. 2013;6(3–4):105–11. Epub 2013/10/29

32. Targeted therapies: one practice's story. https://www.ajmc.com/view/targeted-therapies-one-practices-story. Accessed 12 May 2021

33. Amayiri N, Tabori U, Campbell B, Bakry D, Aronson M, Durno C, et al. High frequency of mismatch repair deficiency among pediatric high grade gliomas in Jordan. Int J Cancer. 2016;138(2):380–5. Epub 2015/08/22

34. Khdair-Ahmad O, Al Husaini M, Ghunaimat S, Ismael T, Amayiri N, Halalsheh H, et al. Constitutional mismatch repair deficiency in children with colorectal carcinoma: a Jordanian center experience. Pediatr Hematol Oncol J. 2021;6(1):18–21.

35. Cantrell MA, Ruble K. Multidisciplinary care in pediatric oncology. J Multidiscip Healthc. 2011;4:171–81. Epub 2011/08/04

36. Fennell ML, Das IP, Clauser S, Petrelli N, Salner A. The organization of multidisciplinary care teams: modeling internal and external influences on cancer care quality. J Natl Cancer Inst Monogr. 2010;2010(40):72–80. Epub 2010/04/14

37. Qaddoumi I, Mansour A, Musharbash A, Drake J, Swaidan M, Tihan T, et al. Impact of telemedicine on pediatric neuro-oncology in a developing country: the Jordanian-Canadian experience. Pediatr Blood Cancer. 2007;48(1):39–43. Epub 2006/10/27

38. Qaddoumi I, Nawaiseh I, Mehyar M, Razzouk B, Haik BG, Kharma S, et al. Team management, twinning, and telemedicine in retinoblastoma: a 3-tier approach implemented in the first eye salvage program in Jordan. Pediatr Blood Cancer. 2008;51(2):241–4. Epub 2008/02/27

39. Copur MS. State of cancer research around the globe. Oncology (Williston Park). 2019;33(5):181–5. Epub 2019/05/17

40. Basbous M, Al-Jadiry M, Belgaumi A, Sultan I, Al-Haddad A, Jeha S, et al. Childhood cancer care in the Middle East, North Africa, and West/Central Asia: a snapshot across five countries from the POEM network. Cancer Epidemiol. 2021;71(Pt B):101727. Epub 2020/06/06

41. UNESCO institute for statistics, gross domestic expenditure on research and development. Calculation according to current PPP$. http://data.uis.unesco.org/?queryid=74#. Accessed 1 May 2021

42. House DR, Marete I, Meslin EM. To research (or not) that is the question: ethical issues in research when medical care is disrupted by political action: a case study from Eldoret, Kenya. J Med Ethics. 2016;42(1):61–5. Epub 2015/10/18

43. Arora RS, Challinor JM, Howard SC, Israels T. Improving care for children with cancer in low- and middle-income countries--a SIOP PODC initiative. Pediatr Blood Cancer. 2016;63(3):387–91. Epub 2016/01/23

44. Yagci-Kupeli B, Ozkan A. Syrian and Turkish children with cancer: a comparison on survival and associated factors. Pediatr Hematol Oncol. 2020;37(8):707–16. Epub 2020/07/25

45. Saab R, Jeha S, Khalifeh H, Zahreddine L, Bayram L, Merabi Z, et al. Displaced children with cancer in Lebanon: a sustained response to an unprecedented crisis. Cancer. 2018;124(7):1464–72. Epub 2018/03/01

46. Mansour A, Al-Omari A, Sultan I. Burden of cancer among Syrian refugees in Jordan. J Glob Oncol. 2018;4:1–6. Epub 2018/10/12

47. Human resources needed for cancer control in low & middle income countries. https://rrp.cancer.gov/programsResources/human_resources_needed.htm. Accessed 21 May 2021
48. Saab R, Obeid A, Gachi F, Boudiaf H, Sargsyan L, Al-Saad K, et al. Impact of the coronavirus disease 2019 (COVID-19) pandemic on pediatric oncology care in the Middle East, North Africa, and West Asia region: A report from the Pediatric Oncology East and Mediterranean (POEM) group. Cancer. 2020;126(18):4235–45. Epub 2020/07/11
49. Global initiative for childhood cancer. https://www.who.int/docs/default-source/documents/health-topics/cancer/who-childhood-cancer-overview-booklet.pdf?sfvrsn=83cf4552 aM

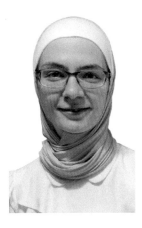

Dua'a Zandaki is a third-year fellow at the Department of Pediatrics at King Hussein Cancer Center. She is interested in the management of children with relapsed leukemia and is working on establishing CAR-T cell therapy at the center. She is also interested in precision medicine and novel therapeutics used in pediatric oncology.

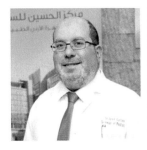

Iyad Sultan is the Chairman of the Department of Pediatrics at King Hussein Cancer Center in Amman, Jordan. After finishing his fellowship in pediatric hematology-oncology at the Medical University of South Carolina, he joined the center in 2005. He treats mainly children with solid tumors and is working on developing a regimen for patients with high-risk neuroblastoma. Dr. Sultan is interested in global oncology, cancer epidemiology, cancer genomics and bioinformatics. He is an advocate for displaced children with cancer. Recently, he helped establish the Cancer Care Informatics program at KHCC. He is teaching Bioinformatics among the precision medicine modules.

Chapter 27
Challenges Associated with Medical Travel for Cancer Patients in the Arab World: A Systematic Review

Wafa K. Alnakhi (ID), **Faryal Iqbal** (ID), **Waleed Al Nadabi** (ID), **and Amal Al Balushi** (ID)

27.1 Introduction

27.1.1 Background, Medical Travel, and Cancer

Medical travel is the practice of traveling abroad to seek healthcare services [1]. This practice has been growing in developing countries and people travel seeking healthcare for different reasons [1]. Since the Gulf Corporate Council countries are high-income countries, on many occasions' governments cover their patients for seeking healthcare overseas. In the UAE, it is estimated that US$ 163 million was spent on treatment abroad for cancer care in 2013 [2]. A recent study by Alnakhi, et al., (2019), which was conducted in the UAE shows that cancer is one of the three top medical conditions that triggered people to travel abroad seeking healthcare.

W. K. Alnakhi (✉)
Health Research & Survey Section/Data Analysis, Research & Studies Department, Strategy & Corporate Development Sector at Dubai Health Authority, Mohammed Bin Rashid University of Medicine and Health Sciences, Dubai, United Arab Emirates
e-mail: wkalnakhi@dha.gov.ae

F. Iqbal
Department of Oncology, Innovation and Research Center, Burjeel Cancer Institute, Burjeel Medical City, Abu Dhabi, United Arab Emirates
e-mail: faryal.iqbal@burjeelmedicalcity.com

W. A. Nadabi
Directorate General of Planning and Studies, Ministry of Health,
Al Khuwair, Sultanate of Oman
e-mail: waleed.alnadabi@moh.gov.om

A. A. Balushi
Oman College of Health Sciences, Nursing Program, Ministry of Health,
Al Khuwair, Sultanate of Oman
e-mail: amal.albalushi@moh.gov.om

© The Author(s) 2022
H. O. Al-Shamsi et al. (eds.), *Cancer in the Arab World*,
https://doi.org/10.1007/978-981-16-7945-2_27

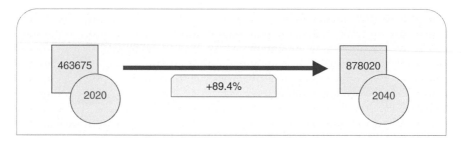

Fig. 27.1 Prediction of new cancer cases from the year 2020 till 2040 in Arab world countries, (0–85+), both sexes [4]. Data used with permission from the source—International Agency for Research on Cancer (IARC) By World Health Organization GLOBOCAN

Moreover, the same study showed the common destinations for seeking medical treatment among Emiratis were the UK, USA, India, and Thailand, with Germany being the top medical travel destination [3].

It has been noticed that the rate of cancer incidence is growing at an alarmingly high rate in Arab countries. According to the Global Cancer Observatory, there will be tremendous inflation in the cancer incidence rate from 4,63,675 in 2020 to 8,78,020 (around 1 million) by 2040 in 22 Arab countries [4].

Due to people's perceptions of their healthcare system and sometimes the unavailability of the treatment domestically, many patients would prefer seeking healthcare services overseas. Although in the Gulf Region, there are many comprehensive cancer centers available such as in the UAE and the Kingdom of Saudi Arabia. However, patients and their families tend to seek a second opinion from advanced specialized regions abroad, despite the reassurances given by their local, American, or Canadian board qualified physicians (Fig. 27.1) [1].

27.2   Factors Associated with Treatment Abroad for Cancer Patients

There are multiple factors that cancer patients would consider when seeking treatment abroad. Some factors are directly related to socio-demographic characteristics and medical conditions, while the rest might be related to the treatment options offered to those patients overseas. Many factors are related to the healthcare systems or services in either patients' home country or the treatment destinations.

(a) *Patients' Characteristics*

Many factors contribute to patients' decision-making, to receive medical care from other destinations. These factors include age, gender, degree of illness, marital status, academic, and income level [3, 5]. Motivations, perceptions, and experiences of the patients will differ by the type and the severity of cancer and whether the treatment had used surgical or medical management [6].

(b) *Treatment Options and Advanced Technology*

Unavailability of specialized treatment in patients' home country is one of the main reasons that push patients to treatment abroad. Moreover, the cost of the treatment and the treatment plan influence patients' decision-making. Given that some patients are covered by their government or health insurance, while some patients pay out of their pockets [6–8].

(c) *Health System and Services*

Quality of the healthcare services provided abroad, physician qualifications and experience, availability of specialized treatment, facility reputation, short waiting time, and skills of medical and administrative staff, all are factors that attract patients to seek treatment overseas. Source of information such as word of mouth from local physicians, family, and friends about the treatment destination are important factors to shape patients' decisions to seek healthcare overseas. In many cases, even if the patients were treated domestically, they would consider overseas treatment for a second opinion [3, 6, 9].

27.3 Risks and Challenges Associated with Medical Travel and Cancer

There are insufficient up-to-date empirical studies that discuss complications and challenges which are associated with the medical travel experience of oncology patients, especially in the Arab world from patients' perspectives. There is a scarcity of studies that looks in depth at the complications and challenges raised from the medical travel experience. In many scenarios, patients might face complications and challenges during or after receiving the treatment overseas. These challenges, if not tackled, could jeopardize patients' health status and quality of life. Quality improvement measures and synergism between the health system of patients' home country and treatment destination are necessary to ensure the best treatment plans are being given to patients. In addition, continuity of care with a proper follow-up care system and palliative care are vital to exist in the patient's home country for best patient outcomes [10]. This systematic review aims to summarize the evidence related to the complications and challenges associated with the medical travel experience for oncology patients in the Arab world.

27.4 Methods

A systematic narrative review was followed, which is according to Booth et al. (2012), a type of review where the literature is reviewed comprehensively and systematically [11]. This methodology helps to descriptively summarize different study designs using summary tables. Additionally, it helps to identify any gaps in the literature. Narrative reviews are usually used to provide a general overview of the existing knowledge, the topic, and to guide the formation of follow-up research questions [12].

The systematic review was conducted in January 2021, and a total of 76 articles were retrieved. After reviewing the articles for eligibility through title and abstract; 23 articles were considered for full-text review, 53 were excluded. Out of 23 articles, 14 were included, and the remaining 9 articles were excluded. Figure 27.2 summarizes the search strategy and selection process using the Preferred Reporting Items for Systematic Reviews and Meta-Analyses (PRISMA) statements [13].

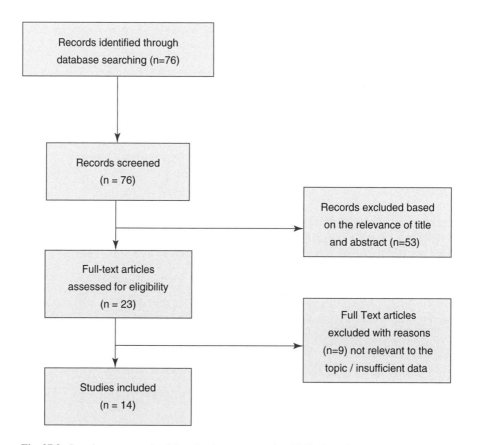

Fig. 27.2 Search strategy and article selection process using PRISMA [13]

Table 27.1 Review protocol

	Inclusion criteria	Exclusion criteria
Population	Patients with malignancy traveling abroad for treatment	Patients who traveled abroad for other medical conditions
Intervention	Any intervention	None
Comparator	None	
Outcomes	Any risks associated with treatment abroad	None
Study	Qualitative, quantitative, and mixed Published in English peer-reviewed articles	Gray literature

27.4.1 Review Protocol

The review protocol is shown in Table 27.1. Several models can be used to guide the search method according to the review by Eriksen and Frandsen (2018) [14]. In this review, PICOS (Population, Intervention, Comparator, Outcome, and Study type) model was used to guide the review process and key term selection.

27.4.2 Search Strategy

Search terms were used in PubMed. Terms appearing in the title and abstract were combined to search for articles that examined patients with malignancy, who traveled abroad and had complications. The scanning of articles through title and abstract was carried out by two groups of researchers (two in each group), who divided the list of articles into half. Each group of researchers reviewed the articles independently and eventually compared their findings with each other. When there is a non-agreement about eligibility, a third researcher is consulted for the final decision. In the second stage, the full-text articles were reviewed and the ones that met the inclusion criteria were included in the review.

27.4.3 Sources of Data

The search engines used for this literature review were limited to PubMed.

27.4.4 Inclusion Criteria

Only studies that were published in English and freely accessible were reviewed. The search was limited to articles published on or after the year 2000. No limits were made for the study design or the setting within which the study was undertaken.

27.4.5 Exclusion Criteria

Any study describing the pathophysiology, or the cost of the disease was excluded. Additionally, articles not discussing the complication or risks associated with traveling abroad for the management of malignancy were excluded.

27.4.6 Data Extraction and Data Synthesis

Data extraction and data synthesis were performed using narrative synthesis. Tables were used simultaneously to summarize group essential information and results about the included studies. The headings of the tables were formulated around the research questions.

27.5 Results and Discussion

Articles included in the review were classified into the following categories:

I. Articles based on primary data collection both qualitative study and quantitative study including, interviews, surveys, case studies.
II. Review articles: literature review and commentary.
III. Study based on secondary sources such as retrospective studies, and secondary data analysis.

The number of participants in the systematic review ranged from n = 1 participant in a case report review study to n = 6557 from administrative dataset. 4 out of 14 of the articles originated from the UAE. Patients traveled to different destinations around the world seeking healthcare services for cancer. Most patients in the systematic review were from Asia, the Mediterranean, and the Middle East regions. Cancer patients traveled seeking healthcare overseas for different reasons ranging from treatment, examination, screening, second opinion, and end-of-life care. Although some studies did not specify or report the type of cancer, patients in this review traveled for different types of cancers. Description of the articles reviewed and the challenges associated with medical travel experience are illustrated in Tables 27.2A and 27.2B.

Table 27.2A Description of included articles

No.	Reference	Country of study	Treatment distention	Patients home country	Target population	Type of cancer	Methods	No. of participants
1	Awano N, Takamoto T, Kawakami J, Genda A, Ninomiya A, Ikeda M, et al. [15]	Japan	Japan	Traveled from different destinations and languages spoken by the patients: Japanese, English, Chinese, Indonesian, Korean, and Mongolian	Patients with cancer who had traveled from abroad to receive second opinions, clinical examination & treatment	Liver cancer, Pancreatic cancer, Lung cancer, Colon cancer, Breast cancer, Intrahepatic cholangiocarcinoma, Malignant lymphoma, Ovarian cancer, Other types of cancer	Retrospective analysis; electronic charts and records	72
2	Hod K, Bronstein Y, Chodick G, Shpilberg O [16].	Israel	Israel	Israeli patients and patients from other destinations e.g., Russia, Ukraine, Kazakhstan, Georgia, Azerbaijan, Tanzania, Uzbekistan, and Qatar.	All hemato-oncology tourists and Israeli patients diagnosed and/or treated at the Institute of Hematology, Assuta Medical Center	Hemato-oncology patients	Retrospective Study; hospital record	Not reported

(continued)

Table 27.2A (continued)

No.	Reference	Country of study	Treatment distention	Patients home country	Type of cancer	Target population	Methods	No. of participants
3	Alnakhi WK, Segal JB, Frick KD, Hussin A, Ahmed S, Morlock L. [3]	UAE	Germany, UK, Thailand, USA, Spain, India, Singapore, Austria, Belgium, France, Swiss, Egypt, South Korea, China, Philippines, KSA, Slovenia, Jordan Czech Republic, Indonesia, Italy, Morocco, Sweden, Turkey,	UAE	Not Specified	Patients from UAE who sought medical treatment overseas	Administrative data	6557
4	Skelton M, Alameddine R, Saifi O, Hammoud M, Zorkot M, Daher M, et al. [17]	Lebanon	Lebanon	Iraq	Thymoma, Testicular cancer, multiple myeloma, liver cancer, Gastric cancer, Brain, Bladder, Adults Wilms tumor, Prostate cancer, Ovarian cancer, lung cancer, Hodgkin Lymphoma, Colon Cancer, Non-Hodgkin Lymphoma, Acute lymphoblastic Leukemia, Acute Myeloid Leukemia, Chronic Myeloid Leukemia	Iraqi patients and caregivers seeking cancer care at a tertiary referral center in Lebanon	Qualitative Study; Patient Interview	60

No.	Reference	Country of study	Treatment distention	Patients home country	Target population	Type of cancer	Methods	No. of participants
5	Joensen BM, Nielsen S, Róin Á [18].	Faroe Island	Urban and rural areas in the Faroe Islands	Urban and rural areas in the Faroe Islands	Patients who had been through a cancer treatment course with a good prognosis volunteered to be interviewed	Not specified	Qualitative Study; Patient's interview	8
6	Galloway T, Horlick S, Cherba M, Cole M, Woodgate RL, Healey Akearok G [19].	Canada	Nunavut (Canada), Patients traveled to southern referral hospitals	Canada	Patients received cancer and/ or end of life care;	Not specified;	Qualitative Study; Interview	10
7	Al-Shamsi HO, Abu-Gheida I, Rana SK, Nijhawan N, Abdulsamad AS, Alrawi S, et al. [10]	UAE	All Over medical treatment Destinations	UAE	Cancer patients returning to the UAE from treatment abroad	Not Specified	Review Study/ Recommendations for cancer patients	Not Reported
8	Young LK, Vimawala S, Ahmad N, Kushnir V, Bonawitz SC, Brody JD, et al. [20]	New Jersey (US)	USA	Liberia (One case) and in general from all over the world	Patients seeking medical care from the US	Head and Neck Cancer	Case Report/ Review	1
9	Alnakhi WK, Segal JB, Frick KD, Ahmed S, Morlock L. [6]	UAE	UAE	USA	Patients & their families from Dubai	Not Specified	Cross-Sectional Study	336
10	Boeger Z [21].	USA	New Zealand/ Australia	Tonga	Healthcare Providers	Breast Cancer	Qualitative Study	20

(continued)

Table 27.2A (continued)

No.	Reference	Country of study	Treatment distention	Patients home country	Target population	Type of cancer	Methods	No. of participants
11	McCarthy AE, Mileno MD [22].	Canada	Not Reported	Not Reported	Immunocompromised travelers	Not Specified	Review	Not Reported
12	Whittaker, A [23].	Thailand	Thailand	Gulf Cooperation Council (GCC)	Patients & families from GCC	Not Specified	Case study	9
13	Al-Shamsi HO, Al-Hajeili M, Alrawi S [1]	UAE	Not Specified	UAE and Saudi Arabic	Cancer Patients	Not Specified	Review; Response to Commentary	Not Reported
14	Oh KM, Jun J, Zhou Q, Kreps G [24].	USA	Korea	USA	Korean American Women aged 40 years or older.	Breast cancer Screening	Qualitative Study (Focused Group Interview)	34

Table 27.2B Summary of the challenges associated with medical treatment overseas

No.	Reference	Summary
1	Awano N, Takamoto T, Kawakami J, Genda A, Ninomiya A, Ikeda M, et al. [15]	• Absence or incomplete referral documents. • Complications or unmet treatment goals. • Risks associated with returning home, continuation, and follow-up care.
2	Hod K, Bronstein Y, Chodick G, Shpilberg O [16].	• Patients present at the treatment destination with an advanced stage of the disease. • Commitment to the treatment plan whether at the treatment destination or the home country.
3	Alnakhi WK, Segal JB, Frick KD, Hussin A, Ahmed S, Morlock L. [3]	• Obtaining healthcare overseas associated with risks, complications, and high cost.
4	Skelton M, Alameddine R, Saifi O, Hammoud M, Zorkot M, Daher M, et al. [17]	• Financial distress when patients paying out of their pockets.
5	Joensen BM, Nielsen S, Róin Á [18].	• Lack of coherence and planning for continuity of care between home country and treatment destination. • Financial and social aspect challenges that may arise during the treatment phase.
6	Galloway T, Horlick S, Cherba M, Cole M, Woodgate RL, Healey Akearok G [19].	• Missing paid work. • Lack of support from family and community. • Language, communication, and cultural barriers at the treatment destination.
7	Al-Shamsi HO, Abu-Gheida I, Rana SK, Nijhawan N, Abdulsamad AS, Alrawi S, et al. [10]	• Interruption of therapy after returning home (during the period of COVID-19). • Disease management and different treatment modalities between patients' home country & treatment destination.
8	Young LK, Vimawala S, Ahmad N, Kushnir V, Bonawitz SC, Brody JD, et al. [20]	• Visa process to the treatment destination.
9	Alnakhi WK, Segal JB, Frick KD, Ahmed S, Morlock L. [6]	• Complications during or after treatment.
10	Boeger Z [21].	• Patients with more unpredictable prognosis are more likely to have challenges with referral and cost of treatment.
11	McCarthy AE, Mileno MD [22].	• Immunocompromised travelers are at high risk of acquiring infection.
12	Whittaker, A [23].	• Patients with long stays overseas produce a considerable burden to their families who support them.
13	Al-Shamsi HO, Al-Hajeili M, Alrawi S [1]	• Delay in initiating the treatment plan due to getting approvals for travel. • Language and cultural barriers in the treatment destination. • Conflict of interests in the treatment destination when accepting patients for financial gains.
14	Oh KM, Jun J, Zhou Q, Kreps G [24].	• Continuation and follow-up care.

In general, few studies and publications are discussing the risks and complications associated with medical travel, especially for oncology patients seeking treatment overseas. Although this systematic review aimed to look at the medical complications that may arise from the medical travel experience for oncology patients; other challenges were found. However, no details of medical challenges such as adverse events, medical errors, incidents, harms, or injuries were reported in these studies. The challenges reported in this systematic review can be grouped into the following themes: a) financial and economic aspects, b) medical care aspects c) social and cultural aspects.

27.5.1 Financial and Economic Aspects

Seeking treatment overseas might be associated with risk for financial distress. Financial distress may arise directly or indirectly. The direct financial risks are linked to the cost of treatment, whereas the indirect financial risks may arise due to the complications of the cancer treatment received overseas [3, 25, 26]. The main financial distress that was highlighted in this review originated from the patients, who are paying out of their pocket rather than those who are sponsored by their governments or insurance agencies. Skelton et al. (2020) discussed the financial distress of Iraqi patients who crossed the border to seek healthcare in Lebanon. Those patients had deficiencies in the healthcare in their home country with limited financial resources and had no choice other than to undergo cancer treatment in a neighboring country. The size of the financial distress increased with the repeated visits to the treatment destination [17]. Other studies highlighted the financial burden of medical travel that impacted both patients and their families, especially with long-stay overseas [18, 19, 23]. On many occasions when patients' companions are not sponsored, cancer patients will support their companions during their treatment journey. Moreover, Galloway, et al. (2020) reported that along with the cost of the travel, patients and their families may have other economic impacts such as missing paid work [19]. In addition, problems with payment might arise post the treatment phase, when the expenses are not covered by patients' insurance agencies [15].

27.5.2 Medical Care Aspects

Based on the findings of this review, challenges may arise at any stage of medical travel experience including pre, during, or post-treatment [15]. In the pre-treatment stage, challenges were linked to incomplete referral documents, along with a lack of information. Information such as pathological findings, laboratory data, a summary of imaging, examination findings, and previous treatment are necessary to oncologists in the treatment destinations to provide a better course of treatment to cancer patients. Another challenge that may arise in this stage pertains to the timelines of treatment and travel. It is crucial to reduce the time between the initial diagnosis at the home country and receiving care at the treatment destinations [1, 16]. A delay in the pre-treatment phase might aggravate the patients' case due to the rapid progress of cancer over time. It is worth mentioning that immunocompromised patients might be at risk of acquiring infection at any stage of medical travel [22].

During the treatment phase, oncology patients receive a variety of treatment options including chemotherapy, radiation, surgery, or palliative care based on the stage of cancer and the treatment plan. Unfortunately, on some occasions, treatment goals are not met in this phase due to complications, side effects, or misdiagnosis in the first place [6, 27].

Additionally, some risks may arise in the post-treatment phase. These risks are associated with returning home, especially when there is no continuation of the treatment or if no proper follow-up care plans. Follow-up care is a concern that was raised in other studies from patients who experienced medical care overseas [24, 28]. Although many cancer patients might be stable during the treatment phase, the health status of the patients might deteriorate after treatment and when patients arrive home, especially patients with unpredictable prognosis [21]. On other occasions, patients might have difficulties committing to the treatment plan, whether during or after the treatment. Lack of coherence and planning in the treatment between patients' home countries and treatment destinations, whether it is due to health system issues or other reasons such as the interruption that occurred during the COVID-19 era will influence the outcomes as discussed by Al-Shamsi, Humaid O., et al. (2020) [10].

27.5.3   Social and Cultural Aspects

Challenges with cultural and social aspects were reported in some of the included reviewed articles [1, 19, 23]. For example, the commentary by Al Shamsi, Al Hajeili, and Alrawi (2018) highlighted the issues of communication between healthcare providers and international patients that could arise due to cultural and language differences. There is a cultural difference regarding disclosing information to patients. Some families, for example, do not prefer and are concerned to disclose the diagnosis and prognosis to their patients to avoid psychological distress. This challenging ethical situation may create a conflict between health care providers and patients' families particularly when healthcare providers do not take patients' and their families' culture into consideration in the treatment plan [1]. Other challenges were discussed in the review related to miscommunication between patients and healthcare providers regarding pain severity and management. For instance, patients from a few cultures might hide their pain during the treatment journey which may cause inappropriate assessment and management of pain by healthcare providers.

Moreover, lack of cultural awareness about patients' traditional ways of coping with illness, dying, and nonverbal communication was also stressed out in the reviewed article [19]. On the other hand, the quality of interpretation was high-lighted in some of the reviewed articles. This was exemplified in having unprofes-sional interpretation, assuming the role of an interpreter by a family member, or when the professional interpreters include their personal views and recommenda-tions in the context which may lead to bias in the decision made by patients and their families around the treatment plan [1, 19].

Moreover, medical travel may cause a social burden. For example, in the study by Whittaker (2015) which aimed to describe the experience of outsourced patients and their families from the Gulf Cooperation Council, the study found that patients who stay for a long period overseas produce a considerable burden to their families who are supporting them [23]. Some instrumental problems such as delaying in issuing the travel visa were pointed out. Young et al. (2019) argued that some patients experienced a delay in initiating the treatment due to the process of obtain-ing a traveling visa from the treatment destination which may not work in favor of the patient's health status [20].

27.6 Strengths and Limitations

Despite the recent studies and publications about medical travel, there are no previ-ous studies solely discussing the challenges and complications associated with medical travel, specifically for oncology patients whether on the international scope or in the Arab world. Therefore, this review can be considered the first systematic review that discusses the challenges and the issues faced by cancer patients during their medical travel experience. This chapter has identified three main aspects that can be addressed to overcome the challenges associated with medical travel in the future. These challenges can be tackled at the different stages of the medical travel experience to have better patient outcomes. In addition, implications from this review can guide future decision-making, and create quality improvement measures and actions related to the challenges associated with medical travel for oncology patients in the three main aspects.

It is also important to acknowledge the limitations of this review. One database was used for this study due to limited access to other databases. In the review, we found that many issues and challenges might accompany the medical travel experi-ence and are not only directly associated with receiving the medical care service, as other aspects of cancer patients' lives are also involved. In this review, we focused only on the challenges associated with the medical travel experience of oncology patients and did not consider the benefits that may come with the experience. Looking at both sides of the medical travel experience, positive and negative, might give a holistic and better picture of the experience. Only articles published in English were included in this review. Other languages and gray literature were not used for this review, although they might add more information to the topic. Due to the limited studies that discuss the challenges and issues of medical travel for cancer patients in the Arab world, it was difficult to narrow the scope of this review to the Arab world only.

27.7 Conclusion

In this chapter, we present the first study to systematically review challenges associated with medical travel for oncology patients seeking healthcare services outside their home country. Some challenges are associated with medical travel including economic and financial, medical care, and social and cultural challenges. In general, there is a scarcity of relevant studies that discuss this topic whether quantitatively, or qualitatively, especially in the Arab world. Such studies are vital to patients, healthcare providers, health insurance, health policymakers, and the different stakeholders involved in the medical travel market. Having sufficient information about the challenges associated with the medical travel experience will assist in creating better synergy between patients' home countries and treatment destination's healthcare systems when dealing with medical travelers. Overall, more research studies are required in this area to inform the different stakeholders involved in the medical travel field to analyze and overcome the challenges associated with this practice. Studies related to the risks and challenges associated with medical travel, will no doubt better characterize the risk profile associated with the medical travel industry at the different phases before, during, and after the medical travel experience for oncology patients.

Conflict of Interest Authors have no conflict of interest to declare.

References

1. Al-Shamsi H, Al-Hajeili M, Alrawi S. Chasing the cure around the globe: medical tourism for cancer care from developing countries. J Glob Oncol. 2018;4:1–3.
2. Abdularoup S. 600 million UAE Dirhams spent on cancer care medical tourism. Ittihad Newspaper. 2014.
3. Alnakhi WK, Segal JB, Frick KD, Hussin A, Ahmed S, Morlock L. Treatment destinations and visit frequencies for patients seeking medical treatment overseas from the United Arab Emirates: results from Dubai Health Authority reporting during 2009–2016. Trop Dis Travel Med Vaccines. 2019;5(1):1.
4. Ferlay J, Laversanne M, Ervik M, Lam F, Colombet M, Mery L, Piñeros M, Znaor A, Soerjomataram I, Bray F. Global cancer observatory: cancer tomorrow. Lyon: International Agency for Research on Cancer; 2020. Available from https://gco.iarc.fr/tomorrow. Accessed 23 Jan 2021
5. Al-Hinai SS, Al-Busaidi AS, Al-Busaidi IH. Medical tourism abroad: a new challenge to Oman's health system-Al Dakhilya region experience. Sultan Qaboos Univ Med J. 2011;11(4):477.
6. Alnakhi WK, Segal JB, Frick KD, Ahmed S, Morlock L. Motivational factors for choosing treatment destinations among the patients treated overseas from the United Arab Emirates: results from the knowledge, attitudes and perceptions survey 2012. Trop Dis Travel Med Vaccines. 2019;5(1):1–7.
7. Kim S, Arcodia C, Kim I. Critical success factors of medical tourism: the case of South Korea. Int J Environ Res Public Health. 2019;16(24):4964.
8. Lunt N, Smith R, Exworthy M. Medical tourism: treatments, markets and health system implications: a scoping review. Paris: Organisation for Economic Co-operation and Development; 2011.

9. Burney IA. The trend to seek a second opinion abroad amongst cancer patients in Oman: challenges and opportunities. Sultan Qaboos Univ Med J. 2009;9(3):260.

10. Al-Shamsi HO, Abu-Gheida I, Rana SK, Nijhawan N, Abdulsamad AS, Alrawi S, Abuhaleeqa M, Almansoori TM, Alkasab T, Alessa EM, McManus MC. Challenges for cancer patients returning home during SARS-COV-19 pandemic after medical tourism-a consensus report by the emirates oncology task force. BMC Cancer. 2020;20(1):1–10.

11. Booth A, Papaioannou D, Sutton A. Systematic approaches to a successful literature review. London: Sage Publications; 2012.

12. Pae CU. Why systematic review rather than narrative review? Psychiatry Investig. 2015;12(3):417.

13. Liberati A, Altman DG, Tetzlaff J, Mulrow C, Gøtzsche PC, Ioannidis JP, Clarke M, Devereaux PJ, Kleijnen J, Moher D. The PRISMA statement for reporting systematic reviews and meta-analyses of studies that evaluate health care interventions: explanation and elaboration. J Clin Epidemiol. 2009;62(10):e1–e34.

14. Eriksen MB, Frandsen TF. The impact of patient, intervention, comparison, outcome (PICO) as a search strategy tool on literature search quality: a systematic review. J Med Libr Assoc. 2018;106(4):420.

15. Awano N, Takamoto T, Kawakami J, Genda A, Ninomiya A, Ikeda M, Matsuno F, Izumo T, Kunitoh H. Issues associated with medical tourism for cancer care in Japan. Jpn J Clin Oncol. 2019;49(8):708–13.

16. Hod K, Bronstein Y, Chodick G, Shpilberg O. Hemato-oncology tourism in Israel: a retrospective review. JCO Glob Oncol. 2020;6:1314–20.

17. Skelton M, Alameddine R, Saifi O, Hammoud M, Zorkot M, Daher M, Charafeddine M, Temraz S, Shamseddine A, Mula-Hussain L, Saleem M. High-cost cancer treatment across borders in conflict zones: experience of Iraqi patients in Lebanon. JCO Glob Oncol. 2020;6:59–66.

18. Joensen BM, Nielsen S, Róin Á. Barriers to quality of care for cancer patients in rural areas: a study from the Faroe Islands. J Multidiscip Healthc. 2020;13:63.

19. Galloway T, Horlick S, Cherba M, Cole M, Woodgate RL, Healey AG. Perspectives of Nunavut patients and families on their cancer and end of life care experiences. Int J Circumpolar Health. 2020;79(1):1766319.

20. Young LK, et al. Review of inbound medical tourism and legal details of obtaining a visa for treatment of head and neck cancer. Head Neck. 2019;41(8):E125–32.

21. Boeger Z. Incorporating mammography into an overseas referral metric: Tongan doctors' assessments of patient eligibility for medical travel. Soc Sci Med. 2020;1(254):112355.

22. McCarthy AE, Mileno MD. Prevention and treatment of travel-related infections in compromised hosts. Curr Opin Infect Dis. 2006;19(5):450–5.

23. Whittaker A. 'Outsourced' patients and their companions: stories from forced medical travellers. Glob Public Health. 2015;10(4):485–500.

24. Oh KM, Jun J, Zhou Q, Kreps G. Korean American women's perceptions about physical examinations and cancer screening services offered in Korea: the influences of medical tourism on Korean Americans. J Community Health. 2014;39(2):221–9.

25. Sheppard CE, Lester EL, Chuck AW, Kim DH, Karmali S, de Gara CJ, Birch DW. Medical tourism and bariatric surgery: who pays? Surg Endosc. 2014;28(12):3329–36.

26. Kim DH, Sheppard CE, de Gara CJ, Karmali S, Birch DW. Financial costs and patients' perceptions of medical tourism in bariatric surgery. Can J Surg. 2016;59(1):59.

27. Hanefeld J, Horsfall D, Lunt N, Smith R. Medical tourism: a cost or benefit to the NHS? PLoS One. 2013;8(10):e70406.

28. Eissler LA, Casken J. Seeking health care through international medical tourism. J Nurs Scholarsh. 2013;45(2):177–84.

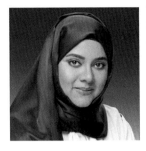

Wafa K. Alnakhi is currently the Acting Head of Health Research and Survey Section at Dubai Health Authority, UAE & Adjunct Clinical Assistance Professor at Mohammed Bin Rashid University of Medicine and Health Sciences, U.A.E. Alnakhi has earned her Doctorate in Public Health from the Health Policy and Management Department from Johns Hopkins University Bloomberg School of Public Health. Her research interest and published work are around medical travel among the Dubai population to understand patients' characteristics, motivational factors, and preferences. Her focus is on improving population health through creating a framework to support health system & services research in the UAE.

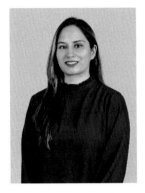

Faryal Iqbal holds an undergraduate degree in Molecular Biology & Biotechnology. Subsequently, she earned postgraduate qualification in Molecular Genetics from Pakistan, where she worked on finding the association between *XRCC1* gene polymorphism and radiation exposure in healthcare workers. She is currently working with an oncology specific research group and serving in the domains of scientific writing, data management, supervision of medical internees, and providing editorial assistance. Ms. Iqbal's research interests and publications encompass genetics and oncology. She intends to support research across the oncology key areas including prevention, diagnosis, and treatment. Her focus is on preparing for future adoption of genomic technology and increased use of genomic information as part of the cancer diagnostic and therapeutic pathways.

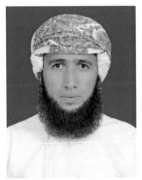

Waleed Al Nadabi is a medical doctor who graduated from Sultan Qaboos University. He further specialized in quality and patient safety and got a master's and PhD degrees from the UK. He held several positions in different hospitals as head of quality and patient safety. Later he became the director of monitoring and evaluation in the Directorate of planning and studies, Ministry of Health, Oman. Currently, he is working as a medical specialist and leading several projects like national health five-year planning, country's cooperation strategy with the World Health Organization as well as other projects.

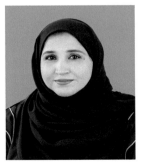

Amal Al Balushi is a lecturer at Oman College of Health Science, Nursing Program, Sultanate of Oman. Dr. Amal leads and teaches Child Health Nursing theory. She also trains undergraduate nursing students during their clinical nursing practice. In 2019, she completed her PhD in Nursing at the University of Maryland-Baltimore, USA. Before joining Oman College of Health Science in 2008, Amal worked as a bedside nurse with the main role of providing nursing care for pediatric patients. The science of family and psychosocial care is her main area of interest. Amal has undergone training in qualitative methods and analysis.

Chapter 28
Radiation Therapy in Arab World

Zeinab Elsayed, Issam Lalya, Hussain AlHussain, and Layth Mula-Hussain

28.1   Background

Radiation Oncology, medical oncology, and surgical oncology are the three main specialties of clinical oncology. Radiotherapy (RT) is an essential pillar of cancer treatment used with curative or palliative intent. It can also be used as a single treatment modality or combined with surgery and/or systemic therapy [2]. Approximately up to 60% of cancer patients receive RT during their course of illness [12]. RT is used with curative intent in about 40% of cases [6].

The League of Arab States, which was formed in 1945, has 22 countries spread over North Africa and the Middle East. These countries are collectively known as the Arab world and have more than 426 million inhabitants [13]. As per the World Bank economic categorization, four countries are Low-Income Countries (LIC), eight countries are Low-Middle Income Countries (LMIC), four countries are Upper-Middle-Income Countries (UMIC), and six countries are High-Income Countries (HIC).

Z. Elsayed
Ain Shams University, Cairo, Egypt
e-mail: z_elsayed@med.asu.edu.eg

I. Lalya
Cadi Ayyad University, Marrakech, Morocco
e-mail: i.lalya@uca.ma

H. AlHussain
King Fahad Medical City, Riyadh, KSA
e-mail: halhussain@kfmc.med.sa

L. Mula-Hussain (✉)
Ninevah University, Mosul, Iraq

Sultan Qaboos Comprehensive Cancer Care and Research Centre, Muscat, Oman
e-mail: l.mulahussain@cccrc.gov.om

© The Author(s) 2022
H. O. Al-Shamsi et al. (eds.), *Cancer in the Arab World*,
https://doi.org/10.1007/978-981-16-7945-2_28

445

Cancer is overgrowing among Arab countries, and by 2030, it is expected that there would be a 1.8-fold increase in cancer cases in this region [4]. Eighty percent of the region's countries have national cancer policies, yet only 45% of the programs function [46, 47]. There is also low research outcome in this field, especially in the preventative cancer control policies [18].

28.1.1 Definition

Radiation oncology is a medical specialty that uses ionizing radiation (X-ray, Gamma-ray, Alpha and Beta particles) to treat malignant diseases and occasionally benign or functional diseases. Ionizing radiation damages cells' DNA and blocks their ability to divide further and proliferate [23]. RT aims to deliver high radiation doses to tumor volumes accurately while minimizing the amount received by surrounding healthy tissues [32]. A distinction must be made between the External Beam Radiation Therapy (EBRT), which is a technique using an irradiation source located outside the patient, most often coming from a linear accelerator, and the brachytherapy, which uses sealed sources placed either inside the target volume (interstitial) or on its contact in a natural cavity (endocavitary) or a duct (endoluminal).

28.1.2 Origin and Development

The discovery of X-rays was announced by Wilhelm Conrad Röntgen, a German mechanical engineer and physicist, on November 30, 1895 [38]. However, there is little doubt that X-rays were produced earlier by Julius Plücker, another German mathematician and physicist, who noticed in 1859 that the passage of a high voltage current through a vacuum tube produced an apple-green fluorescence on the inner wall of the tube. In 1875, Sir William Crookes noted that this apple-green light of Plücker's had its origin at the opposing end of the tube and therefore called this phenomenon the cathode ray [10]. The first therapeutic uses of X-rays in cancer followed its discovery by a few months [19].

Natural radioactivity was discovered by the physicist Antoine-Henri Becquerel while working with uranium salts in 1896. Shortly after that, Marie and Pierre Curie discovered radium and polonium, and in 1902, radium had been used to treat pharyngeal carcinoma. The concept of insertion of radium tubes into tumors (interstitial brachytherapy) had started in 1904 [9]. In the 1920s, Regaud and Ferroux from France established the biologic bases of fractionated radiotherapy [37].

Conceptual, technological, and radiobiological discoveries and innovations over the twentieth century lay the foundations for the safe and effective RT used today [9]. In the last three decades, RT has advanced amazingly, from 2D to 3D and then to Intensity Modulated Radiation Therapy (IMRT) and Stereotactic ABlative Radiotherapy (SABR) with many modalities in between [7].

28.1.3 Members of the Teamwork

28.1.3.1 Radiation Oncologist (RO)

RO is a physician who is a member of a multidisciplinary team (MDT) to treat cancer patients (and some benign diseases) using ionizing radiation [2]. RO should be certified by the appropriate certification board before practicing the specialty [34].

28.1.3.2 Medical Physicist (MP)

MP is a scientist who works closely with physicians, dosimetrists, and therapists and applies knowledge of radiation physics, radiobiology, and radiation safety to perform optimum, safe RT. In addition, MP performs routine Quality Assurance (QA) for radiation equipment and imaging systems and calibration, commissioning, and installation of new RT machines [2]. As per International Atomic Energy Agency (IAEA), "Clinically qualified MP is a physicist working in healthcare who has received adequate academic postgraduate education in medical physics and relevant supervised clinical training" [17].

28.1.3.3 Radiation Therapy Technologist (RTT)

RTT is a technician who uses physics, radiology, patient care, and patient safety to deliver therapeutic ionizing radiation to patients. In addition, RTT is trained and qualified to operate teletherapy machines [2].

28.1.3.4 Radiation Oncology Nurse

Radiation Oncology Nurses have a good overall understanding of general health, cancer medicine, and RT. They help with procedures such as brachytherapy, drug administration, clinical examination, and RT simulation. In addition, they support patients and their families during the treatment journey [2].

28.1.3.5 Radiation Machines Engineer

RT maintenance engineer is responsible for verification that the RT machine performs appropriately and according to both functionality and safety specifications [30].

28.2 History of Radiation Therapy in Arab World

Arab countries started building up radiation services, whether for diagnostic or therapeutic purposes, not far away from its inception. Some radiation machines were used as early as the first quarter of the twentieth century. In Iraq, the first establishment of radiation services was launched with a superficial X-ray therapy machine at the Radiology Institute in Baghdad during the 1920s [30]. In Lebanon, the Hotel-Dieu de France Hospital of the University of St Joseph opened its RT department in 1925. In Morocco, the history of radiotherapy dates back to 1929 by establishing the Bergonié center at the Averroes Hospital in Casablanca. In Egypt, the first RT unit at the Kasr Al-Ainy Hospital (Cairo University Hospital) was established in the 1930s. At that time, just as in other countries worldwide, radiation oncology did not exist as a separate specialty but was a part of the radiology, tumor management, and electrotherapy department at Cairo Faculty of Medicine [49]. Subsequently, RT departments further expanded and grew in other Arab countries.

28.3 Status of Radiation Therapy in Arab World

28.3.1 Human Resources and Treatment Facilities

Worldwide, gaps to RT access have been identified, not only in LMIC as expected, but also in Europe, as access to RT remains limited in many countries [1, 5, 11, 40]. Furthermore, a commonly used benchmark for RT machine availability of 450–500 patients per RT unit per year has been suggested for suitable machine throughput, whereas annual numbers of 200–300 patients per RO, 300–500 per MP, and 100–150 per RTT have also been suggested in several reports [35, 42, 44, 45].

The number of current RT machines in the Arab world was obtained from the Directory of Radiotherapy Centres (DIRAC) database, managed by the IAEA as of April 2021 [20], while population and new cancer cases per country were obtained from GLOBOCAN global cancer statistics 2020 [15]. Data from DIRAC shows that 18 out of the 22 Arab countries have RT facilities, while four countries (Comoros, Djibouti, Palestine, and Somalia) have no information on their facilities. Table 28.1 shows that in 2021, there are 364 Mega-Voltage Machines (MVMs) serving a total population of 427.8 million in 210 RT centers [20]. For the ideal need for MVMs, some equations can be used, similar to the one we mentioned in the previous paragraph. Although that this equation is valid, we think that group II of the World Health Organization (WHO) recommendations, by providing one MVM per one million population, can simply fit the minimal need of our people in the Arab world; However, if we have the facilities to move to group III WHO recommendation, by providing 2 MVMs per one million population, this might be optimal.

Table 28.1 RT status in Arab world countries as in 2021 based on the group II WHO recommendation of 1 MVM/million population

Arab countries	population	New cancer cases	Current MV machines	Ideal RT machines	Ratio of EBRT machine/ million population	Current Brachytherapy equipment	DIRAC data update
Egypt	104,047,786	134,632	120	104	1.15	23	2021
Algeria	44,588,410	58,418	37	44.6	0.83	12	2020
Sudan	44,709,056	27,382	10	44.7	0.2	2	2020
Iraq	40,948,473	33,873	23	40.9	0.56	2	2021
Morocco	37,287,724	59,370	43	37.3	1.15	10	2021
KSA	35,317,914	27,885	34	35.3	0.96	9	2021
Yemen	30,403,164	16,476	1	30.4	0.03	–	2018
Syria	17,299,112	20,959	10	17.3	0.57	2	2020
Somalia	15,893,219	10,134	No information				
Tunisia	11,933,090	19,446	25	11.9	2.1	4	2021
Jordan	10,353,556	11,559	13	10.3	1.26	1	2021
UAE	10,028,579	4,807	6	10	0.6	1	2020
Libya	6,960,374	7,661	6	6.9	0.87	1	2020
Lebanon	6,849,023	11,589	20	6.8	2.94	3	2020
Oman	5,249,890	3,713	2	5.2	0.38	1	2019
Palestine	5,203,412	4,779	No information				
Mauritania	4,756,163	3,079	2	4.7	0.43	1	2019
Kuwait	4,336,507	3,842	5	4.3	1.16	1	2021
Qatar	2,925,692	1,482	3	2.9	1.0	1	2019
Bahrain	1,779,580	1,215	2	1.8	1.11	–	2018
Djibouti	1,000,651	765	No information				
Comoros	885,582	609	No information				

Some Arab countries have comprehensive cancer and research centers, which are gradually becoming more popular, such as the King Hussein Cancer Center in Jordan and the Sultan Qaboos Comprehensive Cancer Care in Oman. Besides the Cyberknife, the Gamma Knife, and the Gantry-based Stereotactic Radiosurgery Units in many Arab countries, Saudi Arabia is going to be the first Arab country to have Proton Therapy Particles through the Saudi Particle Therapy Center that is equipped with ProBeam Cyclotron linked to five treatment units, which is anticipated to start treating patients by 2022.

Cancer patients' data are extracted from 2020 GLOBOCAN, Global Cancer Observatory: Cancer Today, Cancer Today (iarc.fr) in April 2021. Equipment data are extracted from IAEA DIRAC (Directory of Radiotherapy centers [20], Division for Human Health: DIRAC (DIrectory of RAdiotherapy Centres) (iaea.org). Accessed in April 2021. Abbreviations: *MV* Megavoltage, *KSA* Kingdom Saudi Arabia, *UAE* United Arab Emirates.

28.3.2   Education, Training and Certification Programs

Radiation Oncology exposure in many Undergraduate Medical Schools in Arab countries is very limited to a lecture or two with a significant lack of orientation to this particular specialty in many of the Undergraduate Medical Education Curricula [28]. Radiation Oncology Residency Training Program is not one of the many medical specialties offered by the Arab Board of Health Specializations. However, some Arab countries offer national, well-structured radiation oncology training programs.

In Egypt for example, radiation oncology training can be either a pure radiation oncology program or combined with medical oncology training in a clinical oncology program, which is the most popular. Within these programs, candidates are awarded a Master of Science (M.Sc.) degree after 2–3 years of training and a Medical Doctorate (MD) after another three training years. The candidate must pass written, clinical, and oral exams for both degrees and prepare an academic medical thesis. In addition, the Ministry of Health offers a separate fellowship for radiation oncology and another one for medical oncology in a 5-year training program. The Egyptian Children's Cancer Hospital (57357) has already established a 1-year fellowship program in pediatric radiation oncology in collaboration with the Dana-Farber Cancer Institute and Massachusetts General Hospital, Boston, Massachusetts [49].

In Morocco, the teaching of radiation oncology dates back to 1984, with a well-structured program influenced by the curricula of French universities and centers such as Alexis Vautrin and Gustave Roussy Institute. Medical oncology was individualized as a separate specialty since 2004. Training centers are affiliated to the faculties of Medicine and Pharmacy, with six university centers in total and the Military Teaching Hospital Mohamed V in Rabat, and two private university hospitals in Rabat and Casablanca. The National Diploma of Specialty graduates candidates after 4 years of training toward the final specialty exam. In 2016, Morocco requested a national technical cooperation project (MOR6023 'Improving the Quality of Radiotherapy by Developing Human Resources Capacity through Harmonization of Clinical Training in Radiation Oncology') with the IAEA to support the improvement of quality of radiotherapy.

In Lebanon, Saint Joseph University Hotel Dieu de France Radiation Oncology Department has an established residency program in Radiation Oncology. This program consists of one year of training in the general medicine program, 3 years of training at the department, and one year of training in one of the partner departments in France like Institute Gustave Roussy, Villejuif. Moreover, the American University of Beirut also has the first, and only ACME-I accredited Radiation Oncology residency training program that consists of 1 year of preliminary training in either surgery, internal medicine, pediatrics, followed by a 4-year comprehensive radiation oncology training, similar to the United States. This is routinely followed by a fellowship in the center in Northern America, such as the University of Texas MD Anderson Cancer Center, Memorial Sloan Kettering Cancer Center, or other centers.

In Jordan, and since 2004, King Hussein Cancer Center is offering a structured 4-year competency-based program, recognized and accredited by the Jordan Medical Council. In addition, residents have the opportunity to spend 3 months of external training at one of the affiliated cancer centers in either the USA or the UK [25]. In Iraq, The Zhianawa Cancer Center in 2017 celebrated its first board-certified ROs from a 4-year program that launched in 2013, which started back to the 2-year diploma program in oncology and radiation therapy that began in Baghdad in 1984 [29]. In 2018, the Saudi Commission for Health Specialties launched a 5-years robustly structured Radiation Oncology residency and certification program with structure and content built and adapted learning from International Benchmarks, mainly of North American Institutions [41].

MPs in the Arab world graduate from science faculties but with minimal clinical training. They gain their experience from working in different radiation oncology centers and departments. For example, in Egypt, MPs are graduates of biophysics departments within the Faculty of Science in various universities. They receive elective clinical training in radiation oncology and/or clinical oncology departments during their undergraduate studies. To be specialized in radiation oncology physics, they should have at least two years of training in this field within specialized departments [22, 26, 49].

The approximate number of MPs in the Middle East was around 740 in 2017 [33]. In 2009, the Middle East Federation of Organizations of Medical Physics (MEFOMP) was established as a regional organization of the International Organization for Medical Physics (IOMP), initially with 12 participating countries [22, 26]. It has been considered as a milestone that paved the way to establish Medical Physics Associations/Societies in the Middle East countries where there was none before [33].

As regards RTTs in Arab countries, the training programs were limited till recently. Realizing the importance of having adequate qualified RTTs, and as a mandatory step to lower the dependence on foreign personnel, many universities started to establish certified programs in conjunction with cancer hospitals and centers [27]. For many years, RTTs graduated from specialized institutes after studying for two years post-high school graduation in Egypt. However, in recent years, the policy changed to establish specialized universities (both governmental and private) to award graduates a bachelor's degree after the 4-year program in radiographic sciences [49]. Faculty of Health and Rehabilitation Sciences at Princess Nourah University, Saudi Arabia, established in 2011 a 5-years bachelor's degree in Radiological Sciences with four separate tracks that include a dedicated path of Radiation Therapy Program. Another example from Saudi Arabia, College of Applied Medical Sciences, King Saud University, offers a Radiological Sciences Program established in 1979. Graduates are awarded bachelor's degrees and study specialized radiological subspecialties, primarily diagnostic backgrounds [8].

The region has benefited greatly from projects with international organizations such as IAEA, both on the governmental and institutional levels [29]. For example, the American University of Beirut Medical Center has a well-established sister institution-ship and collaboration with the University of Texas MD Anderson Cancer

Center and the Memorial Sloan Kettering Cancer Center, respectively. King Hussein Cancer Center succeeded in collaborating with many reputable international cancer centers, like MD Anderson Cancer Center, Princess Margret Hospital, St June Cancer Center, Sick Hospital Cancer Center, and Moffit Cancer Center, through partnership programs and collaborative agreements [24]. The Children's Cancer Hospital in Egypt (57357), through its outreach division, has successfully collaborated with many regional and international institutions and organizations like Dana Farber Cancer Institute, Joint Commission International (JCI), St. Jude Children's Research Hospital, among many others. Another example was from Tunisia when it implemented modern RT techniques in the Radiation Oncology department of Hannibal Clinic. This project collaborated between the clinic and IAEA and resulted in the first Linear Accelerator (LINAC) 3D conformal radiation treatment in June 2011 [14].

28.3.3 Practice and Licensing

Almost all Arab countries have some form of licensing for ROs, MPs, and RTTs. To be specialized in radiation/clinical oncology, physicians must complete postgraduate studies and training in the specialty field. They are awarded the title after passing a series of written, clinical and oral exams with or without preparing an academic medical dissertation [48] [29]. In Egypt, e.g., physicians who want to practice in this specialty should receive either an M.Sc. or M.D. from an accredited University or obtain the Ministry of Health Fellowship in Radiation Oncology [49]. In addition, all practicing oncologists should get their licenses from the Egyptian medical syndicate.

MPs in Arab countries are licensed based on reviewing their qualifications and not necessarily after passing relevant exams [29]. There are no national or regional certification boards in Middle East countries, however, the International Medical Physics Certification Board (IMPCB), in 2019 onward, started exams in some Arab countries (Saudi Arabia, Jordan, and Qatar), and an increasing number of institutions encourage their MPs to pass these exams [21]. MPs' qualifications in the regulatory bodies have positively impacted MPs' practice in different hospitals. An example is the Radiation Safety Law in Jordan that was implemented in 2015, through which Jordan's Energy and Minerals Regulatory Commission (EMRC) published various reports, including the "Quality Assurance Program for Hospital X-ray Generating Equipment" [29]. The situation for RTTs licensures is similar to MPs regarding certification and accreditation [29].

28.3.4 Professional Societies of Radiation Oncology

The common feature between all countries of the Arab world is the absence of professional societies dedicated to radiation oncology practice and research. Instead, the existing organizations federate all cancer specialists, including medical and surgical oncologists, for example, the Arab Medical Association Against Cancer (AMAAC) and many other national oncology and cancer societies in the Arab world. This fact is maybe the consequence of the limited number of Arab radiation oncology practitioners, not allowing the creation of solid and well-structured societies. Added to this, a permanent feeling of dependence on foreign radiation oncology societies, given the quality of their scientific production, such as good practice guidelines and websites of e-learning and contouring.

In recent years we have seen the development of institutions that will certainly lead in the long term to well-organized societies. For example, the Iraqi Society of Radiation Oncology in 2014 arranged the Best of ASTRO meetings (officially licensed by the American Society of Radiation Oncology—ASTRO) in 2015 in Iraq [29], which was followed by the first Joint Conference Best of ASCO and Best of ASTRO the following year in 2016, in Egypt. The Saudi Assembly of Radiation Oncology was established in 2018 as a National Radiation Oncology Professional Community Group of Practice, and the National College of Radiation Oncology Professors in 2020 in Morocco with the sole mission of unifying the radiation oncology teaching program in Morocco, as well as the harmonization of practices. The most significant step would be to create a regional big society, from the MENA region, or ideally from the whole Arab world.

28.3.5   Research in Radiation Oncology

Scientific research in radiation oncology in the Arab world is limited to participation in the enrollment of patients for international multicentric randomized trials and the publication of treatment planning and dosimetric studies in high indexed journals.

In Morocco, the Institute of Research in Cancer was created in 2014 by the Lalla Salma Foundation, the Ministry of Higher Education and Scientific Research, and the University Sidi Mohamed Ben Abdellah in Fes. Among research laboratories affiliated with this institute, there is a nuclear physics laboratory whose activity is still rudimentary.

Radiation Oncology research activity in Saudi Arabia has gained momentum in terms of volume and international collaboration over the period from 2010 to 2019; however, the resulting level of evidence has not improved over time, which calls for an effort to contribute to the literature as a priority, allocate adequate resources, and apply appropriate measures to enhance research productivity and quality [3].

The basic research unit, the clinical trials unit, and the biobank at the Egyptian Children's Cancer Hospital 57357 facilitate high-quality research through efficient coordination and successful implementation of basic research and clinical trials in collaboration with international pediatric cancer centers, which resulted in many international publications in the field of pediatric radiation oncology.

28.3.6 Pediatric Radiation Oncology

RT is an essential part of childhood cancer treatment. However, the presence of a dedicated pediatric cancer center/hospital in Arab countries is uncommon. Most Arab countries have centers that treat both adults and pediatric patients or pediatric oncology departments within hospitals. A unique example of a specialized pediatric cancer hospital is the Egyptian Children's Cancer Hospital (57357). It was established in 2007 and was inspired by the St. Jude Research Hospital model in Memphis, Tennessee, in the USA. In addition to the Egyptian people, many Arab countries have contributed generously to make it one of the largest hospitals in capacity (320 beds). The King Fahad National Centre for Children's Cancer and Research is the only standalone children's cancer center in Saudi Arabia.

28.4 Future of Radiation Therapy in Arab World

28.4.1 Overcoming the Challenges

RT is an essential component of effective cancer treatment, yet the worldwide availability of RT facilities is unacceptably low [5]. Twelve of the 22 countries are classified as LMIC or LIC, according to the World Bank. These countries face the same challenges as other LMIC worldwide. As shown by [27], the availability of RT facilities was significantly influenced by economic status and correlated positively with GDP per capita. Based on group II WHO recommendations of at least one MVM/million population as a minimum supply, the Arab countries need about 427 MVMs to be in a minimally acceptable situation [36]. According to the most recent DIRAC data (Table 28.1), Arab countries currently possess 362 MVMs. This represents about 85% of the actual needs. This may look better than many other countries in Africa and Asia-Pacific (34% and 61%, respectively) [50]. Still, these facilities are not equally distributed among countries. High-income countries already have around 135% of their MVM needs, while UMIC and LMIC have 75.5% and 72.5% of their needs, respectively [27].

Optimal delivery of RT requires well-trained ROs, qualified MPs and RTTs, competent nurses, and non-medical staff. Unfortunately, some Arab countries are still lacking competency-based residency training programs. On the other hand, many Arab countries still have clinical oncology programs, with radiation oncology and medical oncology curricula over a minimal time. Lack of Work-Place Based Assessment and training on communication skills is another character of training programs in countries with high patient volume and a small number of supervising well-trained staff; Egypt is an example.

MPs working in the clinical environment are health professions per the International Labor Organization and WHO classification. However, they receive primarily theoretical education with very minimal clinical exposure during their undergraduate studies. Other challenges include a lack of incentives and opportunities for personal and professional development, unlike the opportunities offered to the doctors. Undergraduate Medical Physics Bachelor's Degrees are available in a limited number of universities in the Arab countries, for example, at King Abdulaziz University and Umm Al-Qura University, in Saudi Arabia. Otherwise, most MPs usually have a General Physics or Engineering undergraduate Bachelor's Degree then pursue their Master's Program in Medical Physics.

Postgraduate Medical Physics Certification is based chiefly on Master and Ph.D. studies. However, a limited number of Arab countries have established institution-based Medical Physics Clinical Residency Training, like King Hussein Cancer Center, Jordan, and King Faisal Specialist Hospital, Saudi Arabia. In addition, the Saudi Commission for Health Specialties established a National-wide Medical Physics Clinical Residency Training, awaiting to be launched.

Traditionally, highly qualified young staff from LMIC emigrate to HIC for training. Later, they choose to stay abroad with subsequent "brain drain" with more load on the already suffering health system [2]. There is an urgent need to fill the gaps in MVM availability, human resources, knowledge, and clinical experience in our region. However, the analysis of RT needs is focused more on the equipment and infrastructure with less attention to qualified professionals [51].

Needs assessment and gap analysis are essential for any improvement plan. This requires accurate registry and documentation systems. According to a recent publication, 17 of the 22 countries have population-based cancer registries [43]. However, data about radiotherapy facilities and human resources are lacking in many countries. Data derived from DIRAC is self-reported with no auditing or confirmation. In addition, this data does not consider the details of RT techniques [27].

28.4.2 Capacity Building

The IAEA has the longest track record for human capacity building in the field of radiation oncology in LMICs [2]. Training of an entire team, including ROs, MPs, RTTs, and occasionally nurses and maintenance engineers, has always been a part of any Technical Cooperation (TC) project to start a new RT facility [39]. Radiation oncology departments worldwide offered training opportunities to many LMIC trainees. The problem with these programs is the high cost and the eventual result of "brain drain." Most professional societies offer training courses and programs abroad, but the curricula of high-income countries are not applicable in home countries most of the time [16]. Some of the successful examples of training options include the American Society for Radiation Oncology's (ASTRO)/Association of Residents in Radiation Oncology's (ARRO)'s Global Health Scholar Program and the American College of Radiology Foundation's Goldberg-Reeder Resident Travel Grant [2]. There is a need for an adequate number of competency-based and well-structured radiation oncology programs in all Arab world countries to fill their national need. Some practical roadmaps can be followed in this regard, like the

"Specialty Portfolio in Radiation Oncology: A global certification roadmap for trainers and trainees" [31].

Telemedicine is an area that is gaining increasing attention. It can overcome many barriers of traditional training, such as time and distance barriers. It is challenging to provide care to cancer patients during the COVID-19 while protecting both patients and staff from infection. The use of video consultations and remote networking can save time, decrease physical contact and save resources.

Arab countries continue to collaborate with regional and international organizations for knowledge and skills transfer. With the new interest in career development in global health, there are many successful examples of twinning partnerships between regional institutes and international universities and organizations. An example from Morocco can be given here, in 1984, the first two Moroccan radiation oncology professors started a training program at the faculties of medicine of Rabat and Casablanca, which allowed the graduation of hundreds of Moroccan and African radiation oncologists. Since 2005, and thanks to the support of the Lalla Salma Foundation in partnership with the Ministry of Health, Morocco has made a giant technological leap by the acquisition of more than 40 linear accelerators equipped with the most advanced technologies to deliver high precision treatments.

28.5   Conclusion

Arab countries share language, culture, and history, but they have variable economic characteristics, with significant variation in radiotherapy services across different countries. There are many gaps in the current radiation oncology facilities. Many Arabic countries still lack systems of accurate and up-to-date data registries. Information about the status of RT in our region is mainly derived from sources like DIRAC. Training programs across many countries are sub-optimal. To face these challenges, Arab countries must collaborate both on the regional and international levels. Governments and international organizations need to invest in RT resources and help the less advantageous countries. Many successful and inspiring examples that other countries can follow are present.

28.5.1   Strengths and Limitations

This chapter describes many RT-related issues that can be used as a baseline for future studies. The authors tried to explore some dimensions of this field through the published literature and their expertise and networks. However, many Arab countries do not have well-established systems that document all aspects of cancer care, from infrastructure to workforce and outcomes. Data on RT infrastructure was derived from DIRAC, which is a self-reporting source with no verification. Also, data about cancer incidence was retrieved from GLOBOCAN estimates, which may not reflect the real-life registries. Information about other parts such as training programs, certification and licensing relied on personal communication between the authors and colleagues from different Arab countries, again with no external verification.

Conflict of Interest Authors have no conflict of interest to declare.

References

1. Abdel-Wahab M, Bourque J-M, Pynda Y, Iżewska J, Van der Merwe D, Zubizarreta E, Rosenblatt E. Status of radiotherapy resources in Africa: an International Atomic Energy Agency analysis. Lancet Oncol. 2013;14(4):e168–75. https://doi.org/10.1016/S1470-2045(12)70532-6.
2. Abdel-Wahab M, Nitzsche-Bell A, Olson A, Polo A, Shah MM, Zubizarreta E, Patel S. Radiation oncology in global health. In: Mollura DJ, Culp MP, Lungren MP, editors. Radiology in global health: strategies, implementation, and applications. Cham: Springer International Publishing; 2019. p. 349–60.
3. Alghamdi MA, et al. Scholarly activity of radiation oncologists in high-income developing countries: Saudi Arabia as an example. JCO Glob Oncol. 2021;7:378–83. https://doi.org/10.1200/GO.20.00449.
4. Arafa MA, Rabah DM, Farhat KH. Rising cancer rates in the Arab world: now is the time for action. East Mediterr Health J. 2020;26(6):638–40. https://doi.org/10.26719/emhj.20.073.
5. Atun R, Jaffray DA, Barton MB, Bray F, Baumann M, Vikram B, et al. Expanding global access to radiotherapy. Lancet Oncol. 2015;16(10):1153–86. https://doi.org/10.1016/s1470-2045(15)00222-3.
6. Baskar R, Lee KA, Yeo R, Yeoh K-W. Cancer and radiation therapy: current advances and future directions. Int J Med Sci. 2012;9(3):193–9. https://doi.org/10.7150/ijms.3635.
7. Blake M. I.4 advances in radiotherapy and radiotherapy innovations. J Thorac Oncol. 2019;14(11):S1157. https://doi.org/10.1016/j.jtho.2019.09.098.
8. CAMS. College of Applied Medical Sciences. 2021. Retrieved from https://cams.ksu.edu.sa/en/departments/radiological-sciences.
9. Connell PP, Hellman S. Advances in radiotherapy and implications for the next century: a historical perspective. Cancer Res. 2009;69(2):383–92. https://doi.org/10.1158/0008-5472.Can-07-6871.
10. Crookes W. Priority in the therapeutic use of X-rays, quoted by Grubbe, E.H. Radiology. 1933;21:156–62.
11. Datta NR, Samiei M, Bodis S. Radiation therapy infrastructure and human resources in low-and middle-income countries: present status and projections for 2020. Int J Radiat Oncol Biol Phys. 2014;89(3):448–57. https://doi.org/10.1016/j.ijrobp.2014.03.002.
12. Delaney G, Jacob S, Featherstone C, Barton M. The role of radiotherapy in cancer treatment: estimating optimal utilization from a review of evidence-based clinical guidelines. Cancer. 2005;104(6):1129–37. https://doi.org/10.1002/cncr.21324.
13. Elbanna S, Abdelzaher DM, Ramadan N. Management research in the Arab world: what is now and what is next? J Int Manag. 2020;26(2):100734. https://doi.org/10.1016/j.intman.2020.100734.
14. Frikha H, Chaouache K, Abdessaied S, Elhattab I, Bousselmi S, Ksouri W, et al. Implementation of a radiation therapy center in low and middle-income countries. the case of collaborative project to implement modern radiotherapy center in Tunisia. Int J Radiat Oncol Biol Phys. 2019;105(1):E445–6.
15. GLOBOCAN. Population fact sheets. 2020. Retrieved from https://gco.iarc.fr/today/fact-sheets-populations.

16. Gospodarowicz M. Global access to radiotherapy—work in progress. JCO Glob Oncol. 2021;7:144–5. https://doi.org/10.1200/go.20.00562.

17. Guidelines for the certification of clinically qualified medical physicists. Vienna: International Atomic Energy Agency; 2021.

18. Hamadeh RR, Borgan SM, Sibai AM. Cancer research in the Arab world: a review of publications from seven countries between 2000-2013. Sultan Qaboos Univ Med J. 2017;17(2):e147–54. https://doi.org/10.18295/squmj.2016.17.02.003.

19. Hellman S. Roentgen Centennial Lecture: discovering the past, inventing the future. Int J Radiat Oncol Biol Phys. 1996;35(1):15–20. https://doi.org/10.1016/s0360-3016(96)85006-1.

20. IAEA. DIRAC (DIrectory of RAdiotherapy Centres). 2021. Retrieved from https://dirac.iaea.org/Query/Countries.

21. IMPCB. International Medical Physics Certification Board. 2021. Retrieved from https://www.impcbdb.org/.

22. IOMP. The International Organisation for Medical Physics. 2021. Retrieved from https://www.iomp.org/.

23. Jackson SP, Bartek J. The DNA-damage response in human biology and disease. Nature. 2009;461(7267):1071–8. https://doi.org/10.1038/nature08467.

24. Khader J. Improving cancer outcomes through international collaboration in developing countries: King Hussein cancer center as a unique experience. J Glob Oncol. 2018;4(Supplement 2):161s. https://doi.org/10.1200/jgo.18.43300.

25. Khader J, Al-Mousa A, Al Khatib S, Wadi-Ramahi S. Successful development of a competency-based residency training program in radiation oncology: our 15-year experience from within a developing country. J Cancer Educ. 2020;35(5):1011–6. https://doi.org/10.1007/s13187-019-01557-8.

26. MEFOMP. Middle east federation of organizations of medical physics. 2021.

27. Mousa AG, Bishr MK, Mula-Hussain L, Zaghloul MS. Is economic status the main determinant of radiation therapy availability? The Arab world as an example of developing countries. Radiother Oncol. 2019;140:182–9. https://doi.org/10.1016/j.radonc.2019.06.026.

28. Mula-Hussain L. Undergraduate oncology education: mini-literature review with single institution experience from Iraq. In: Dubaybo B, editor. ACCESS Health Journal - Proceedings of the 7th international conference on health issues in Arab communities. Dearborn: The Arab Community Center for Economic and Social Services; 2015. p. 183–94.

29. Mula-Hussain L, Shamsaldin AN, Al-Ghazi M, Muhammad HA, Wadi-Ramahi S, Hanna RK, Alhasso A. Board-certified specialty training program in radiation oncology in a war-torn country: challenges, solutions and outcomes. Clin Transl Radiat Oncol. 2019;19:46–51. https://doi.org/10.1016/j.ctro.2019.08.002.

30. Mula-Hussain L, Wadi-Ramahi SJ, Zaghloul MS, Al-Ghazi M. Radiation oncology in the Arab world. In: Laher I, editor. Handbook of healthcare in the Arab world. Cham: Springer International Publishing; 2019. p. 1–19.

31. Mula-Hussain L, Wadi-Ramahi S, Li B, Ahmed S, de Moraes FY. Specialty portfolio in radiation oncology: a global certification roadmap for trainers and trainees (Handbook – Logbook). Qatar: Qatar University Press; 2021.

32. Murray LJ, Robinson MHJM. Radiotherapy: technical aspects. Medicine. 2016;44(1):10–4.

33. Niroomand-Rad A, Tabakov S, Duhaini I, Mahdavi R, Rasuli B, Naji N, et al. Status of medical physics education, training, and research programs in middle east. Med Phys Educ Train. 2017;5(2):16.

34. Pawlicki T, Hayman J, Ford E. Safety is no accident: a framework for quality radiation oncology and care. Arlington, VA: American Society for Radiation Oncology; 2019.

35. Planning National Radiotherapy Services: A Practical Tool. Vienna: International Atomic Energy Agency; 2011.

36. Porter A, Aref A, Chodounsky Z, Elzawawy A, Manatrakul N, Ngoma T, Orton C, Van't Hooft E. and Sikora K. A global strategy for radiotherapy: a WHO consultation. Clin Oncol. 1999;11(6):368–70.

37. Regaud C, Ferroux R. Discordance des effets de rayons X, d'une part dans le testicule, par le peau, d'autre parts dans le fractionment de la dose. Compt Rend Soc Biol. 1927;97:431–4.
38. Röntgen WG. Ueber eine neue Art von Strahlen. Sitzungsberichte der physikalisch-medicinischen Gesellschaftzu Wurzburg. Sitzung. 1895;30:132–41.
39. Rosenblatt E, Acuña O, Abdel-Wahab M. The challenge of global radiation therapy: an IAEA perspective. Int J Radiat Oncol Biol Phys. 2015;91(4):687–9. https://doi.org/10.1016/j.ijrobp.2014.12.008.
40. Rosenblatt E, Fidarova E, Zubizarreta E, Barton MB, MacKillop W, Jones GW, et al. Radiation therapy utilization in middle-income countries. Int J Radiat Oncol Biol Phys. 2016;96(2, Supplement):S37. https://doi.org/10.1016/j.ijrobp.2016.06.102.
41. SCHS. Saudi Commission for Health Specialties. 2021. Retrieved from https://www.scfhs.org.sa/Pages/default.aspx.
42. Setting Up a Radiotherapy Programme. Vienna: International Atomic Energy Agency; 2008.
43. Siddiqui AA, Amin J, Alshammary F, Afroze E, Shaikh S, Rathore HA, Khan R. Burden of cancer in the Arab world. In: Laher I, editor. Handbook of healthcare in the Arab world. Cham: Springer International Publishing; 2020. p. 1–26.
44. Silbermann M, Pitsillides B, Al-Alfi N, Omran S, Al-Jabri K, Elshamy K, et al. Multidisciplinary care team for cancer patients and its implementation in several Middle Eastern countries. Ann Oncol. 2013;24(Suppl 7):vii41–7. https://doi.org/10.1093/annonc/mdt265.
45. Slotman BJ, Cottier B, Bentzen SM, Heeren G, Lievens Y, van den Bogaert W. Overview of national guidelines for infrastructure and staffing of radiotherapy. ESTRO-QUARTS: work package 1. Radiother Oncol. 2005;75(3):349–54. https://doi.org/10.1016/j.radonc.2004.12.005.
46. WHO. World Health Organization. Cancer control: a global snapshot in 2015. 2015.Retrieved from https://www.who.int/cancer/Cancer_Control_Snapshot_in_2015.pdf.
47. World Health Organization. Global health estimates 2020: deaths by cause, age, sex, by country and by region, 2000–2019. Geneva: WHO; 2020.
48. Zaghloul MS. Radiation oncology facilities in Africa: what is the most important: equipment, staffing, or guidelines? Int J Radiat Oncol Biol Phys. 2008;71(5):1600–1.; author reply 1601. https://doi.org/10.1016/j.ijrobp.2008.03.053.
49. Zaghloul MS, Bishr MK. Radiation oncology in Egypt: a model for Africa. Int J Radiat Oncol Biol Phys. 2018;100(3):539–44. https://doi.org/10.1016/j.ijrobp.2017.10.047.
50. Zubizarreta E, Van Dyk J, Lievens Y. Analysis of global radiotherapy needs and costs by geographic region and income level. Clin Oncol (R Coll Radiol). 2017;29(2):84–92. https://doi.org/10.1016/j.clon.2016.11.011.
51. Zubizarreta EH, Fidarova E, Healy B, Rosenblatt E. Need for radiotherapy in low and middle income countries – the silent crisis continues. Clin Oncol. 2015;27(2):107–14. https://doi.org/10.1016/j.clon.2014.10.006.

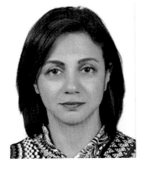

Zeinab Elsayed is a medical graduate of Ain Shams University (ASU) in Cairo, where she also obtained both M.Sc. & Ph.D. in Clinical Oncology. Dr. Elsayed got a second M.Sc. in Advanced Oncology from Ulm University (Germany) and became a FAIMER Fellow (Foundation for Advancement of International Medical Education and Research). Dr. Elsayed is an Oncology Professor & the Director of the Extended Modular Program for UG at ASU. She is an active member of EORTC-QOL and HN Groups, an author of Cochrane Hepatobiliary and Thoracic Groups, a member of Guidelines International Network (G-I-N) (LMIC-WG) & has published in national and international medical journals.

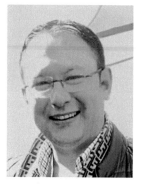

Issam Lalya was born in 1983 in Casablanca, Morocco is a military doctor, specialist in radiation oncology since 2012, and associate professor at Cadi Ayyad University in Marrakech since 2016 and Mohammed-V University in Rabat since 2021. He authored and co-authored numerous publications in highly indexed journals, including three in the New England Journal of Medicine (NEJM). He is mainly involved in the implementation and teaching of innovative radiation therapy techniques (Intensity Modulated Radiation Therapy, Stereotactic Radiotherapy) and postdoctoral education in many fields of oncology.

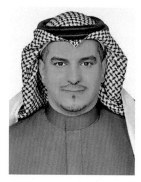

Hussain AlHussain graduated from King Saud University in 2004, then did his Radiation Oncology Residency (2007–2011) and Sub-Specialty Fellowship in Head, Neck, Neuro-Oncology and Stereotactic Radiosurgery (2012–2013), both at the University of Ottawa, Canada. He has been a Fellow of the Royal College of Physicians of Canada since 2011 and received his Master of Healthcare Management from McGill University and CPHQ Certification in Healthcare Quality. Dr. AlHussain is a consultant Radiation Oncologist at the King Fahad Medical City (2013–Present), and he is the Executive Director of Accreditation, Saudi Commission for Health Specialties (2018–Present).

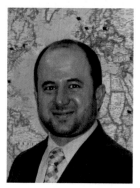

Layth Mula-Hussain was born, raised, and gained his medical degree in Mosul, Iraq. He did radiation oncology specialization and further training and education in Jordan, Germany, and Canada. Currently, he is an ESTRO Fellow & a consultant physician at the Sultan Qaboos Comprehensive Cancer Care and Research Center in Muscat, Oman. Layth was the Founding Director of the first radiation oncology board program in Iraq (2013–2017). He acted as an Expert within imPACT IAEA (2013 & 2021) and was an ASCO International Affairs Steering Committee member (2016–2019). He authored/co-authored five books, six chapters, 50+ manuscripts and did 100+ scientific presentations.

Chapter 29
Cancer Care During War and Conflict

Rola El Sayed, Zahi Abdul-Sater, and Deborah Mukherji

29.1 Introduction

A humanitarian crisis is a situation of human emergency causing physical, economical or environmental damage that overwhelms a community's potential to tend to its population's needs [1]. Although crises may be natural: geophysical (earthquakes, volcanoes), meteorological (storms), hydrological (floods), climatic (droughts), or biologic (epidemics), the most commonly encountered humanitarian emergencies are man-made [2].

Conflicts are defined as violent struggles between at least two groups resulting in at least 25 battle-related deaths per calendar year [3]. They usually develop within the context of long-standing inequalities and social quarrels that intensify with the breakdown of civil authority [4]. In a battle for power and resources, where predatory social domination fuels existing tensions, and fluid local identities are manipulated, sectarian differences arise, intensifying societal fragmentation [5]. Conflicts torment populations, causing loss of lives and infrastructure plus profound health effects. Civilians face dislocation and migration or stay becoming victims of violence, political turmoil, hunger and illness [6].

Multiple countries of the Arab world are in a state of humanitarian crisis because of armed conflict. Conflicts distress the entire region, affecting countries of active

R. E. Sayed
Conflict Medicine Program, Global Health Institute, Division of Hematology-Oncology, American University of Beirut, Beirut, Lebanon

Z. Abdul-Sater
Global Health Institute, American University of Beirut, Beirut, Lebanon
e-mail: za44@aub.edu.lb

D. Mukherji (✉)
Department of Internal Medicine, Division of Hematology Oncology, American University of Beirut, Beirut, Lebanon
e-mail: Dm25@aub.edu.lb

© The Author(s) 2022
H. O. Al-Shamsi et al. (eds.), *Cancer in the Arab World*,
https://doi.org/10.1007/978-981-16-7945-2_29

461

combat as well as adjacent host countries with already frail economies. These countries include Syria, Iraq, Lebanon, Somalia, Sudan, Yemen, Libya and the occupied Palestinian Territory [7]. The past decade has witnessed a surge in numbers of people in humanitarian crises with non-resolution of present conflicts, as well as the uprising of new conflicts [8]. The more protracted conflicts are, the larger the health-related deficit grows as countries fall short on medical supplies, equipment, infrastructure, and personnel.

A devastating impact on health systems, daily life, and well-being of civilians is noted, with an increase both in communicable and Non-Communicable Diseases (NCDs) such as cancer in conflict-affected zones as well as in host countries to displaced populations [9–11]. With the escalation of the humanitarian situation, the number of civilian casualties renders too high, and international response becomes vital. The WHO Constitution, formulated in 1946 [12], mandates protection of human rights as well as the security and maintenance of proper healthcare. Its commission emphasizes the fundamentality of providing all human beings with "the right to the highest attainable standard of health" [13]. Furthermore, the United Nations ascertains "the global community's responsibility for everyone's welfare" with a doctrine of the "responsibility to protect" [14]. Although humanitarian action often provides short-term requirements of food, shelter and trauma relief, longer-term humanitarian aid focuses mainly on communicable diseases, with relative control of infectious diseases. Nevertheless, an increase in NCDs, cancer particularly, has been noticed in the context of ageing populations and collapsing health systems [15, 16].

Available studies in the region led by international collaborators show an increased incidence of NCDs with increased disease burden and increased morbidity, elaborated by higher disability-adjusted life years, and higher mortality [11]. As part of 2015's established Sustainable Development Goals (SDG), the United Nations focused on ensuring healthy lives and promoting well-being for all at all ages (SDG 3) [17]. SDG 3.4 further elaborated the need to reduce by one-third premature mortality from NCD by the year 2030, including cancer, through prevention and treatment [17]. Moreover, the World Health Assembly in 2019 discussed a 5-year global action plan to promote the health of refugees and migrants, focusing on aid organization and delivery, with the strengthening of health policies and information systems [18]. The humanitarian community, based on collaborations between international and local organizations, re-directed forces towards coordinated humanitarian reform to fill the gaps achieving a more comprehensive, effective, and sustainable needs-based relief effort. The humanitarian reform aims to dramatically enhance humanitarian response capacity, predictability, accountability, and partnership. It is empirical to identify and integrate key interventions for NCD care into humanitarian programmes, to conceptualize and empower local healthcare systems through capacity building and strengthening. Thereby, available resources and the resilience of populations can be harnessed to attain present as well as future well-being.

In 2018, cancer incidence was estimated at 18.1 million people worldwide, with cancer mortality reaching 9.6 million [19]. Surveys showed cancer to be the culprit of 30% of all premature deaths from NCD in young adults, with lung cancer being the most common (11.6%) and most lethal (18.4%) [19]. However, numbers differ significantly according to the socioeconomics and Human Development Index (HDI) of countries. Despite all efforts to control the growing incidence of NCD and their corresponding premature deaths, specifically due to cancer, responsible for about 70% of all deaths, SDG 3.4 is far from being achievable given the currently slowing progress [20, 21]. In 2020, 1 out of 6 individuals dies because of cancer. These numbers are expected to increase by about 60% over the next two decades, with the greatest increase in Low- and Middle- Income Countries (LMICs), significantly burdening already struggling health systems [22]. By 2040, the predicted global cancer incidence will reach about 29–37 million cases, and LMICs will be the most affected, harbouring about 67% of all new cases [19]. Not only is cancer incidence not equitable, but also cancer death seems to affect more countries of the lowest socio-economic status, even more so, conflict-affected countries.

Cancer care in this region has been long considered too costly and complex, with a lack of consensus on cost-effective interventions as well as an inability of host health systems to expand cancer services [23]. Patients already diagnosed or with a new possible diagnosis of cancer face deficiencies in healthcare facilities, resources, and treating specialists [24, 25]. They are often forced to migrate seeking expensive cross-border therapy that occasionally proves to be unaffordable; given limited international aid available [26]. In an attempt to decrease NCDs and premature death rates, thereby achieve SDG 3.4, as well as integrate SDG 3.8 tackling universal health coverage where the provision of medical assistance and access to quality healthcare services including cancer care is available to all, the international community established the need to accelerate action against cancer and decrease its imposed global health burden, especially in territories most in need [17, 27]. In this review, we discuss the challenges facing cancer care in conflict situations, with a focus on vulnerable populations where humanitarian assistance is fundamental to fill the gaps, build local capacities, and strengthen healthcare systems to improve health-related outcomes at all stages of disease: primary prevention, screening and early diagnosis, multi-modality management and importantly palliative care.

29.2 Challenges Facing Cancer Care in Conflict-Affected Regions

"Cancer is a deeply personal disease, with tremendous physical, emotional and financial strains, on individuals, communities and countries", a statement eloquently made by Mr. Tedros Adhanom Ghebreyesus, director of WHO [22]. Cancer can affect anyone anywhere in the world, regardless of wealth, social status, security, or humanitarian situation. Given its immense burden on global health, with a growing number of cases as a function of increased life expectancy worldwide, the international community rushed to accelerate global cancer control, with more effective means of prevention, screening, diagnosis, management, surveillance as well as palliation. However, cancer care remains uneven and inequitable across the globe.

What seems easily attainable in high-income countries (HICs) leading the way for the "moon-shot" approach of cancer care, having easy access to new expensive technology and drugs, is far from attainable in countries struggling with conflicts that prohibit them from accessing basic healthcare, where even the "groundshot" approach to cancer care may be difficult to provide due to extremely limited resources [28]. Inequity in access to effective means of diagnosis and management is mirrored in the much higher estimated mortality rates amongst vulnerable populations of conflict-affected countries of the Arab world. Underprivileged populations in conflict regions are faced with multiple challenges that delay diagnosis, hinder care, and make screening almost impossible. Treatable diseases become incurable with late diagnoses causing advanced stages, lower-quality care, and incomplete treatments, all of which are detrimental to patient outcomes [29–31].

Because of destroyed health facilities, non-operational infrastructure, exodus of medical staff and experts corresponding to the progressive Arab world brain drain [32], as well as the lack of much-needed diagnostic material, medications, or technology due to insufficient funds [33], people find no option but to seek medical care in other regions, cities and very often other countries. Displaced populations embark on paths loaded with military checkpoints and expensive "out-of-pocket" payments every step of the way, and despite selling all their worldly possessions, they still fall short of successfully managing to access appropriate care [24, 34]. Humiliation, violence, abuse, morbidity, and death are no strangers to refugees and migrants. International and national stakeholders are attempting to improve healthcare. However, it remains beyond the capacities of host countries or regions to manage the magnitude of such influx of ill people, especially when it comes to complex entities such as cancer requiring multi-disciplinary action and close follow-up [35, 36]. Optimal management of cancer requires the integration of multi-modal interventions including surgery, chemotherapy, radiation therapy, targeted and biologic treatment as well as immunotherapy, much of which is not available in conflict-affected LMICs of the Arab world.

In the presence of frail social, economic, and political instabilities, in addition to already burdened and fragmented healthcare systems, host countries are overwhelmed. From social taboos of insecure cancer patients fearing discrimination, to governmental labelling of malignancies as "helpless", and international organizations such as the UN limiting financial support to individual cases [37], curability and treatment-quality rates remain low. Patients, if ever reach the clinic, get deferred, never continue the requested work-up, or fail to find the needed support to access and complete treatment [36]. In another scenario, the continuity of care of a patient already on active treatment is compromised after displacement. With no data documentation and no transfer of medical records, patients are confronted with significant delays and imposed repetition of work-up, indicating potentially avoidable waste of resources [31]. The absence of national policies to regulate healthcare and cancer access for these patients is just the start of the wider problem. Humanitarian aid may be targeting sound investment in immediate cancer control; yet substantial global heterogeneity in leading cancer types ought to be taken into consideration, and regional responses must be contextualized accordingly to the epidemiologic burden of disease [19, 38, 39]. Therefore, the presence of proper tumour registries, population-based guidelines, and need-based research is of utmost importance, all of which are deficient in LMICs of the Arab world. Figure 29.1 summarizes the challenges leading to poor cancer care in the region.

Cancer occurs in more than 300,000 children annually worldwide, and the rate is expected to increase, more so in LMICs. Most paediatric cancers have a cure rate that can reach up to ≥80% in some HICs [40, 41]. The burden of paediatric cancer has shown wide inequality among countries, as children in countries with low HDIs are significantly less likely to access care or receive successful treatment with high morbidity and mortality rates [42]. Why would a child be deprived of possibly curable treatment because he or she was born in an inconvenient time and place?

In conclusion, delays in effective cancer control become increasingly costly with increased morbidity, preventable life loss, as well as significant economic and social burdens. Highly effective National Cancer Control Plans (NCCPs) based on affordable and feasible interventions are suggested as an integral component of Universal Health Coverage (UHC) that would fall under the banner of SDG 3.8 promoting access to high-quality essential healthcare services [43, 44]. UHC aims to protect people and improve their outcomes [45], through the strengthening of existing healthcare systems, as well as local capacity building [46]. Cancer diagnosis and management have developed rapidly in recent years. However, in many crisis-affected countries of the Arab World, cancer control strategies, if existent, are inefficient, uninformed, do not adhere to best practices, and are not adapted to national health systems' capacities with an inappropriate allocation of available resources.

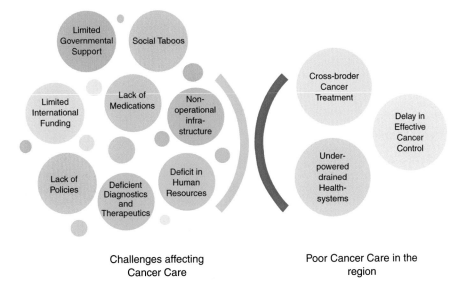

Fig. 29.1 Challenges leading to poor cancer care in the region

Implementation of NCCPs through collaboration with national and local organizations would strategize priorities and cancer care investments so as to efficiently fulfil unmet needs, reduce suffering, save lives as well as aid in promoting economic productivity through evidence-based policies [47–49]. Coordination of governmental figures such as ministries, public health institutes or social securities, private insurance companies as well as health providers, civil society stakeholders and several voluntary organizations is inevitable for proper healthcare workers' training, not to forget the creation and monitoring of national policies and specific population-based guidelines.

Finally, it is worth mentioning the ongoing COVID-19 pandemic that has affected the entire globe [50]}. It has been a particularly tough challenge for cancer patients who are immunosuppressed, immunocompromised or simply fatigued and in need of assistance in daily-living activities. All these characteristics render cancer patients more vulnerable to infectious diseases [51, 52]. Strategic planning, capacity building and policy creating have been paused, with attention re-focused towards virus containment. Some diagnostic and even therapeutic modalities are halted. Furthermore, travel difficulties and long waiting periods are driving patients away from consulting with their primary physicians. An international cross-sectional study was done in 54 countries across six continents to evaluate the impact of the pandemic on cancer care worldwide. It showed a devastating impact, with reported harm from interruption of cancer-specific care reaching 36.52%, up to 80% in some centres, and worse in lower-resource countries. Challenges included patients missing therapy in >10% of cases, medication restriction in 10% of cases and overwhelmed medical systems in 20% of cases {[53]}.

Despite all these challenges, some conflict-affected economically drained communities in the region managed to issue pragmatic need-based recommendations for daily practice in cancer patient care during the COVID-19 pandemic, as well as establish proper means for distant/telemedicine and tele-education, so as to follow and manage cancer patients according to the best updated data with extremely limited resources [54, 55].

29.3 Potential for Development & Improvement of Cancer Care in the Arab World

Countries in the region find themselves facing immense challenges of intractable conflicts with a pertinent increase in cancer burden. In addition, with the absence of standard guidelines or clear national policies for much-needed developmental reforms in the provision of cancer care to citizens as well as refugees and displaced people, the international society shed light on the importance of the establishment of NCCPs [56]. NCCPs are based on the principle of governance to provide the population's needs and set norms with focused agendas for strategic investments in local resource-stratified healthcare [57]. Given the scarcity of cancer registries, the lack of quality cancer prevalence data as well as the absence of proper conflict-adapted population-based studies to inform programming and care delivery, strategic planning for cancer care development seemed to be a difficult target [58]. Therefore, international aid emphasized the importance of strengthening the quality of tumour registries, quality of data collection as well as the importance of crisis-contextualized research. Means of electronic data collection were sought and implemented by multiple NGOs, helping make documentation and transfer of medical information easier for better continuity of care [59–61]. Technology was also noted to be of utmost importance in communication among healthcare workers, improving coordination, multi-disciplinary care, and implementing distant training and education, staying in line with all international information updates.

Despite shouldering a significant proportion of the global cancer burden, these countries of the Arab World notably lag in knowledge yield and production of resource-stratified evidence-based cancer research [62–64]. Table 29.1 as well as Fig. 29.2 retrieved from Abdul-Sater et al. [65] show an example of barriers to cancer research and researcher training needs in the region [65]. These gaps in obtaining population-based research impede nations from reaching target care goals, more so with drastic impact in conflict-affected settings. In fact, focusing on creating unified health research structural regulatory frameworks that embark on

Table 29.1 Themes, subthemes, and their share of mentions of research barriers form participants' responses [65]. Used with permission from Abdul-Sater, Zahi, Elsa Kobeissi, Marilyne Menassa, Talar Telvizian, and Deborah Mukherji. "Research Capacity and Training Needs for Cancer in Conflict-Affected MENA Countries". Annals of Global Health 86, no. 1 (2020)

Theme	Sub-theme	Number of mentions	Number of mentions (%)
Research infrastructure	Amenities (facilities and equipment)	20	10.99%
	Research resources	12	6.59%
	Data poverty	10	5.49%
	Cancer registration	9	4.95%
Support	Financial support	32	17.58%
	Institutional support	4	2.20%
	Governmental support	3	1.65%
Logistics	Research participation	11	6.04%
	Travel	6	3.30%
	Workload and time	5	2.75%
	Collaboration	5	2.75%
	Training	3	1.65%
Human resources		17	9.34%
Political economy	Politics	9	4.95%
	Security	7	3.85%
Culture and conducive environment		15	8.24%
Others		14	7.69%

a

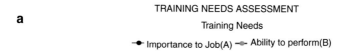

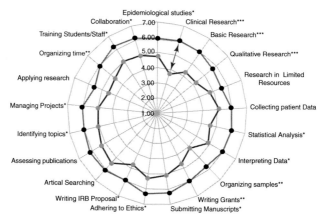

P Value <0.01(*): <0.001 (**); <0.0001 (***)

PERCEIVED BARRIERS TO CONDUCTING RESEARCH ON CANCER AND ATTENING TRAINING

b   Research Barriers   **c**   Training Barriers

Fig. 29.2 (**a**) Radar chart highlighting the difference between the importance to job and ability to perform regarding activities related to cancer research and care. Tree map chart showing the themes mapped from participants; responses to the research (**b**) and training (**c**) barriers. Used with permission from Abdul-Sater, Zahi, Elsa Kobeissi, Marilyne Menassa, Talar Telvizian, and Deborah Mukherji. "Research Capacity and Training Needs for Cancer in Conflict-Affected MENA Countries". Annals of Global Health 86, no. 1 (2020)

building research capacity through training of researchers and healthcare professionals, helps identify actual population needs. They bridge the gaps to the provision of high-quality cancer care [66], as well as develop profound networks and enhance communication among physicians, technicians, healthcare workers, social workers, civilians, media, academia, policymakers, governmental organizations as well as national and international non-governmental stakeholders [67, 68]. These networks facilitate access to information, as well as dissemination and implementation of knowledge by addressing questions that cannot be otherwise addressed in non-crisis settings.

Task Forces have emphasized the absolute necessity for priority-setting and policymaking at all stages of the cancer continuum [69, 70]. For example, specific exposure-related cancers, more common in these regions, can be approached more conclusively. Hepatocellular carcinoma related to hepatitis viruses B and C (HBV, HCV), cervical cancer related to human papillomavirus (HPV), lymphomas as well as head and neck tumours related to Ebstein-Barr virus, are all diseases that can either be prevented by vaccination (HBV, HPV) or caught at an earlier more curable stages by screening [71]. Nation-wide screening and early detection programmes can help minimize cancer burden, especially in common malignancies such as lung, breast and colon cancer [72]. Awareness campaigns regarding tumour-related signs and symptoms, as well as tobacco-cessation programmes and informing of the whereabouts of screening/detection programmes should be incorporated in all physician clinics and media.

In presence of proper guidance and informed planning, cancer care in conflict-affected regions should not be dreaded. Infrastructure can be provided [73], if not in regions of active conflicts, then in neighbouring countries, or in "cease-fire safe-grounds" with properly equipped specialized care centres such as in Kurdistan [74]. Eventually, there is truth to health being a bridge to peace where death and morbidity can trigger humanity [75, 76]. As for cost and cost-effectiveness, cancer care can be economically yielding rather than expensive. Taken up in the momentum, with investments properly placed into systems not individuals, seven million cancer deaths can be avoided in LMICs by 2030, at a cost of US\$ 2.70 per person in low-income countries, and US\$ 3.95 per person in LMICs [22]. When financial costs are calculated from estimated purchases, and programmes for pre-specified numbers of citizens and refugees are based on registries and databases for treatment, screening, and early primary detection, inefficient primary care and cumbersome clinical pathways leading to more advanced stages with greater costs and worse outcomes can be evaded [27]. Budgets for expensive targeted therapy or immunotherapy that benefit minorities can be deterred and privatized, focusing on effective chemotherapeutic agents or curative surgical interventions.

Neglecting the incorporation of palliative care in cancer control agendas remains a pertinent concern. Only half of the countries worldwide seem to include palliative care in their NCD plans [77]. Palliative care is an essential part of comprehensive cancer care. It revolves around the prevention, early identification, and relief of any suffering of cancer patients on the physical, psycho-social, and emotional levels, with proper control of symptoms, most importantly pain [47, 49, 78, 79]. Palliative care preserves patient dignity, improves the quality of life and improves survival [80, 81]. It includes home care sparing patients and families costly lengthy hospital admissions, while simultaneously preventing hospital overcrowding and cutting down healthcare expenses [82, 83]. Perhaps it is worthy to ensure adequate opioid pain relief and oral morphine supply whose availability barely reaches 10% in LICs and 29% in MICs [84].

Once more, we need to emphasize the importance of sustaining cancer care during the COVID-19 pandemic. Cancer patients have been particularly affected by the pandemic, not only because of their vulnerable immune status and the possibility of severe adversities but also because their diagnosis, management and follow-up have been deferred until after the storm abides. Different care strategies and approach algorithms have been suggested by major health institutions of the Arab world regarding resource allocation, screening methods and general diagnostic and management recommendations in the outpatient and inpatient settings of patients with suspected cancer as well as those on active treatment with high-risk of COVID-19 infection [54]. Awareness campaigns indicating the importance of preventive measures and reporting symptoms have been shown to play a significant role. Furthermore, online consultations replaced clinic visits in the era of "social distancing", and oral treatments prevailed over lengthy chemotherapy sessions whenever possible. Nevertheless, many people needing hospital admission remain and they cannot wait long. Otherwise, the recession phase (phase III) of COVID-19 will not only witness overcrowding of hospitals due to ill COVID-positive patients but also sick cancer patients. Studies discussed hospital system re-organization to include COVID-free areas where cancer care can be safely provided along new situation-adapted guidelines [85]. On the other hand, when it comes to networking, education and multi-disciplinary opinions, healthcare workers have shown remarkable adaptability with an unprecedented "webinar fever" and innumerable free online courses and discussions that have simply brought the entire world closer together.

29.4 Conclusion

Cancer care in conflict-affected regions of the Arab World is very heterogeneous, inequitable, and uneven, with an increasing cancer burden. Obstacles to quality cancer care are numerous and finding one purpose-oriented care model fitting all is impossible. International organizations attempt to empower local capacities, all while trying to fulfil SDGs 3.4 and 3.8. Improvement of cancer care and delivery of cost-effective and sustainable high-quality care must be based on local knowledge and evidence-based regional resource-dependent research-informed guidelines, within the context of a regulatory body and policies focused on dynamic priority-setting.

Cancer prevention, screening, early detection, and optimal management provision within a groundshot approach are pivotal to achieving targeted milestones. Palliative care, moreover, needs to be incorporated into pragmatic cancer control plans, due to its important role in the improvement of survival as well as the quality of life. International and national collaborations are essential, and funding can only be provided within organized frameworks. Although COVID-19 put all plans on pause, and adversely affected cancer care across the globe, especially conflict-affected countries of the region; however, it helped improve communication among national and international collaborators and stakeholders, all while enhancing access to the most updated knowledge.

29.5   Funding Information

The authors are funded through the UK Research and Innovation GCRF Research for Health in Conflict in the Middle East and North Africa (R4HC-MENA) project, developing capability, partnerships and research in the Middle and North Africa ES/P010962/1.

Conflict of Interest   Authors have no conflict of interest to declare.

References

1. WorldVision. What is a humanitarian disaster? Accessed 28 Aug 2020.
2. Watts S, Siddiqi S, Mediterranean World Health Organization, Regional Office for the Eastern. Social determinants of health in countries in conflict: a perspective from the eastern Mediterranean region. Nasr City, Cairo: World Health Organization Regional Office for the Eastern Mediterranean; 2008.
3. Pettersson T. Armed conflicts, 1946–2014. J Peace Res. 2015;52:536–50.
4. Krug EG, Mercy JA, Dahlberg LL, Zwi AB. The world report on violence and health. Lancet. 2002;360:1083–8.
5. Chourou B, Unesco. Promoting human security: ethical, normative and educational frameworks in the Arab states. Paris: UNESCO; 2005.
6. de Waal A. Who are the Darfurians? Arab and African identities, violence and external engagement. Afr Aff. 2005;104:181–205.
7. World-Bank-Group. By the numbers: the cost of War and Peace in the Middle East. 2016. https://www.worldbank.org/en/news/feature/2016/02/03/by-the-numbers-the-cost-of-war-and-peace-in-mena
8. UN. A record number of people will need help worldwide during 2020: UN Humanitarian Overview, 4 December 2019, section Humanitarian Aid; 2019.
9. GBD 2015 Eastern Mediterranean Region Collaborators. Danger ahead: the burden of diseases, injuries, and risk factors in the Eastern Mediterranean Region, 1990-2015. Int J Public Health. 2018;63:11–23.
10. GBD 2015 Eastern Mediterranean Region Cancer Collaborators. Burden of cancer in the Eastern Mediterranean Region, 2005-2015: findings from the global burden of disease 2015 study. Int J Public Health. 2018;63:151–64.
11. GBD 2016 DALYs and HALE Collaborators. Global, regional, and national disability-adjusted life-years (DALYs) for 333 diseases and injuries and healthy life expectancy (HALE) for 195 countries and territories, 1990-2016: a systematic analysis for the global burden of disease study 2016. Lancet. 2017;390:1260–344.
12. International Health, Conference. Constitution of the World Health Organization, 1946. Bull World Health Organ. 2002;80:983–4.
13. World Health Organization. A conceptual framework for action on the social determinants of health. Geneva: World Health Organization; 2010.
14. Brock G. International commission on intervention and state sovereignty (ICISS). In: Chatterjee DK, editor. Encyclopedia of global justice. Dordrecht: Springer Netherlands; 2011.

15. Akik C, Ghattas H, Mesmar S, Rabkin M, El-Sadr WM, Fouad FM. Host country responses to non-communicable diseases amongst Syrian refugees: a review. Confl Heal. 2019;13:8.
16. Naja F, Shatila H, El Koussa M, Meho L, Ghandour L, Saleh S. Burden of non-communicable diseases among Syrian refugees: a scoping review. BMC Public Health. 2019;19:637.
17. UN, United Nations. Transforming our world: the 2030 agenda for sustainable development. eSocialSciences; 2015.
18. WHO. Promoting the health of refugees and migrants Draft global action plan, 2019–2023. In *Seventy-Second World Health Assembly*, edited by World Health Organization Report by Director-General, 13. Health and migration programme; 2019.
19. Ferlay J, Colombet M, Soerjomataram I, Mathers C, Parkin DM, Piñeros M, Znaor A, Bray F. Estimating the global cancer incidence and mortality in 2018: GLOBOCAN sources and methods. Int J Cancer. 2019;144:1941–53.
20. Bennett JE, Stevens GA, Mathers CD, Bonita R, Rehm J, Kruk ME, Riley LM, Dain K, Kengne AP, Chalkidou K, Beagley J, Kishore SP, Chen W, Saxena S, Bettcher DW, Grove JT, Beaglehole R, Ezzati M. NCD countdown 2030: worldwide trends in non-communicable disease mortality and progress towards sustainable development goal target 3.4. Lancet. 2018;392:1072–88.
21. WHO. Non-communicable diseases progress monitor 2020. In, edited by Surveillance Noncommunicable diseases, Monitoring and Reporting, 230; 2020a.
22. WHO. WHO report on cancer: setting priorities, investing wisely and providing care for all. Geneva: WHO Headquarters (HQ); 2020b. p. 160.
23. UNHCR. Health sector, humanitarian response strategy: Jordan 2019–2020. Geneva: UNHCR; 2019. p. 19. https://data2.unhcr.org/en/documents/download/68348.
24. Sahloul E, Salem R, Alrez W, Alkarim T, Sukari A, Maziak W, Atassi MB. Cancer care at times of crisis and war: the Syrian example. J Glob Oncol. 2017;3:338–45.
25. Yusuf MA, Hussain SF, Sultan F, Badar F, Sullivan R. Cancer care in times of conflict: cross border care in Pakistan of patients from Afghanistan. Ecancermedicalscience. 2020;14:1018.
26. Skelton M, Alameddine R, Saifi O, Hammoud M, Zorkot M, Daher M, Charafeddine M, Temraz S, Shamseddine A, Mula-Hussain L, Saleem M, Namiq KF, Dewachi O, Sitta GA, Abdul-Sater Z, Telvizian T, Faraj W, Mukherji D. High-cost cancer treatment across borders in conflict zones: experience of Iraqi patients in Lebanon. JCO Glob Oncol. 2020;6:59–66.
27. Ilbawi A, Slama S. Cancer care for refugees: time to invest in people and systems. Lancet Oncol. 2020;21:604–5. 'Indicators and a Monitoring Framework for the Sustainable Development Goals: Launching a data revolution for the SDGs'. *Indicators and a Monitoring Framework for the Sustainable Development Goals: Launching a data revolution for the SDGs.*
28. Gyawali B, Sullivan R, Booth CM. Cancer groundshot: going global before going to the moon. Lancet Oncol. 2018;19:288–90.
29. Aarts MJ, Kamphuis CBM, Louwman MJ, Coebergh JWW, Mackenbach JP, van Lenthe FJ. Educational inequalities in cancer survival: a role for comorbidities and health behaviours? J Epidemiol Community Health. 2013;67:365.
30. Bergeron-Boucher MP, Oeppen J, Holm NV, Nielsen HM, Lindahl-Jacobsen R, Wensink MJ. Understanding differences in cancer survival between populations: a new approach and application to breast Cancer survival differentials between Danish regions. Int J Environ Res Public Health. 2019;16(17):3093.
31. Brand NR, Qu LG, Chao A, Ilbawi AM. Delays and barriers to cancer care in low- and middle-income countries: a systematic review. Oncologist. 2019;24:e1371–e80.
32. El Saghir NS, Anderson BO, Gralow J, Lopes G, Shulman LN, Moukadem HA, Yu PP, Hortobagyi G. Impact of merit-based immigration policies on brain drain from low- and middle-income countries. JCO Glob Oncol. 2020;6:185–9.
33. Malaker K. Cancer care in poverty. J Glob Oncol. 2018;4:240s.
34. Mukherji D, Skelton M, Alameddine R, Saifi O, Hammoud MS, Daher M, Charafeddine M, Faraj W, Temraz SN, Shamseddine A, Mula-Hussain LYI, Saleem M, Namiq KF, Dewachi O, Sitta GA. Financial toxicity associated with conflict-induced cross-border travel for cancer care: experience of Iraqi patients in Lebanon. J Clin Oncol. 2018;36(15):6562.

35. Al Qadire M, Aljezawi M, Al-Shdayfat N. Cancer awareness and barriers to seeking medical help among Syrian refugees in Jordan: a baseline study. J Cancer Educ. 2019;34:19–25.
36. El Saghir NS, de Celis ESP, Fares JE, Sullivan R. Cancer Care for Refugees and Displaced Populations: Middle East conflicts and global natural disasters. Am Soc Clin Oncol Educ Book. 2018;38:433–40.
37. International, Amnesty. Agonizing choices-Syrian refugees in need of healthcare in Lebanon; 2014. p. 1–138.
38. Bray F, Ferlay J, Soerjomataram I, Siegel RL, Torre LA, Jemal A. Global cancer statistics 2018: GLOBOCAN estimates of incidence and mortality worldwide for 36 cancers in 185 countries. CA Cancer J Clin. 2018;68:394–424.
39. UNDP. Human development report 2019, beyond income, beyond averages, beyond today: inequalities in human development in the 21st century. Washington DC: UNDP; 2019. p. 1–366.
40. Lam CG, Howard SC, Bouffet E, Pritchard-Jones K. Science and health for all children with cancer. Science. 2019;363:1182.
41. WHO. Cancer in children; 2018.
42. Saab R, Jeha S, Khalifeh H, Zahreddine L, Bayram L, Merabi Z, Abboud M, Muwakkit S, Tarek N, Rodriguez-Galindo C, El Solh H. Displaced children with cancer in Lebanon: a sustained response to an unprecedented crisis. Cancer. 2018;124:1464–72.
43. GBD 2019 Collaborators. Universal Health Coverage. Measuring universal health coverage based on an index of effective coverage of health services in 204 countries and territories, 1990-2019: a systematic analysis for the global burden of disease study 2019. Lancet. 2020;396:1250–84.
44. UHC2030. SDG Indicator 3.8.1: measure what matters. 2018. https://www.uhc2030.org/blog-news-events/uhc30-news/sdg-indicator-3-8-1-measure-what-matters-465653/.
45. Maruthappu M, Watkins J, Noor AM, Williams C, Ali R, Sullivan R, Zeltner T, Atun R. Economic downturns, universal health coverage, and cancer mortality in high-income and middle-income countries, 1990-2010: a longitudinal analysis. Lancet (London, England). 2016;388:684–95.
46. Cometto G, Buchan J, Dussault G. Developing the health workforce for universal health coverage. Bull World Health Organ. 2020;98:109–16.
47. World Health Organization. Cancer control: knowledge into action: WHO guide for effective programmes: module 3: early detection. Geneva: World Health Organization; 2007a.
48. World Health, Organization. National cancer control programmes: policies and managerial guidelines. Geneva: World Health Organization; 2002.
49. World Health Organization. Palliative care. Geneva: World Health Organization; 2007b.
50. Raymond E, Thieblemont C, Alran S, Faivre S. Impact of the COVID-19 outbreak on the management of patients with cancer. Target Oncol. 2020;15(3):249–59. https://doi.org/10.1007/s11523-020-00721-1.
51. Liang W, Guan W, Chen R, Wang W, Li J, Xu K, Li C, Ai Q, Lu W, Liang H, Li S, He J. Cancer patients in SARS-CoV-2 infection: a nationwide analysis in China. Lancet Oncol. 2020;21(3):335–7.
52. Onder G, Rezza G, Brusaferro S. Case-fatality rate and characteristics of patients dying in relation to COVID-19 in Italy. JAMA. 2020;323:1775–6.
53. Jazieh AR, Akbulut H, Curigliano G, Rogado A, Alsharm AA, Razis ED, Mula-Hussain L, Errihani H, Khattak A, De Guzman RB, Mathias C, Alkaiyat MOF, Jradi H, Rolfo C, on behalf of the International Research Network on COVID-19 Impact on Cancer Care. Impact of the COVID-19 pandemic on cancer care: a global collaborative study. JCO Glob Oncol. 2020;2020(6):1428–38.
54. Al-Shamsi HO, Alhazzani W, Alhuraiji A, Coomes EA, Chemaly RF, Almuhanna M, Wolff RA, Ibrahim NK, Chua M, Hotte SJ, Meyers BM, Elfiki T, Curigliano G, Eng C, Grothey A, Xie C. A practical approach to the management of cancer patients during the novel coronavirus disease 2019 (COVID-19) pandemic: an international collaborative group. Oncologist. 2020;25(6):e936–45. https://doi.org/10.1634/theoncologist.2020-0213.

55. Bitar N, Kattan J, Kourie HR, Mukherji D, El Saghir N. The Lebanese Society of Medical Oncology (LSMO) statement on the care of patients with cancer during the COVID-19 pandemic. Future Oncol (London, England). 2020;16:615–7.
56. Prager GW, Braga S, Bystricky B, Qvortrup C, Criscitiello C, Esin E, Sonke GS, Martínez GA, Frenel JS, Karamouzis M, Strijbos M, Yazici O, Bossi P, Banerjee S, Troiani T, Eniu A, Ciardiello F, Tabernero J, Zielinski CC, Casali PG, Cardoso F, Douillard JY, Jezdic S, McGregor K, Bricalli G, Vyas M, Ilbawi A. Global cancer control: responding to the growing burden, rising costs and inequalities in access. ESMO Open. 2018;3:e000285.
57. Sayani A. Health equity in national cancer control plans: an analysis of the Ontario cancer plan. Int J Health Policy Manag. 2019;8:550–6.
58. Abdul-Khalek RA, Guo P, Sharp F, Gheorghe A, Shamieh O, Kutluk T, Fouad F, Coutts A, Aggarwal A, Mukherji D, Abu-Sittah G, Chalkidou K, Sullivan R. The economic burden of cancer care for Syrian refugees: a population-based modelling study. Lancet Oncol. 2020;21:637–44.
59. Ariffin NA, Ismail A, Kadir IKA, Kamal JIA. Implementation of electronic medical records in developing countries: challenges & barriers. Int J Acad Res Progress Educ Dev. 2018;7:187–99.
60. Asan O, Nattinger AB, Gurses AP, Tyszka JT, Yen TWF. Oncologists' views regarding the role of electronic health records in care coordination. JCO Clin Cancer Inform. 2018;2:1–12.
61. Manca DP. Do electronic medical records improve quality of care? Yes. Can Fam Physician. 2015;61:846–51.
62. Benamer HTS, Bakoush O. Arab nations lagging behind other middle Eastern countries in biomedical research: a comparative study. BMC Med Res Methodol. 2009;9:26.
63. El Rassi R, Meho LI, Nahlawi A, Salameh JS, Bazarbachi A, Akl EA. Medical research productivity in the Arab countries: 2007-2016 bibliometric analysis. J Glob Health. 2018;8:020411.
64. Sweileh WM, Zyoud S'e H, Al-Jabi SW, Sawalha AF. Contribution of Arab countries to breast cancer research: comparison with non-Arab middle Eastern countries. BMC Womens Health. 2015;15:1–7.
65. Abdul-Sater Z, Kobeissi E, Menassa M, Telvizian T, Mukherji D. Research capacity and training needs for cancer in conflict-affected MENA countries. Ann Glob Health. 2020;86(1):142. https://doi.org/10.5334/aogh.2809.
66. El Achi N, Papamichail A, Rizk A, Lindsay H, Menassa M, Abdul-Khalek RA, Ekzayez A, Dewachi O, Patel P. A conceptual framework for capacity strengthening of health research in conflict: the case of the Middle East and North Africa region. Glob Health. 2019;15:81.
67. Ali R, Finlayson A. Building capacity for clinical research in developing countries: the INDOX cancer research network experience. Glob Health Action. 2012;5:17288.
68. Kohrt BA, Mistry AS, Anand N, Beecroft B, Nuwayhid I. Health research in humanitarian crises: an urgent global imperative. BMJ Glob Health. 2019;4:e001870.
69. Adewole I, Martin DN, Williams MJ, Adebamowo C, Bhatia K, Berling C, Casper C, Elshamy K, Elzawawy A, Lawlor RT, Legood R, Mbulaiteye SM, Odedina FT, Olopade OI, Olopade CO, Parkin DM, Rebbeck TR, Ross H, Santini LA, Torode J, Trimble EL, Wild CP, Young AM, Kerr DJ. Building capacity for sustainable research programmes for cancer in Africa. Nat Rev Clin Oncol. 2014;11:251–9.
70. Brown R, Kerr K, Haoudi A, Darzi A. Tackling cancer burden in the Middle East: Qatar as an example. Lancet Oncol. 2012;13:e501–8.
71. de Martel C, Georges D, Bray F, Ferlay J, Clifford GM. Global burden of cancer attributable to infections in 2018: a worldwide incidence analysis. Lancet Glob Health. 2020;8:e180–e90.
72. Shah SC, Kayamba V, Peek RM Jr, Heimburger D. Cancer control in low- and middle-income countries: is it time to consider screening? J Glob Oncol. 2019;5:1–8.
73. Sirohi B, Chalkidou K, Pramesh CS, Anderson BO, Loeher P, El Dewachi O, Shamieh O, Shrikhande SV, Venkataramanan R, Parham G, Mwanahamuntu M, Eden T, Tsunoda A, Purushotham A, Stanway S, Rath GK, Sullivan R. Developing institutions for cancer care in low-income and middle-income countries: from cancer units to comprehensive cancer centres. Lancet Oncol. 2018;19:e395–406.

74. Skelton M, Mula-Hussain LYI, Namiq KF. Oncology in Iraq's Kurdish Region: navigating cancer, war, and displacement. J Glob Oncol. 2018;4:1–4.
75. World Health Organization. Consultation on health as a bridge for peace, development World Health Organization. Adviser on Health policy in, and W. H. O. Task force on Health in development. "Report of the consultation on Health as a bridge for peace, 15 May 1996, WHO, Geneva.". Geneva: World Health Organization; 1996.
76. Schneider ML. Health as a bridge for peace. World Health. 1987:4–6.
77. World Health Organization, Regional Office for South-East, Asia. National capacity for prevention and control of non-communicable diseases in WHO SEAR - Results from NCD country capacity survey 2019. New Delhi: World Health Organization, Regional Office for South-East Asia; 2020.
78. Kaasa S, Loge JH, Aapro M, Albreht T, Anderson R, Bruera E, Brunelli C, Caraceni A, Cervantes A, Currow DC, Deliens L, Fallon M, Gómez-Batiste X, Grotmol KS, Hannon B, Haugen DF, Higginson IJ, Hjermstad MJ, Hui D, Jordan K, Kurita GP, Larkin PJ, Miccinesi G, Nauck F, Pribakovic R, Rodin G, Sjøgren P, Stone P, Zimmermann C, Lundeby T. Integration of oncology and palliative care: a lancet oncology commission. Lancet Oncol. 2018;19:e588–653.
79. White RE, Parker RK, Fitzwater JW, Kasepoi Z, Topazian M. Stents as sole therapy for oesophageal cancer: a prospective analysis of outcomes after placement. Lancet Oncol. 2009;10:240–6.
80. Haun MW, Estel S, Rücker G, Friederich HC, Villalobos M, Thomas M, Hartmann M. Early palliative care for adults with advanced cancer. Cochrane Database Syst Rev. 2017;6:Cd011129.
81. Knaul FM, Farmer PE, Krakauer EL, De Lima L, Bhadelia A, Jiang Kwete X, Arreola-Ornelas H, Gómez-Dantés O, Rodriguez NM, Alleyne GAO, Connor SR, Hunter DJ, Lohman D, Radbruch L, Del Rocío Sáenz M, Madrigal R, Atun KM, Foley J, Frenk DT, Jamison, and M. R. Rajagopal. Alleviating the access abyss in palliative care and pain relief-an imperative of universal health coverage: the lancet commission report. Lancet. 2018;391:1391–454.
82. Desrosiers T, Cupido C, Pitout E, van Niekerk L, Badri M, Gwyther L, Harding R. A hospital-based palliative care service for patients with advanced organ failure in sub-Saharan Africa reduces admissions and increases home death rates. J Pain Symptom Manag. 2014;47:786–92.
83. World Health Organization. Integrating palliative care and symptom relief into primary health care: a WHO guide for planners, implementers and managers. Geneva: World Health Organization; 2018.
84. UN. Narcotic drugs: estimated world requirements for 2018; statistics for 2016. New York: International Narcotics Control Board; 2017. p. 1–476.
85. Tuech J-J, Gangloff A, Di Fiore F, Benyoucef A, Michel P, Schwarz L. The day after tomorrow: how should we address health system organization to treat cancer patients after the peak of the COVID-19 epidemic? Oncology. 2020;98:1–9.

Suggested Books for Reading

Laher I. Handbook of healthcare in the Arab World. Cham: Springer; 2020.
Ngwa W, Nguyen P. Global oncology. Harvard Global Health Catalyst summit lecture notes. Bristol: IOP Publishing; 2017.
Silbermann M. Cancer care in countries and societies in transition. individualized care in focus. Cham: Springer; 2016.
WHO. WHO report on cancer. Setting priorities, investing wisely and providing care for all. Geneva: WHO; 2020.
WHO, Regional Office of the Eastern Mediterranean. Social determinants of health in countries in conflict. A perspective from the Eastern Mediterranean Region. Cairo: WHO, Regional Office of the Eastern Mediterranean; 2008.

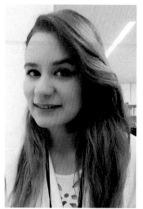

Rola El Sayed, MD, is currently a thoracic oncology sub-specialty trainee at the Center Hospitalier de l' Université de Montreal since March 2021. Dr. El Sayed finished her training in general and internal medicine at the Lebanese University in Beirut, Lebanon, and was awarded her Postgraduate Medical Diploma in Hematology-Oncology from the American University of Beirut Medical Center in June 2020. She continued with a 6-month position as a clinical research associate working on the Cancer in Conflict Program of the Research for Cancer in Conflict (R4HC MENA) collaboration at the Global Health Institute, American University of Beirut.

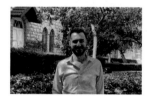

Zahi Abdul-Sater is the Head of research programs and coordinator of the Conflict Medicine Program at the Global Health Institute at the American University of Beirut (AUB-GHI). He is also an assistant professor of Public Health at Phoenicia University in Lebanon. He joined AUB-GHI in 2017 as a postdoctoral fellow after finishing his PhD in Biochemistry and Molecular Biology at Indiana University in the USA. Dr. Abdul Sater is interested in global cancer research and in developing innovative approaches to building capacity for medical research in the Middle East and North Africa.

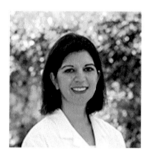

Deborah Mukherji joined the faculty of the American University of Beirut Medical Center in June 2012 as a medical oncologist with a special interest in genitourinary and gastrointestinal oncology. Dr. Mukherji completed her advanced specialty training in Medical Oncology at Guys and St Thomas's NHS Foundation Trust, London UK and was awarded a Postgraduate Diploma in Oncology from the Institute of Cancer Research, University of London in 2011. Dr. Mukherji leads the Cancer in Conflict Workstream of the Research for Cancer in Conflict (R4HC MENA) collaboration at AUB.

Printed in the United States
by Baker & Taylor Publisher Services